eXtreme
Lateral
Interbody
Fusion (XLIF®)

eXtreme
Lateral
Interbody
Fusion (XLIF®)

EDITED BY

J. Allan Goodrich, MD

Associate Clinical Professor,
Department of Orthopaedic Surgery, Medical College of Georgia;
Augusta Orthopaedic Clinic, Augusta, Georgia

Ildemaro J. Volcan, MD

Associate Clinical Professor,
Department of Neurological Surgery, Medical College of Georgia;
West Augusta Spine Specialists, LLC, Augusta, Georgia

QUALITY MEDICAL PUBLISHING, INC.
St. Louis, Missouri
2008

PUBLISHER   Karen Berger
EDITORIAL DIRECTOR   Michelle Berger
PROJECT MANAGER   Sara Blackwell
MANUSCRIPT EDITOR   Rebecca Sweeney
ASSISTANT EDITOR   Julie Dill
VICE PRESIDENT OF PRODUCTION AND MANUFACTURING   Carolyn G. Reich
ART DIRECTION, BOOK, AND COVER DESIGN   Amanda Yarberry Behr
SELECT ILLUSTRATIONS   Robert Margulies
GRAPHICS TECHNICIAN   Brett Stone
PRODUCTION   Sandy Hanley
LAYOUT ARTIST/COMPOSITOR   Elaine Kitsis

Quality Medical Publishing, Inc.
2248 Welsch Industrial Court
St. Louis, Missouri 63146
Telephone: 1-800-348-7808
Web site: *http://www.qmp.com*

LIBRARY OF CONGRESS CATALOGING-IN-PUBLICATION DATA

Extreme lateral interbody fusion / edited by J. Allan Goodrich, Ildemaro J. Volcan.
     p. ; cm.
  Includes bibliographical references and index.
  ISBN 978-1-57626-277-1 (hardcover)
1. Spinal fusion. 2. Spine—Endoscopic surgery. I. Goodrich, J. Allan.
II. Volcan, Ildemaro J.
  [DNLM: 1. Lumbar Vertebrae—surgery. 2. Spinal Fusion—methods. 3. Surgical Procedures, Minimally Invasive—methods. 4. Thoracic Vertebrae—surgery. WE 750 E96 2008]
  RD768.E98 2008
  617.5′60597—dc22

                               2008021683

QM/QM/LG
5   4   3   2   1

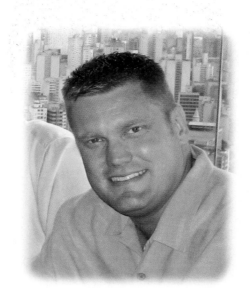

In Memory of

ERIC A. THOMAS, MD

November 11, 1971 – March 22, 2008

The members of the Society of Lateral Access Surgery (SOLAS) would like to dedicate this book to one of our founding members, Dr. Eric A. Thomas, a man who definitively had an impact on our lives, both professionally and personally.

Dr. Thomas (ET) loved the craft of surgery and especially enjoyed taking care of others. His passion and dedication for teaching helped positively transform the Marquis Visit Program, a surgeon education program with a focus on XLIF, with his high-quality standards and personal touch. ET was generous, and he openly shared his clinical expertise not only with surgeons, but with other health care professionals as well. He was the consummate teacher.

Dr. Eric A. Thomas will be remembered as a truly remarkable gentleman, surgeon, teacher, and an inspiring friend. His love for life and his passion for patient care will be his lasting legacies.

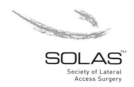

SOLAS™
Society of Lateral
Access Surgery

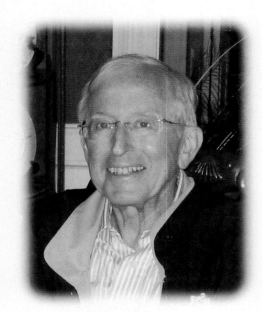

Dedicated to

SAMUEL M. GOODRICH, MD

To my brother, Sam, a dedicated physician for over 40 years who is adored by his patients and respected by his colleagues. A devoted son and a loving husband and father, he was recently diagnosed with pancreatic cancer and continues to fight with both courage and dignity. This book is in special recognition for all you have done for me.

To my parents, Ellis and Frieda Goodrich, who at an early age emphasized the importance of education and encouraged me to pursue a career in medicine. To my brothers, Sam and Ike, both outstanding physicians and role models, whose support has been invaluable throughout my medical training and practice. I cannot thank you enough. To my children, David and Amanda, who have been both understanding and tolerant over the years. To my grandson, Seth, who makes me look forward to every upcoming day. And especially to my wife, Martha, who has tried to keep me level-headed and has encouraged me to continue to follow my dreams in medicine. She deserves a medal of honor in perseverance.

Finally, to my patients and colleagues who continue to educate me in the craft of spinal surgery. I am forever grateful.

J.A.G.

In Dedication

To Daisy, my wife of 36 years, who has been my friend and companion, and the best cheerleader on my team. Her encouragement to pursue dreams and excel in our activities has been the energy that keeps me going. To my children, Beatriz Carolina, Ildemaro Javier, and Isabel Cristina, who have filled my life with challenges, love, and happiness. I hope they pursue their dreams as well. To my father, Dr. Ramon Volcan, who encouraged me to follow in his footsteps, and to my mother, Dorina Volcan, who filled my young life with love, principle, and dedication. To my parents-in-law, Luis Antonio and Hilda Pellicer, who have loved me as one of their own. To my grandchildren, Annabel Cristina, Andrew, Daisy Marie, and Miguel Juaquin—I love you more than I can express with words. To my siblings and other beloved relatives, who have each, in their own way, made a positive impact on my life. Thank you for your love, advice, and encouragement.

Finally, to my patients, who have taught me so much throughout my career and inspire me to excel on a daily basis.

I.J.V.

Contributors

Behrooz A. Akbarnia, MD
Clinical Professor, Department of Orthopaedics, University of California–San Diego, San Diego; Medical Director, San Diego Center for Spinal Disorders, La Jolla, California

Neel Anand, MD, Mch Orth
Director, Orthopaedic Spine Surgery; Director, Minimally Invasive Spinal Surgery, Institute for Spinal Disorders, Cedars-Sinai Medical Center, Los Angeles, California

John A. Anson, MD
Assistant Clinical Professor, Department of Neurosurgery, University Medical Center; Director, Nevada Neurosciences Institute, Department of Neurosurgery, Las Vegas, Nevada

Kent N. Bachus, PhD
Director, Orthopaedic Research Laboratory, Department of Orthopaedics, University of Utah Orthopaedic Center, Salt Lake City, Utah

Ramin Bagheri, MD
Clinical Instructor, Department of Orthopaedic Surgery, University of California–San Diego, San Diego, California

Eli M. Baron, MD
Neurosurgeon and Spine Surgeon, Institute for Spinal Disorders, Cedars-Sinai Medical Center, Los Angeles, California

R. Shay Bess, MD
Colorado Spine and Scoliosis Institute, Lonetree, Colorado

Darrel S. Brodke, MD
Professor and Vice Chairman, Department of Orthopaedics, University of Utah, Salt Lake City, Utah

Andrew Cappuccino, MD, BES
Director of Buffalo Spine Surgery, Buffalo, New York

Norman B. Chutkan, MD
Chairman, Department of Orthopaedics, Medical College of Georgia, Augusta, Georgia

Bernard Allan Cohen, PhD, FASNM, DABNM
Managing Director, Neurological Monitoring Associates, LLC, Milwaukee, Wisconsin

G. Bryan Cornwall, PhD, PEng
Vice President, Research and Clinical Resources, NuVasive, Inc., San Diego, California

Etevaldo Coutinho, MD
Department of Minimal Invasive Spine Surgery, Santa Rita Hospital, São Paulo, Brazil

Vedat Deviren, MD
Associate Professor, Department of Orthopaedic Surgery, University of California–San Francisco, San Francisco, California

Paul Fuchs, DO
Orthopedic Spine Surgeon, Department of Orthopedic Surgery, Lee Memorial Health Systems, Fort Myers, Florida

Ihab Gharzeddine, MD
Spine Surgeon, Department of Minimal Invasive Spine Surgery, Santa Rita Hospital, São Paulo, Brazil

David P. Goodrich, RN, BSN
Nurse Case Manager, Heartland Hospice, Augusta, Georgia

J. Allan Goodrich, MD
Associate Clinical Professor, Department of Orthopaedic Surgery, Medical College of Georgia; Augusta Orthopaedic Clinic, Augusta, Georgia

Kelli M. Howell, MS
Director of Clinical Resources, NuVasive, Inc., San Diego, California

Jonathan A. Hyde, MD
Spine Surgeon, Department of Orthopaedic Surgery, Mount Sinai Medical Center, Miami Beach, Florida

H. Brad Jones, Jr., MD
Brown and Radiology Associates, Augusta, Georgia

Stuart S. Kaplan, MD
Chief of Neurosurgery, Department of Neurosurgery; Head, Gamma Knife Center, Sunrise Hospital and Medical Center; The Nevada Neurosciences Institute, Department of Neurosurgery, Las Vegas, Nevada

Chad M. Kessler, MD
Orthopaedic Surgeon, Georgia Bone and Joint, LLC; Piedmont Hospital, Department of Orthopaedic Spine Surgery, Newnan, Georgia

Michael J. Lee, MD

Assistant Professor, Department of Orthopaedics and Sports Medicine, University of Washington Medical Center, Seattle, Washington

Juliano T. Lhamby, MD

Spine Surgeon, Department of Minimal Invasive Spine Surgery, Santa Rita Hospital, São Paulo, Brazil

Kyle Malone, MS

Director of Research, The NNI Research Foundation, Las Vegas, Nevada

Robert A. McGuire, MD

Professor and Chairman, Department of Orthopedics and Rehabilitation, University of Mississippi Medical Center, Jackson, Mississippi

Daniel K. Park, MD

Department of Orthopaedic Surgery, Rush University Medical Center, Chicago, Illinois

Murat Pekmezci, MD

Assistant Clinical Professor, Department of Orthopaedic Surgery, University of California–San Francisco, San Francisco, California

Mark D. Peterson, MD

Orthopedic Spine Surgeon, Sourthern Oregon Orthopedics, Inc., Medford, Oregon

Frank M. Phillips, MD

Professor, Department of Orthopaedic Surgery, Rush University Medical Center, Chicago, Illinois

Luiz Pimenta, MD, PhD

Assistant Professor, Department of Neurosurgery, University of California–San Diego, San Diego, California; Chief, Department of Minimal Invasive and Reconstructive Surgery, Santa Rita Hospital, São Paulo, Brazil

John J. Regan, MD

Director, Department of Orthopaedics, Cedars-Sinai Medical Center, Los Angeles; Medical Director, Spine Group Beverly Hills, Beverly Hills, California

W. Blake Rodgers, MD

President, Spine Midwest, Inc.; Medical Director, St. Mary's Health Center Spine Center, Jefferson City, Missouri

Thomas D. Schaffa, MD

Assistant Doctor Gastro Surgery, Hospital Servidor Público; Access Surgeon, Department of Minimal Invasive and Reconstructive Surgery, Santa Rita Hospital, São Paulo, SP, Brazil

William D. Smith, MD
Chief of Neurosurgery, University Medical Center of Southern Nevada; Director of Clinical Neurosurgery, The NNI Research Foundation, Las Vegas, Nevada

Bobby Tay, MD
Associate Professor, Department of Orthopaedic Surgery, University of California–San Francisco, San Francisco, California

William R. Taylor, MD
Professor of Surgery, Division of Neurosurgery, University of California–San Diego, San Diego, California

†Eric A. Thomas, MD
Spine Orthopaedic and Rehabilitation Center, Albuquerque, New Mexico

Jonathan A. Tuttle, MD
Department of Neurosurgery, Medical College of Georgia, Augusta, Georgia

Alexander R. Vaccaro, MD, PhD
Professor, Department of Orthpaedics and Neurosurgery, The Rothman Institute, Philadelphia, Pennsylvania

Richard E. Vance, BSME
Research Engineer, Department of Orthopedics, University of Utah, Salt Lake City, Utah

Ildemaro J. Volcan, MD
Associate Clinical Professor, Department of Neurological Surgery, Medical College of Georgia; West Augusta Spine Specialists, LLC, Augusta, Georgia

†Deceased.

Foreword

Minimally invasive techniques were long thought to be incompatible with spine surgery. Perhaps one reason for this belief is that there is an inherent reluctance to embrace new technologies and procedures when conventional surgeries can achieve the same surgical results. This reluctance can be a major obstacle for surgeons who choose to adopt new techniques. In my practice, however, minimally invasive techniques are the standard, not the exception. I have learned over the years that minimally invasive procedures not only simplify the processes of conventional surgeries, but they also make preserving the surrounding tissues possible. In no other procedure does this resonate as true as with lateral access surgery.

My experience with lateral access surgery began with an appreciation of the advantages of approaching the spine from the side—there is no need for posterior muscle, bony, and ligamentous dissection; the risks associated with anterior vascular dissection are avoided altogether because such a dissection is not necessary; and access to the diseased disc is typically straightforward.

I worked with access surgeon Dr. Thomas Schaffa, my longtime friend and colleague, on perfecting a minimally invasive technique for spine surgeries. Our experiences revealed that we could produce the safest and most reproducible results by using finger dissection to achieve retroperitoneal access. This insight—along with my collaboration with NuVasive®, Inc. (San Diego, CA) to design the appropriate surgical techniques, access instruments, and implants—resulted in the extreme lateral interbody fusion (XLIF®) procedure as it is defined today. I am delighted to see that the XLIF technique has been so widely adopted, and I believe that this book validates the exceptional clinical results that Dr. Schaffa and I found in our own practice.

This book marks a new era in minimally invasive techniques; we are literally turning spine surgery on its side. I look forward to watching how lateral access surgery will continue to evolve—from our early attempts to treat the degenerative disc to more advanced indications such as revisions, deformities, and motion preservation. I encourage you to participate in this revolution by becoming involved with the Society of Lateral Access Surgery (SOLAS™). For more information, please visit *www.lateralaccess.org*.

Obrigado,

Luiz Pimenta, MD, PhD
Hospital Santa Rita
São Paulo, Brazil

Preface

The practice of spine surgery is changing, fueled in large part by innovations in technology that offer surgeons superior options for treating challenging spinal pathologies and improving outcomes for their patients. Traditional techniques and approaches—those demanding significant dissections with inherent morbidities, including blood loss and prolonged recoveries—are giving way to new, less invasive procedures. Minimally invasive surgical techniques require smaller incisions and less dissection; they are swiftly and dynamically transforming the practice of spine surgery. Patient expectations have also changed—they insist on quick recoveries with minimal scarring. The extreme lateral interbody fusion (XLIF®, NuVasive®, Inc., San Diego, CA) technique is an innovative approach that plays an important role in this changing scenario. XLIF offers the potential for reduced tissue trauma, decreased blood loss, enhanced healing, improved cosmesis, and reduced morbidity.

Although the popularity of the XLIF technique is rapidly growing worldwide, a comprehensive reference that describes the procedure and details its clinical applications for the thoracic and lumbar spine has been lacking. This book exists to fill that void. We were joined in our endeavor by an amazing group of contributors, all of whom are experts in the XLIF approach; these individuals add tremendous depth to this project and provide an astounding amount of expertise. In fact, many of these individuals are the pioneers who blazed the trails to develop the XLIF approach.

eXtreme Lateral Interbody Fusion (XLIF®) is divided into two sections. Part I provides the fundamentals of the XLIF technique, a historical overview, and the relevant applied anatomy and biomechanics. In addition, fundamentals that guide the decision-making process are also explored in depth, with specific information given about radiology, the clinical evaluation of low back and leg pain, principles of direct and indirect decompression, and bone grafting options for lumbar spine fusions. We regard Part I as essential reading for the surgeon who is just beginning to learn the basic technique and for the experienced surgeon whose goal is to refine and enhance his or her skills.

Part II focuses on surgical techniques and clinical applications. The first chapter in the section details the step-by-step technique for the lumbar XLIF approach. Subsequent chapters focus on the safety of the procedure and potential complications. Of particular note are the clinical application chapters (Chapters 11 through 17), which provide information on how the XLIF approach can be used to treat a variety of spine conditions, including a degenerated/collapsed disc, junctional disease of the lumbar spine, degenerative spondylolisthesis and scoliosis, complex deformity, and revision surgery. Each clinical application chapter includes information on pathophysiology of the disease entity, clinical presentation, treatment options, XLIF application, postoperative management, and most conclude with case studies, which show the excellent results that can be achieved with the XLIF approach. Part II concludes with a section on other lateral approach applications, including XLIF in the outpatient setting, thoracic disc herniations, corpectomy, and total disc replacement.

A wealth of information is contained within these pages; numerous photographs, medical illustrations, and clinical cases have been included to enhance the educational experience. The book is filled with key information, tips, and surgical nuances to assist surgeons with developing the finesse necessary to avoid complications in the pursuit of surgical excellence.

It is our sincere hope that this book will provide a solid foundation of knowledge and assist surgeons at all levels by providing guidance to the beginner, insight to the experienced, and a source of stimulation to the most proficient, who continue to refine their skills. We have been given an opportunity to advance the art and science of spine surgery, but the ultimate reward of this book is that in sharing our knowledge, we are helping to improve outcomes for patients now and in the years to come.

ACKNOWLEDGMENTS

We would like to acknowledge the work of Luiz Pimenta, who realized the potential applications of minimally invasive lateral surgery of the spine. It was Dr. Pimenta who first merged the extreme lateral approach with neuromonitoring to provide safe access to the thoracic and lumbar spine above L5, and who helped to design appropriate access instruments and implants to take advantage of the approach. Dr. Pimenta is an innovator, mentor, and excellent teacher. He is an unusually humble and talented individual, and is eager to assist others as they master the XLIF approach. He has been extremely supportive and nurturing of this project, and his advice and guidance will always be appreciated.

At NuVasive, Kelli Howell has been the engine running the vehicle—the book itself. Her tireless efforts, including organizing the project, reviewing chapters, communicating with numerous authors, and keeping us (almost) on schedule, will never be forgotten. Her work, along with the support of Pat Miles, made this publication possible. Paul Cory has been more than a NuVasive representative in our region. He is a gentleman and friend, and his diligent efforts have provided tremendously positive experiences with the XLIF procedure. He is a pleasure to work with, and we look forward to many more positive cases in the future.

We would also like to thank Michelle Berger, Sara Blackwell, and the entire Quality Medical Publishing team, who have worked with us under tight deadlines to ensure this publication is the best it can be. Their combined efforts and expertise are truly appreciated.

J. Allan Goodrich, MD
Ildemaro J. Volcan, MD

Contents

PART II

Surgical Techniques and Clinical Applications

Lateral Techniques

Part I

Fundamentals

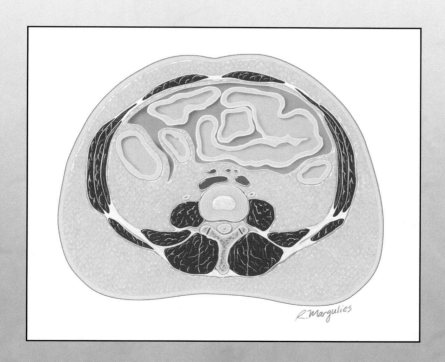

R. Margulies

1

Historical Background of Minimally Invasive Spine Surgery*

John J. Regan

Since the earliest recorded history, numerous pathologies have affected the spine. The earliest report of operative treatment of the spinal column is from Paulus of Aegina[1] in the seventh century. He advocated and conducted the direct removal of osseous tissue at the site of the pathology. A wide variety of approaches and techniques for the operative treatment of the spine have since been developed.

At one time, it was believed that speed was the critical, determining factor of a patient's surgical outcome. However, in the late 1800s, William S. Halsted noted that this outcome could be optimized if certain principles were applied during surgery. Although Halsted was known to work quickly, he nevertheless stressed the importance of minimal tissue disruption, meticulous hemostasis, and the proper closure of anatomic layers as essential factors for achieving optimal results. These were among the first principles of what is today known as *minimally invasive surgery*.

The popularity of minimally invasive surgery has grown recently, as surgeons face economic pressures from the competitive health care climate and continue to strive to optimize patient satisfaction. Developments in multiple surgical disciplines have led to reduced operative times and complications, minimal intraoperative tissue traumas, shorter hospital stays, the decreased use of narcotics postoperatively, and enhanced outcomes. Successful early ambulation after surgery and the advantages that outpatient procedures provide for the patient, hospital, and physician have resulted in a rapid progression toward minimally invasive surgical procedures.[2-6]

*Modified from Leonard MA, Samartzis D, Perez-Cruet MJ. Historical background of minimally invasive spine surgery. In Perez-Cruet MJ, Khoo LT, Fessler RG, eds. An Anatomic Approach to Minimally Invasive Spine Surgery. St Louis: Quality Medical Publishing, 2006, pp 3-23. With permission from Quality Medical Publishing, Inc.

GENERAL ADVANCEMENTS

The development of two fundamental techniques, endoscopy and microsurgery, has been essential to the evolution of minimally invasive spine surgery. Although it may seem that such technical advancements are new, many of these innovations were actually conceived more than 100 years ago.

The evolution of the endoscope began in 1806, when Philip Bozzini developed an endoscopic device, the *Lichtleiter,* in which a beeswax candle was used for illumination to facilitate the exploration of various body cavities.[7] In 1853, Desormeaux used a lens and an alcohol-based fluid, which allows better clarity and light conduction, on the endoscope for direct-light focus and increased intensity, respectively.[8,9] The first endoscopic procedure was performed by Bevan in 1868 to treat esophageal pathology.[8] Later, Nitze[10] developed a cystoscope that consisted of a working channel, illumination, and an optical lens for reflection. In 1902, the first laparoscopic surgery was performed,[11] and in 1911, Lespinasse, a urologist working in Chicago, performed the first cranial neuroendoscopic procedure when he fulgurated the choroid plexus in two infants with hydrocephalus.[12] In 1931, Burman[13] first reported on the use of endoscopy for the spine, which he termed *myeloscopy,* and in 1938, Pool[14] reported on his use of myeloscopy to inspect the nerve roots and spinal cord in patients with disc herniation, hypertrophied ligamentum flavum, benign and malignant neoplasms, and arachnoiditis. As the years progressed, the endoscope was improved and used for various diagnostic and therapeutic purposes. The development of a large variety of endoscopic instruments has made numerous endoscopic procedures possible. In 1997, Foley and Smith[15] attached an endoscope to a tubular retractor system, and the concept of *microendoscopic discectomy,* or *MED,* was born.

Although tubular retractors have been used for 20 years for cranial neurosurgery,[16] their introduction to spine surgery helped to usher in a new era in minimally invasive spine surgery. In 1998, the METRx-MD™ System (Medtronic Sofamor Danek, Memphis, TN) was introduced; the system used the same tubular retractors as with MED, but allowed the use of the microscope. This spawned the development of other tubular retractor systems and the advancement toward split-blade retractors, the first of which—the MaXcess® System (NuVasive®, Inc., San Diego, CA)—was introduced in 2003 for use in posterior and lateral approaches to the spine. The split-blade design obviates the need for endoscopes and instead allows direct visualization, aided by the attachment of fiberoptic light (Fig. 1-1).

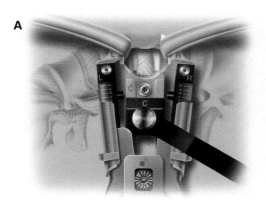
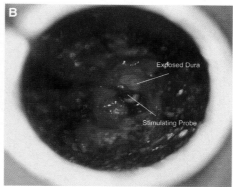

FIG. 1-1 **A,** Visualization through the split-blade exposure of the MaXcess System. **B,** Visualization through a tubular retractor system.

ADVANCEMENTS IN THE LUMBAR AND THORACIC SPINE

Although minimally invasive techniques can be applied to all regions of the spine, the history of the cervical applications is outside the scope of this book; only the thoracic and lumbar areas are discussed in this chapter. The focus is largely on the treatment of disc herniations and spondylosis, because much of the progress in the field of minimally invasive spine surgery was made while treating patients with these more common degenerative spinal diseases. However, these advancements were quickly adapted to treat virtually all other conditions that involve the spine.

THE LUMBAR SPINE

In 1857, Virchow[17] described traumatic intervertebral disc rupture, and in 1911, Middleton and Teacher[18] expanded on Virchow's first account when they reported their autopsy findings of traumatic disc rupture. Also in 1911, Goldthwait[19] speculated that lumbar disc herniations were responsible for sciatica. The first lumbar laminectomy in the United States reportedly occurred in 1829 and was performed by Smith to treat progressive paresis stemming from a previous fracture.[20] Using this laminectomy approach, in 1908 Oppenheim and Krause,[21] and later, in 1913, Elsberg[22] resected what were, in all likelihood, herniated lumbar discs. In 1929, Dandy[23] reported the first definitive description of operative treatment for lumbar disc disease, recognizing that the disease has a traumatic origin (Fig. 1-2). In 1934, the influential description by Mixter and Barr[24]—of neurologic deficits associated with a herniated lumbar disc and subsequent treatment with a lumbar discectomy via a laminectomy—stressed the practicality of operative intervention to address such lumbar pathology. In 1939, Love[25] advanced the practice of lumbar disc surgery when he reported on his technique that involved removing herniated discs through a minimally inva-

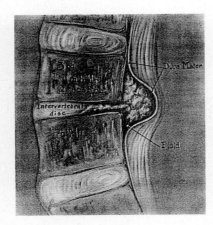

FIG. 1-2   Posterior protrusion from a disrupted intervertebral disc, causing spinal canal compromise and cauda equina compression. (From Dandy W. Loose cartilage from intervertebral disk simulating tumor of the spinal cord. Arch Surg 19:660-672, 1929.)

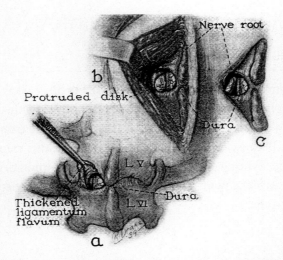

FIG. 1-3   Nerve root decompression viewed through a minimally invasive laminotomy. **A,** Initial exposure and removal of the ligamentum flavum. **B,** The nerve root and herniated disc fragment are identified. **C,** The relaxed nerve root is shown after decompression via removal of the herniated disc fragment. (From Love J. Protruded intervertebral disks with a note regarding hypertrophy of ligamenta flava. JAMA 113:2029-2034, 1939.)

sive interlaminar approach that typically required no bone removal (Fig. 1-3). Adaptations of this technique form the basis for the microlumbar discectomy that is still in use today. In 1973, Scoville and Corkill[26] reported on early mobilization of the postoperative discectomy patient. Before these findings, patients were usually bedridden for days after undergoing a discectomy, with instructions for severely restricting their activities for weeks or months. Striving to promote intraoperative visual acuity and reduce tissue trauma, Caspar[27] and Yasargil[28] simultaneously introduced the use of an operating microscope and microsurgical techniques in 1977 for the treatment of lumbar disc disease. In addition, Caspar's 1977 paper described instruments and techniques that bear a striking resemblance to those used

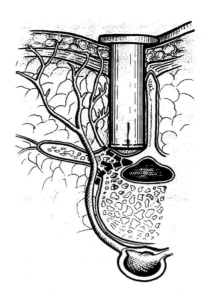

FIG. 1-4   The retractor introduced by Caspar in 1977, with striking similarities to the technique of microendoscopic discectomy introduced by Foley and Smith in 1997. (From Caspar W. A new surgical procedure for lumbar disc herniation causing less tissue damage through a microsurgical approach. In Wüllenweber R, Brock M, Hamer J, et al, eds. Advances in Neurosurgery. Berlin: Springer-Verlag, 1977, pp 74-80.)

two decades later by Foley and Smith[15] in their description of MED (Fig. 1-4). Williams[29] further supported and popularized microdiscectomy in the 1970s by advocating minimizing the skin incision and removing only the herniated disc fragment through an intralaminar window, not unlike Love's technique. During the 1990s, an explosion in the number of endoscopic procedures and techniques occurred in numerous fields, and spine surgery was no exception. The use of an endoscope for lumbar discectomy was introduced by Mayer and Brock in 1993.[30] In the mid-1990s, a transforaminal endoscopic microdiscectomy was reported that provided direct visualization of the epidural space via entry under the pars and superior articular facet.[31] In 1997, Foley and Smith[15] illustrated the development and application of the MED system. Shortly thereafter, the METRx-MD system was introduced, allowing surgeons to take advantage of the tubular retractors that could be used with either the endoscope or the microscope. Based on the success of these systems in treating herniated discs,[32] a minimally invasive technique for the treatment of lumbar stenosis was developed; this technique avoids many of the consequences of the traditional laminectomy, including the formation of excessive scar tissue, disruption of the posterior bony elements, subsequent instability of the spine, and ensuing biomechanical alterations.[33]

In an attempt to further decrease tissue trauma and enhance postoperative outcome, other minimally invasive surgical procedures have been developed to address lumbar disc herniation. In 1941, Jansen and Balls[34] first isolated chymopapain, a proteolytic enzyme extracted from papaya latex. After in-depth animal experimentation, chymopapain was injected into humans, and the subsequent results were reported by Smith[35] in 1964. This process, aptly called *chemonucleolysis,* leads to the depolymerization of the nucleus pulposus by liberating chondroitin and keratin sulfates through the hydrolysis of the noncollagenous proteins of mucopolysaccharide. The efficacy of chemonucleolysis in randomized prospective clinical trials compared with open techniques remains controversial; chemonucleolysis has not demonstrated significant clinical benefit and has also been associated with allergic reactions and paralysis.[36-39] In 1975, Hijikata[40] demonstrated a percutaneous nucleotomy by using arthroscopic techniques for disc removal via intradiscal access to treat posterior or posterolateral lumbar disc herniations. Automated percutaneous discectomy (APD) was developed in 1985 by Onik et al[41]; this technique involved the insertion of a 2 mm probe for rapid, safe removal of the disc material. In the late 1980s, percutaneous laser discectomy was introduced by Choy et al[42] and has since gained considerable attention. As with APD, this technique uses a percutaneous approach to the disc, but then uses a laser that has varying intensities to absorb the nucleus pulposus. Stereotactic lumbar microdiscectomy has also been suggested, as well as intraoperative magnetic resonance imaging (MRI) for discectomies.[43,44]

Whether or not these advancements were better than the traditional open procedure is a subject of debate; however, each technique represents how clinicians continue to strive to make surgery for their patients with herniated lumbar discs as minimally invasive as possible. In addition to the progress made for the treatment of herniated lumbar discs, advancements have also been developed that make lumbar spine fusions less invasive. Posterior lumbar interbody fusion (PLIF) was proposed by Cloward in 1953[45] to treat degenerative disc disease or spondylolisthesis. Since that time, the procedure has been modified and advocated by many others. It has proved effective in treating select patients who require fusion, but has remained essentially as invasive as when Cloward first proposed it.[46-52] In 2002, Foley and Gupta[53] reported on their experiences with a percutaneous, minimally invasive PLIF. Based on previous reports on the success of a unilateral PLIF,[54,55] Isaacs et al[56] reported their experiences with a modification of Foley and Gupta's technique in which they incorporated a unilateral, less invasive approach. In addition, continuous developments in image-guided computer and fluoroscopic technologies have greatly facilitated the safe and expeditious application of instrumentation.

As an alternative to PLIF for patients requiring fusion, an anterior lumbar interbody fusion (ALIF) has been described. Since ALIF was first reported, the preferred route to the anterior lumbar spine has been via a retroperitoneal approach.[57-59] In recent years, several authors have modified the retroperitoneal approach to make it less invasive.[60-63] In 1998, McAfee et al[64] described a minimally invasive endoscopic retroperitoneal approach that allowed a small skin incision and less tissue disruption. In the early 1990s, the use of laparoscopic procedures to address various pathologies of the spine began and gained immense momentum. Laparoscopic spine surgery was first reported in 1991 by Obenchain[65] in his description of a lumbar discectomy of L5-S1. In 1995, Zucherman et al[66] performed laparoscopic instrumented interbody fusion of the spine. Since then, the use of the laparoscope for spinal procedures has become significantly more common.[67-74] However, such procedures have a steep learning curve, and higher complication rates are reported, compared with traditional open procedures. In addition, such techniques lack any appreciable increased benefit; as a result, laparoscopic anterior lumbar interbody fusion is a less attractive option than traditional open methods.[75-79]

In an effort to find a less invasive way to treat discogenic back pain, Saal and Saal[80] developed an intradiscal electrothermal therapy (IDET) in the late 1990s. Fundamentally, the IDET approaches the nucleus pulposus in a similar manner as the aforementioned procedures; a navigable catheter with a temperature-controlled thermal resistive coil is introduced to heat and alter the disc material. However, clinical results have been mixed,[81,82] and the procedure has fallen out of use in recent years.

More recently, building on the experience of lateral transpsoas retroperitoneal endoscopic approaches, a direct lateral mini-open approach to the lumbar spine was popularized by Luiz Pimenta. This extreme lateral interbody fusion approach (XLIF®, NuVasive, Inc.) relies on a lateral-based split-blade Retractor (MaXcess), a real-time nerve root monitoring system (NeuroVision®, NuVasive, Inc.), and a laterally placed interbody cage (CoRoent® XL, NuVasive, Inc.). Unlike anterior retroperitoneal approaches, mobilization of the iliac vessels is not necessary, accounting primarily for the rise in popularity of this procedure.

THORACIC SPINE

In 1779, Pott[83] was one of the first to propose surgical intervention for an ailment of the thoracic spine. In his writings on paraplegia, he recommended draining the tuberculum abscess. Since then, patients with an assortment of ailments affecting the thoracic spine have undergone a wide variety of surgical approaches in an attempt to minimize the morbidity of this procedure. Surgery for the anterior column of the thoracic spine poses certain challenges not seen in either the cervical or lumbar region. Certain anatomic structures complicate the anterior exposure when operating on either the thoracic or cervical region. For this reason, early surgical approaches to the thoracic spine were like approaches to the cervical spine in that they were posterior in nature and resulted in the same relatively poor outcomes, prompting surgeons to seek alternate approaches. However, unlike the cervical spine, which is easy to approach anteriorly, the contents of the chest make anterior approaches to the thoracic spine challenging. When surgeons first devised alternate approaches to treat lesions of the thoracic spine, the presence of the spinal cord posteriorly and the thoracic cavity contents anteriorly had to be addressed. A number of approaches were in development that varied in how they responded to these two limitations, all with the intention of making surgery of this nature as minimally invasive as possible. The history of the treatment of thoracic disc herniations provides an excellent example of how surgeries of the thoracic spine have evolved over the past century.

The first reported case of a herniated thoracic disc was made by Key in 1838.[84] In 1911, Middleton and Teacher[18] provided additional evidence that disc herniations occur in the thoracic spine. The first known case of operative treatment of a thoracic herniated disc was described in 1922 by Adsen,[85] who performed disc removal after a laminectomy. For much of the next several decades, the procedure of choice was a posterior approach, but the results were dismal.[86-88] The lateral extracavitary approach was first described by Menard[89] in 1894 to treat Pott's disease and was later adapted to treat disc herniations.[90] Cauchoix and Binet[91] reported on their initial experience with a transsternal approach to the upper thoracic spine in 1957. In 1969, Perot and Munro[92] and Ransohoff et al[93] adapted the transthoracic technique of Hodgson and Stock[94] and simultaneously reported on a transthoracic approach to treat thoracic disc herniations. In 1978, Patterson and Arbit[95] described the transpedicular approach in an attempt to avoid entering the thoracic cavity. In the late 1990s, Stillerman et al[96,97] introduced the slightly less invasive, transfacet, pedicle-sparing approach. In 1995, McCormick[98] described the retropleural approach, which avoided entering the thoracic cavity and disrupting the facet joint. Jho[99] introduced the posterior microendoscopic approach to treat thoracic disc herniations in 1997.

Although the evolution of these approaches details significant advances in making surgery for thoracic disc herniations much less invasive, such approaches were still somewhat invasive. In an attempt to minimize operative morbidity, thoracoscopic video-assisted spine surgery (VATS) was developed and first performed in the early 1990s simultaneously by Mack et al[100] in the United States and Rosenthal et al[101] in Europe. Initially, thoracoscopic spine procedures were implemented to treat disc herniations or for tumor biopsies. However, in the ensuing years, thoracoscopy was used to address scoliosis, anterior interbody fusion, drainage of disc space abscess, and vertebrectomy for tumors.[102-107] In a series of 100 consecutive cases, Anand and Regan[108] developed a classification system to identify and treat thoracic disc disease using endoscopic thoracic techniques.

More recently, the XLIF mini-open approach has been described for accessing the anterior thoracic spine with minimal morbidity. Detailed descriptions are found in Chapters 19 through 21.

FUTURE DIRECTIONS

The recent development of methods used to preserve motion—not to fuse the spine—has led to significant interest in artificial disc replacement of the lumbar and cervical spine. Intervention in the earlier stages of the degenerative disc cascade will undoubtedly lead to biologic solutions using stem cell technology. Posterior interspinous systems have been developed to treat spinal stenosis and may also be efficacious in the treatment of symptomatic degenerative disc disease. Alternatively, pilot Food and Drug Administration (FDA) trials for nuclear disc replacements have been completed. These technologies lend themselves to minimally invasive and percutaneous surgical approaches and offer patients the hope of treating earlier-stage degenerative disc disease with motion preservation and restoring disc physiology and biomechanics. Even total disc replacement will have a minimally invasive approach option in the lumbar spine, with the advent of a laterally placed device through the XLIF approach.

CONCLUSION

The field of spine surgery has undergone significant growth in the last two decades. A considerable part of this growth has been devoted to the development of less invasive techniques and technologies that minimize approach-related trauma to the patient. Refinements of standard techniques of lumbar and cervical discectomy and fusion using microsurgical techniques—combined with improvements in anesthesia—have resulted in the application of these procedures in the outpatient setting. The evolution of surgical techniques and treatment methodologies is a testament to the optimal quality of care that physicians seek to offer their patients. Advances in minimally invasive spine surgery have led to significantly improved outcomes, reduced complication rates, shortened hospital stays, and lower costs. As with any new technology, surgeons are responsible for learning and using these new techniques in a manner that, when applied, avoids further complications for their patients. Some procedures, such as laparoscopy and IDET, do not stand the test of time as a result of the steep learning curve or lack of sufficient outcome data. Others, such as mini-TLIF and XLIF, minimize the learning curve by involving conventional techniques and may offer practical options for an even wider range of minimally invasive spine surgeries.

REFERENCES

1. Knoeller SM, Seifried C. History of spine surgery. Spine 25:2838-2843, 2000.
2. Nichol JM. Surgery of infancy. Br Med J 2:753-756, 1909.
3. Detmer DE, Buchanan-Davidson DJ. Ambulatory surgery. In Rutkow IM, ed. Socioeconomics of Surgery. St Louis: CV Mosby, 1989, pp 30-50.
4. Dubois F, Icard P, Berthelot G, et al. Coelioscopic cholecystectomy. Preliminary report of 36 cases. Ann Surg 211:60-62, 1998.
5. Durant GD. Ambulatory surgery centers: surviving, thriving into the 1990s. Med Group Manage J 36:16-20, 1989.
6. Sulvetta MB. Achieving cost control in the hospital outpatient department. Health Care Financ Rev Annu Suppl 12:95-106, 1991.
7. Bush RB, Leonhardt H, Bush RB IV, et al. Dr. Bozzini's Lichtleiter. A translation of his original article (1806). Urology 3:119-123, 1974.
8. Rosenthal DJ, Dickman CA. The history of thoracoscopic spine surgery. In Dickman CA, Rosenthal DJ, Perin NI, eds. Thoracoscopic Spine Surgery. New York: Thieme, 1999, pp 1-5.
9. Smythe WR, Kaiser LR. History of thoracoscopic surgery. In Kaiser LR, Daniel TM, eds. Thoracoscopic Surgery. Boston: Little Brown, 1993, pp 1-16.
10. Nitze M. Eine neue Beobachtungs—und Untersuchungsmethode für Harnrohre, Harnblase und Rectum. Wien Med Wochenschr 24:649-652, 1879.
11. Kelling G. Uberoesophagoskopie, gastroskopie, and kalioskope. Munch Med Wochenschr 52: 21-24, 1902.
12. Gerzeny M, Cohen AR. Advances in endoscopic neurosurgery. AORN J 67:957-961, 963-965, 1998.
13. Burman M. Myeloscopy or the direct visualization of the spinal canal and its contents. J Bone Joint Surg Am 12:695-696, 1931.
14. Pool JL. Direct visualization of dorsal nerve roots of cauda equina by means of a myeloscope. Arch Neurol Psychiatr 39:1308-1312, 1938.

15. Foley KT, Smith MM. Microendoscopic discectomy. Tech Neurosurg 3:301-307, 1997.

16. Kelly PJ. State of the art and future directions of minimally invasive stereotactic neurosurgery. Cancer Control 2:287-292, 1995.

17. Virchow R. Untersuchungen über die Entwicklung des Schadelgrundes im gesunden und krankhaften Zustande. Berlin: Reimber, 1857.

18. Middleton G, Teacher JH. Injury of the spinal cord due to rupture of an intervertebral disc during muscular effort. Glasgow Med J 6:1-66, 1911.

19. Goldthwait JE. The lumbosacral articulation. An explanation of many cases of "lumbago," "sciatica," and paraplegia. Boston Med Surg J 164:365-372, 1911.

20. Keller T, Holland MC. Some notable American spine surgeons of the 19th century. Spine 22:1413-1417, 1997.

21. Oppenheim H, Krause F. Über Einklemmung und Strangulation der Cauda equina. Dtsch Med Wochenschr 35:697-700, 1909.

22. Elsberg CA. Experiences in spinal surgery: observations upon 60 laminectomies for spinal disease. Surg Gynecol Obstet 16:117-120, 1913.

23. Dandy W. Loose cartilage from intervertebral disk stimulating tumor of the spinal cord. Arch Surg 19:660-672, 1929.

24. Mixter WJ, Barr JS. Rupture of the intervertebral disc with involvement of the spinal canal. N Engl J Med 211:210-215, 1934.

25. Love J. Protruded intervertebral disks with a note regarding hypertrophy of ligament flava. JAMA 113:2029-2034, 1939.

26. Scoville WB, Corkill G. Lumbar disc surgery: technique of radical removal and early mobilization. Technical note. J Neurosurg 39:265-269, 1973.

27. Caspar W. A new surgical procedure for lumbar disc herniation causing less tissue damage through a microsurgical approach. In Wüllenweber R, Brock M, Hamer J, et al, eds. Advances in Neurosurgery. Berlin: Springer-Verlag, 1977, pp 74-80.

28. Yasargil MG. Microsurgical operation of herniated lumbar disc. In Wüllenweber R, Brock M, Hamer J, et al, eds. Advances in Neurosurgery. Berlin: Springer-Verlag, 1977, p 81.

29. Williams RW. Microlumbar discectomy: a conservative surgical approach to the virgin herniated lumbar disc. Spine 3:175-182, 1978.

30. Mayer HM, Brock M. Percutaneous endoscopic discectomy: surgical technique and preliminary results compared to microsurgical discectomy. J Neurosurg 78:216-225, 1993.

31. Mathews HH. Transforaminal endoscopic microdiscectomy. Neurosurg Clin North Am 7:59-63, 1996.

32. Palmer S. Use of a tubular retractor system in microscopic lumbar discectomy: 1 year prospective results in 135 patients. Neurosurg Focus 13:1-5, 2002.

33. Palmer S, Turner R, Palmer R. Bilateral decompression of lumbar spinal stenosis involving a unilateral approach with microscope and tubular retractor system. J Neurosurg 97(2 Suppl): 213-217, 2002.

34. Jansen EF, Balls AK. Chymopapain: a new crystalline proteinase from papaya latex. J Biol Chem 137:459-460, 1941.

35. Smith L. Enzyme dissolution of the nucleus pulposus in humans. JAMA 187:137-140, 1964.

36. Crawshaw C, Frazer AM, Merriam WF, et al. A comparison of surgery and chemonucleolysis in the treatment of sciatica. A prospective randomized trial. Spine 9:195-198, 1984.

37. Ejeskar A, Nachemson A, Herberts P, et al. Surgery versus chemonucleolysis for herniated lumbar discs. A prospective study with random assignment. Clin Orthop Relat Res 174:236-242, 1983.

38. Muralikuttan KP, Hamilton A, Kemohan WG, et al. A prospective randomized trial of chemonucleolysis and conventional disc surgery in single level lumbar disc herniation. Spine 17:381-387, 1992.

39. van Alphen HAM, Brackman R, Bezemer PD, et al. Chemonucleolysis versus discectomy: a randomized multicenter trial. J Neurosurg 70:869-875, 1989.

40. Hijikata S. Percutaneous nucleotomy. A new concept technique and 12 years' experience. Clin Orthop Relat Res 238:9-23, 1989.

41. Onik G, Helms CA, Ginsburg L, et al. Percutaneous lumbar discectomy using a new aspiration probe. AJR Am J Roentgenol 6:290, 1985.

42. Choy DS, Case RB, Fielding W, et al. Percutaneous laser nucleolysis of lumbar disks. N Engl J Med 317:771-772, 1987.

43. Koutrouvelis PG, Lang E. Stereotactic lumbar microdiscectomy. Neurosurg Clin North Am 7:49-57, 1996.

44. Woodard EJ, Leon SP, Moriarty TM, et al. Initial experience with intraoperative magnetic resonance imaging in spine surgery. Spine 26:410-417, 2001.

45. Cloward RB. The treatment of ruptured lumbar intervertebral discs by vertebral body fusion. I. Indications, operative technique, after care. J Neurosurg 10:154-168, 1953.

46. Lin PM. A technical modification of Cloward's posterior lumbar interbody fusion. Neurosurgery 1:118-124, 1977.

47. Branch CL Jr. The case for posterior lumbar interbody fusion. Clin Neurosurg 43:252-267, 1996.

48. Ma GW. Posterior lumbar interbody fusion with specialized instruments. Clin Orthop Relat Res 193:57-63, 1985.

49. Steffee AD, Sitkowski DJ. Posterior lumbar interbody fusion and plates. Clin Orthop Relat Res 227:99-102, 1988.

50. Brantigan JW, Steffee AD. A carbon fiber implant to aid interbody lumbar fusion. Two-year clinical results in the first 26 patients. Spine 18:2106-2107, 1993.

51. Suk SI, Lee CK, Kim WJ, et al. Adding posterior lumbar interbody fusion to pedicle screw fixation and posterolateral fusion after decompression in spondylolytic spondylolisthesis. Spine 22:210-219; discussion 219-220, 1997.

52. Lowe TG, Tahemia AD, O'Brien MF, et al. Unilateral transforaminal posterior lumbar interbody fusion (TLIF): indications, technique, and 2-year results. J Spinal Disord Tech 15:31-38, 2002.

53. Foley KT, Gupta SK. Percutaneous pedicle screw fixation of the lumbar spine: preliminary clinical results. J Neurosurg 97(1 Suppl):S7-S12, 2002.

54. Blume HG, Rojas CH. Unilateral lumbar interbody fusion (posterior approach) utilizing dowel grafts: experience in over 200 patients. J Neurol Orthop Surg 2:171-175, 1981.

55. Rosenberg WS, Mummaneni PV. Transforaminal lumbar interbody fusion: technique, complications, and early results. Neurosurgery 48:569-574, 2001.

56. Isaacs RE, Khoo LT, Perez-Cruet MJ, et al. Minimally invasive microendoscopic posterior lumbar interbody fusion with instrumentation. Presented at the Annual Meeting of the American Association of Neurological Surgeons, Chicago, April 2002.

57. Sacks S. Anterior interbody fusion of the lumbar spine. J Bone Joint Surg Br 47:211-223, 1965.

58. Loguidice VA, Johnson RG, Guyer RD, et al. Anterior lumbar interbody fusion. Spine 13:366-369, 1988.

59. Knox BD, Chapman TM. Anterior lumbar interbody fusion for discogram concordant pain. J Spinal Disord 6:242-244, 1993.

60. Dewald CJ, Millikan KW, Hammerberg KW, et al. An open, minimally invasive approach to the lumbar spine. Am Surg 65:61-68, 1999.

61. Mayer HM. The ALIF concept. Eur Spine J 9(Suppl 1):S35-S43, 2000.

62. Mayer HM. A new microsurgical technique for minimally invasive anterior lumbar interbody fusion. Spine 22:691-699; discussion 700, 1997.

63. Fraser RD, Gogan WJ. A modified muscle-splitting approach to the lumbosacral spine. Spine 17:943-948, 1992.

64. McAfee PC, Regan JJ, Geis WP, et al. Minimally invasive anterior retroperitoneal approach to the lumbar spine. Emphasis on the lateral BAK. Spine 23:1476-1484, 1998.

65. Obenchain TG. Laparoscopic lumbar discectomy: a case report. J Laparoendosc Surg 1:145-149, 1991.

66. Zucherman JF, Zdeblick TA, Baily SA, et al. Instrumented laparoscopic spinal fusion: preliminary results. Spine 20:2029-2034; discussion 2034-2035, 1995.

67. Cloyd DW, Obenchain TG. Laparoscopic lumbar discectomy. Semin Laparosc Surg 3:95-102, 1996.

68. Cloyd DW, Obenchain TG, Savin M. Transperitoneal laparoscopic approach to lumbar discectomy. Surg Laparosc Endosc 5:85-89, 1995.

69. Slotman GJ, Stein SC. Laparoscopic lumbar diskectomy: preliminary report of a minimally invasive anterior approach to the herniated L5-S1 disk. Surg Laparosc Endosc 5:363-369, 1995.

70. Slotman GJ, Stein SC. Laparoscopic laser lumbar diskectomy. Operative technique and case report. Surg Endosc 9:826-829, 1995.

71. Slotman GJ, Stein SC. Laparoscopic L5-S1 diskectomy: a cost-effective, minimally invasive general surgery–neurosurgery team alternative to laminectomy. Am Surg 62:64-68, 1996.

72. Slotman GJ, Stein SC. Laminectomy compared with laparoscopic diskectomy and outpatient laparoscopic diskectomy for herniated L5-S1 intervertebral disks. J Laparoendosc Adv Surg Tech A 8:261-267, 1998.

73. Stein S, Slotman GJ. Laser-assisted laparoscopic lumbar diskectomy. N Engl J Med 91:175-176, 1994.

74. Zelko JR, Misko J, Swanstrom L, et al. Laparoscopic lumbar discectomy. Am J Surg 169:496-498, 1995.

75. Chung SK, Lee SH, Lim SR, et al. Comparative study of laparoscopic L5-S1 fusion versus open mini-ALIF, with a minimum 2-year follow-up. Eur Spine J 12:613-617, 2003.

76. Escobar E, Transfeldt E, Garvey T, et al. Video-assisted versus open anterior lumbar spine fusion surgery: a comparison of four techniques and complications in 135 patients. Spine 28:729-732, 2003.

77. Kaiser MG, Haid RW Jr, Subach BR, et al. Comparison of the mini-open versus laparoscopic approach for anterior lumbar interbody fusion: a retrospective review. Neurosurgery 51:97-103; discussion 103-105, 2002.

78. Liu JC, Ondra SL, Angelos P, et al. Is laparoscopic anterior lumbar interbody fusion a useful minimally invasive procedure? Neurosurgery 51(Suppl 5):S155-S158, 2002.

79. Sasso RC, Kenneth Burkus J, LeHuec JC. Retrograde ejaculation after anterior lumbar interbody fusion: transperitoneal versus retroperitoneal exposure. Spine 28:1023-1026, 2003.

80. Saal JA, Saal JS. Intradiscal electrothermal treatment for chronic discogenic low back pain. Spine 25:2622-2627, 2000.

81. Ercelen O, Bulutcu E, Oktenoglu T, et al. Radiofrequency lesioning using two different time modalities for the treatment of lumbar discogenic pain: a randomized trial. Spine 28:1922-1927, 2003.

82. Saal JA, Saal JS. Intradiscal electrothermal treatment for chronic discogenic low back pain: prospective outcome study with a minimum 2-year follow-up. Spine 27:966-973; discussion 973-974, 2002.

83. Pott P. Remarks on that Kind of Palsy of the Lower Limbs Which is Frequently Found to Accompany a Curvature of the Spine. London: J Johnson, 1779.

84. Key C. Mr. Aston Key on paraplegia. Guy's Hospital Reports 3:17-34, 1838.

85. Zeidman SM, Rosner MK, Poffenbarger JG. Thoracic disc disease, spondylosis, and stenosis. In Benzel EC, Stillerman CV, eds. The Thoracic Spine. St Louis: Quality Medical Publishing, 1999, pp 297-303.

86. Hawk WA. Spinal compression caused by ecchondrosis of the intervertebral fibrocartilage: with a review of the recent literature. Brain 59:204-224, 1936.

87. Horwitz NH, Rizzoli HV. Postoperative Complications in Neurosurgical Practice. Baltimore: Williams & Wilkins, 1967.

88. Logue V. Thoracic intervertebral disc prolapse with spinal cord compression. J Neurol Neurosurg Psychiatr 15:227-241, 1952.

89. Menard V. Étude Pratique sur le Mal de Pott. Paris: Masson et Cie, 1900.

90. Maiman DJ, Larson SJ, Luck E, et al. Lateral extracavitary approach to the spine for thoracic disc herniation: report of 23 cases. Neurosurgery 14:178-182, 1984.

91. Cauchoix J, Binet J. Anterior surgical approaches to the thoracic spine. Ann R Coll Surg Engl 27:237-243, 1957.

92. Perot PL Jr, Munro DD. Transthoracic removal of midline thoracic disc protrusions causing spinal cord compression. J Neurosurg 31:452-458, 1969.

93. Ransohoff J, Spencer F, Siew F, et al. Transthoracic removal of thoracic disc. Report of three cases. J Neurosurg 31:459-461, 1969.

94. Hodgson A, Stock FE. Anterior spinal fusion, a preliminary communication on the radical treatment of Pott's disease and Pott's paraplegia. Br J Surg 44:266-275, 1956.

95. Patterson RHJ, Arbit E. A surgical approach through the pedicle to protruded thoracic discs. J Neurosurg 48:768-772, 1978.

96. Stillerman CB, Chen TC, Couldwell WT, et al. Experience in the surgical management of 82 symptomatic herniated thoracic discs and review of the literature. J Neurosurg 88:623-633, 1998.

97. Stillerman CB, Chen TC, Couldwell WT, et al. Transfacet pedicle-sparing approach. In Benzel EC, Stillerman CB, eds. The Thoracic Spine. St Louis: Quality Medical Publishing, 1999, pp 338-345.

98. McCormick PC. Retropleural approach to the thoracic and thoracolumbar spine. Neurosurgery 37:908-914, 1995.

99. Jho HD. Endoscopic microscopic transpedicular thoracic discectomy. Technical note. J Neurosurg 87:125-129, 1997.

100. Mack MJ, Regan JJ, Bobechko WP, et al. Application of thorascopy for diseases of the spine. Ann Thorac Surg 56:736-738, 1993.

101. Rosenthal DJ, Rosenthal DR, de Simone A. Removal of a protruded thoracic disc using microsurgical endoscopy. A new technique. Spine 19:1087-1091, 1994.

102. Clay RS, Court TH. The history of the microscope compiled from original instruments and documents, up to the introduction of the achromatic microscope. London: Charles Griffin, 1932.

103. Dickman CA, Mican CA. Multilevel anterior thoracic discectomies and anterior interbody fusion using a microsurgical thoracoscopic approach. Case report. J Neurosurg 84:104-109, 1996.

104. Dickman CA, Rosenthal D, Karahalios DG, et al. Thoracic vertebrectomy and reconstruction using a microsurgical thoracoscopic approach. Neurosurgery 38:279-293, 1996.

105. Goldstein JA, McAfee PC. Minimally invasive endoscopic surgery of the spine. J South Orthop Assoc 5:251-262, 1996.

106. McKenna RJ Jr, Maline D, Pratt G. VATS resection of a mediastinal neurogenic dumbbell tumor. Surg Laparosc Endosc 5:480-482, 1995.

107. Parker LM, McAfee PC, Feder IL, et al. Minimally invasive surgical techniques to treat spine infections. Orthop Clin North Am 27:183-199, 1996.

108. Anand N, Regan JJ. Video-assisted thoracoscopic surgery for thoracic disc disease: classification and outcome study of 100 consecutive cases with a 2-year minimum follow-up period. Spine 27:871-879, 2002.

2

Basic Concepts:
Applied Anatomy of Extreme
Lateral Interbody Fusion

J. Allan Goodrich ▪ Ildemaro J. Volcan
Thomas D. Schaffa ▪ David P. Goodrich

Surgical procedures, whether open or minimally invasive, cannot be performed safely or successfully without a thorough knowledge of the relevant anatomy. Specific knowledge of the bony structures, soft tissues, and vascular and neurologic structures is of the utmost importance. Orthopaedic and neurosurgeons are, in general, quite familiar with posterior approaches to the lumbar spine. Anterior access is usually obtained with the assistance of a vascular or general surgeon who is adept at mobilizing the great vessels and protecting these throughout the procedure. With the introduction of the extreme lateral interbody fusion (XLIF®, NuVasive®, Inc., San Diego, CA) approach—a retroperitoneal, transpsoas approach to anterior column stabilization of the thoracolumbar spine (Fig. 2-1)—a review of the contents and boundaries of the retroperitoneal space is appropriate.

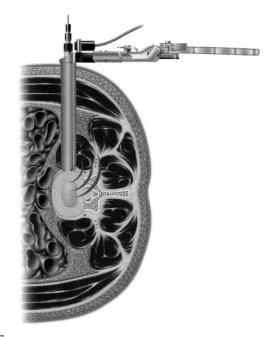

FIG. 2-1 Axial illustration of XLIF's retroperitoneal, transpsoas access to the lumbar spine using the MaXcess® (NuVasive, Inc.) Retractor.

The retroperitoneal space is the area of the posterior abdominal wall located between the posterior parietal peritoneum and the posterior part of the transversalis fascia. Located within this space are embryologically related organs such as the adrenal glands, kidneys, and ureters, all of which are referred to as the *retroperitoneal viscera*. Also within the retroperitoneal space is the neurovascular apparatus, formed by the aorta and its branches, the inferior vena cava and its tributaries, the lymphatic vessels and the lymph nodes, and the lumbar plexus, with its branches and the sympathetic trunk.

The retroperitoneal space is covered anteriorly by the parietal peritoneum (Fig. 2-2) and posteriorly by the transversalis fascia. The retroperitoneal space extends from the twelfth thoracic vertebra and the twelfth rib cephalad to the base of the sacrum, the iliac crest, and the pelvic diaphragm caudally. The lateral borders extend from an imaginary line from the tip of the twelfth rib down to the junction of the anterior and posterior halves of the iliac crest.

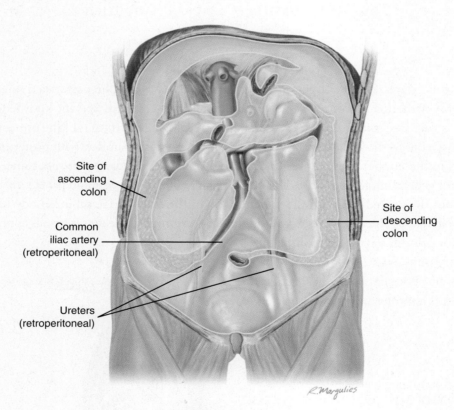

FIG. 2-2 The peritoneum.

MUSCULAR ANATOMY

The anterior lateral abdominal muscles include the external oblique, internal oblique, transversus abdominis, and rectus abdominis. The XLIF approach involves careful dissection through the oblique muscles—the most superficial of these is the external oblique, which arises from eight fleshy digitations of the external surface and lower borders of the eight inferior ribs. From these attachments, the muscular fibers pass in various directions. Those from the lowest ribs pass nearly vertically to insert into the anterior half of the outer lip of the iliac crest. The middle and upper fibers are directed downward and forward to terminate in tendinous fibers that spread out into a broad aponeurosis joining the opposite side.

The internal oblique is smaller and lies beneath the external oblique. It is irregularly quadrilateral and situated at the anterior, lateral, and posterior part of the abdomen. It arises from the outer half of Poupart's ligament, from the anterior two thirds of the middle tip of the crest of the ileum, and from the lumbar fascia. From this origin, fibers diverge in different directions. From Poupart's ligament, fibers arch downward and anteriorly across the spermatic cord, inserting conjointly with the transversus abdominis into the crest of the pubis and pectineal line. Fibers from the anterior superior iliac spine are horizontal in direction, and those from the anterior portion of the iliac crest pass obliquely upward and inward, terminating in an aponeurosis that continues forward to the linea alba. The posterior fibers ascend almost vertically, inserting into the lower borders of the lower four rib cartilages.

The only two structures that pass between the external and internal oblique muscles are the iliohypogastric and ilioinguinal branches of the first lumbar nerve root, which are pure sensory fibers. The transversalis muscle is so named because of the direction of its fibers. It lies immediately beneath the internal oblique and arises from the outer third of Poupart's ligament, the inner lip (anterior two thirds) of the iliac crest, and the inner suture of the six lower rib cartilages, interdigitating with the diaphragm and a broad aponeurosis from the spinous and transverse processes of the lumbar vertebrae.[1] All three of these abdominal muscles are traversed with the lateral dissection in the XLIF approach to the lumbar spine.

The psoas major muscle is the key muscle dissected during the XLIF approach. It functions as a hip flexor, abductor, and lateral rotator. It extends from the posterior mediastinum to the thigh on either side of the lumbosacral spine and arises from the sides of the vertebral bodies, intervertebral discs, and anterior base of the transverse processes of the last thoracic and all lumbar vertebrae (see Fig. 2-3). The muscle originates from tendinous arches between vertebrae and travels across the pelvic brim, diminishing in size as it passes beneath

Poupart's ligament, where it terminates in a tendon joined by fibers of the iliacus muscle to insert into the lesser trochanter of the femur. Within the substance of the psoas major lies the lumbar plexus, which receives contributions from T12 to L5. The genitofemoral nerve pierces the psoas and can be visualized on the anterior surface of the muscle. The sympathetic chain can be identified along the lateral surface of the vertebral body, just anterior to the tendinous origin of the psoas. Anterior to this muscle are the peritoneum, kidneys, renal vessels, ureters, spermatic vessels, and the colon. The medial border of the psoas muscle encompasses the lumbar vertebrae, the lumbar arteries, and the sympathetic ganglia with communicating branches with the spinal nerves.

APPLIED NEUROANATOMY

The union of neuromonitoring with the XLIF approach made lateral access spine surgery possible. The ability to locate the neural elements allows repositioning of the approach dilator and the subsequent docking of the retractor system. However, there is no substitute for a thorough knowledge of the normal location of the neural elements within the spinal canal, as well as their exit zones and paths through the psoas muscle. A review of the pertinent anatomy is extremely warranted.

In the adult, the spinal cord generally terminates at the L1-2 level. The spinal nerve is formed by ventral (motor) and dorsal (sensory) roots, which pierce the dura separately as they exit through the intervertebral foramen. The dorsal root is thicker and larger than the ventral root and has a bulbous enlargement within the neuroforamen, the dorsal root ganglion. After uniting as the spinal nerve, both ventral and dorsal branches form. Sympathetic fibers from the lateral columns of the lower thoracic and lumbar cord travel along the ventral branch. The dorsal primary rami divide into medial and lateral branches. The medial branch descends posteriorly at the back of the transverse and superior articular processes to supply sensory fibers to two facet joint levels. Therefore each facet receives sensory innervation from two different spinal nerve segments. The medial branch continues posteriorly to innervate the dorsal muscles of the back (such as multifidus and interspinalis). Medial branches also supply the interspinous and supraspinous ligaments. The lateral branches of the dorsal primary rami supply small branches to the sacrospinal muscles and cutaneous structures in the lumbar area. Although the nucleus pulposus of the disc is devoid of nerve endings, the posterior anulus fibrosus shares free nerve endings with the fibrous tissue that binds to the posterior longitudinal ligament.

The lumbar plexus is formed by the ventral rami of the first three lumbar nerves and part of the fourth lumbar nerve (Fig. 2-3). It is narrow above and broad below, and it is generally situated in the posterior substance of the psoas muscle.[2] The first lumbar spinal nerve (L1) gives off the iliohypogastric and ilioinguinal nerves, which travel superficially to the retroperitoneal space and provide sensory innervation to the area of the groin. The genitofemoral nerve—formed from the L1 and L2 spinal nerves—penetrates the lateral border of the psoas to lie on its anterior fascia and sends branches to the genital and femoral areas. The lateral cutaneous nerve of the thigh is formed from the L2 and L3 spinal nerves and innervates the skin of the anterolateral and lateral surfaces of the thigh. The femoral nerve is formed by the L2, L3, and L4 spinal nerves, exits in the angle between the iliacus and psoas muscles, and travels to the thigh to innervate the quadriceps. The obturator nerve comprises branches of the L2, L3, and L4 spinal nerves, which, together with a branch of L4 that joins L5 to form the lumbosacral trunk, appear at the medial border of the psoas muscle and cross the ala of the sacrum. The obturator nerve provides motor innervation to the adductor muscles of the thigh and cutaneous sensory innervation of the inner thigh. The sympathetic trunk enters the abdomen with the psoas, behind the medial crural ligament. The trunk is closely attached to the medial psoas muscle as it descends along the vertebral bodies and intervertebral discs to enter the abdomen.

The lumbar plexus nerves are often encountered in the posterior psoas when approaching the L4-5 disc. Care should be taken to use NeuroVision® dynamic EMG (NuVasive, Inc.) guidance through the muscle; this system allows the surgeon to locate and avoid neural structures in the path of the approach by entering slightly anterior to the identified locations of nerves, thereby achieving a safe and effective access channel.

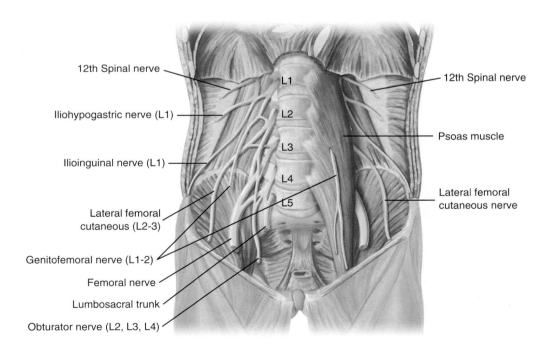

FIG. 2-3   The psoas muscle and lumbar plexus.

Vascular Anatomy

The arterial supply in the lumbar spine arises directly from the aorta. Four paired lumbar arteries emerge directly from the posterior aspect of the aorta, anterior to the bodies of the upper four lumbar vertebrae. The venous supply matches the arterial pattern, draining internal and external venous tributaries into the inferior vena cava. These segmental vessels curve posteriorly around the spine in the valley or midportion of the vertebral bodies, supplying the vertebrae and ligaments (Fig. 2-4, *A*).[3] Lateral access to the lumbar disc spaces need not approach the location of the segmental vessels, but care should be taken to ensure that the disc exposure is not exaggerated unnecessarily.

Bifurcation of the aorta and vena cava into the left and right common iliac vessels generally occurs at the L4-5 disc level, but this may vary with more caudal bifurcations (Fig. 2-4, *B*). To avoid injury on either the ipsilateral or contralateral side of the approach, the surgeon should always keep the location of these vessels in mind when he or she approaches the disc laterally. Targeting the lateral center of the disc space in an XLIF approach generally avoids an encounter with the anterior vasculature. Exceptions include the presence of anomalous vasculature and procedures in patients who have undergone previous surgeries. The locations of the blood vessels are shown in the MRIs and axial illustrations on pages 24 through 26.

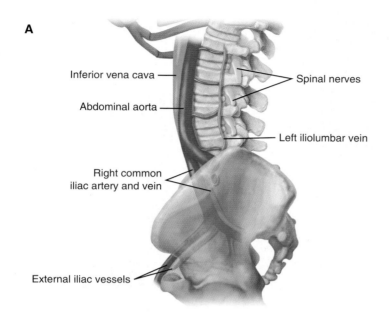

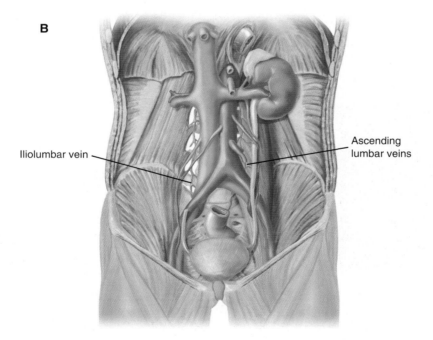

FIG. 2-4   A and **B,** The major lumbar vasculature.

L1-2 BLOOD VESSEL LOCATIONS

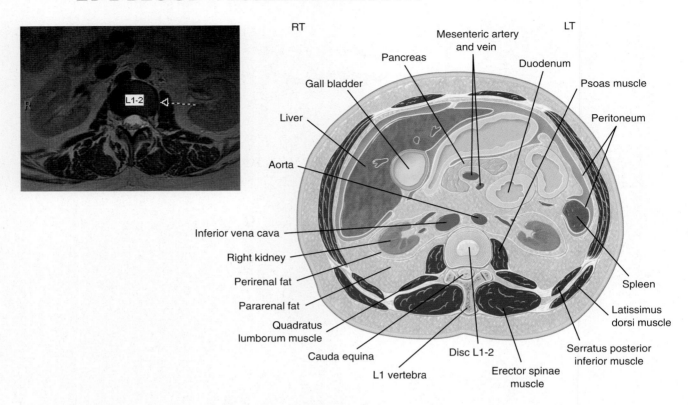

L2-3 BLOOD VESSEL LOCATIONS

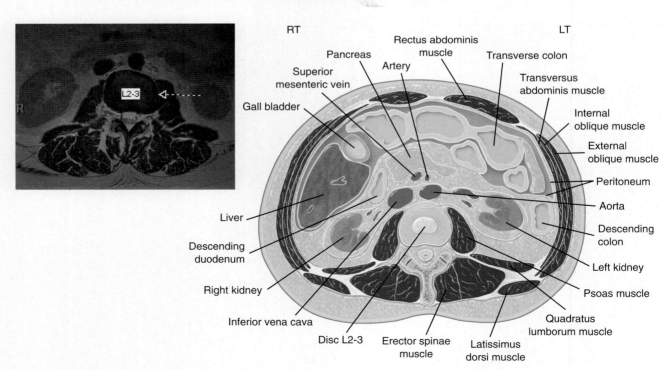

L3-4 BLOOD VESSEL LOCATIONS

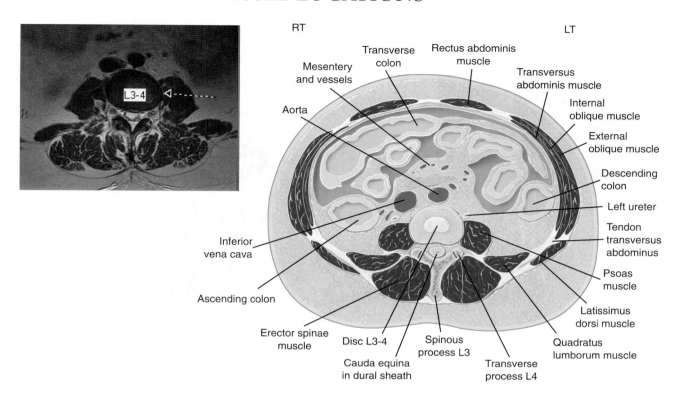

L4-5 BLOOD VESSEL LOCATIONS

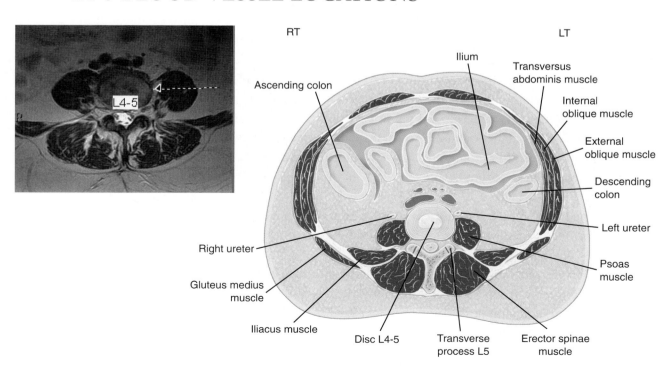

L5-S1 BLOOD VESSEL LOCATIONS

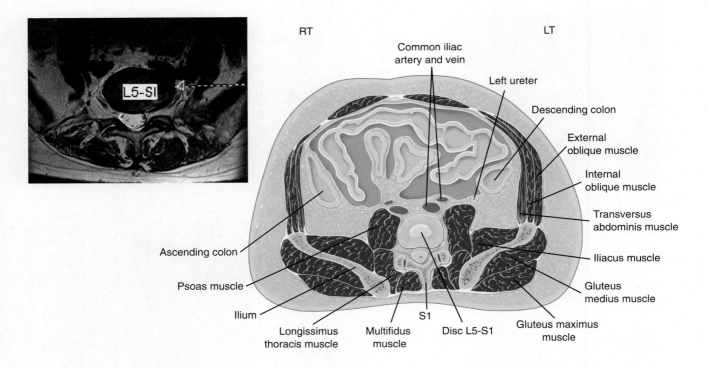

OSTEOLOGY

There are five vertebrae in the lumbar spine. The anterior portions—or vertebral bodies—are the primary load-bearing structures, and the posterior features—including the pedicles, facet joints, and spinous and transverse processes—protect the neural elements and act as the origins and insertions of muscle groups. The superior and inferior articular processes are connected by an isthmus called the *pars interarticularis.* The facet joints are true synovial joints, with superior and inferior portions projecting from adjacent vertebrae. They function to stabilize motion between vertebral segments. Each joint is enclosed by a capsule that consists of both an outer, dense connective tissue and an inner layer of elastic fiber, similar to ligamentum flavum.

The transverse process projects laterally from the junction of the facet and lamina, which provides a good landmark for the surgeon when he or she enters the retroperitoneal space.

The intervertebral foramina provide passages for each exiting nerve root and are bordered by the pedicles superiorly and inferiorly, the disc and body anteriorly, and the lamina and anterior facet joint posteriorly. They are longer in a vertical direction and are largest at L1-2; the overall configuration resembles an inverted teardrop.

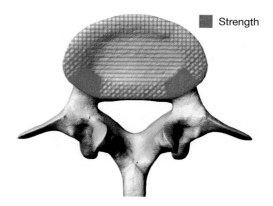

FIG. 2-5   The endplate and areas of relative strength. The red areas indicate the strongest regions.

Lumbosacral transitional vertebrae are commonly encountered radiographically. In a study by Eyo et al,[4] 37% of the radiographs reviewed demonstrated transitional changes. Sacralization or incorporation of the fifth lumbar vertebra was more common than lumbarization of the first sacral vertebra, by a 2:1 ratio. In the Eyo et al[4] study, these changes were found more often in males (46%) than in females (29%). Transitional changes may affect the ability to access the L4-5 interspace for XLIF procedures, as may advanced degenerative collapse of L5-S1.

The vertebral body itself is covered by a thick cortex that is at its thickest posteriorly and peripherally, which creates a solid base of support for cages. In addition, the trabecular pattern of the central cancellous portion tends to follow the lines of force that these cages place on the spine.

ENDPLATE ANATOMY (RING APOPHYSIS)

The vertebral endplates in the lumbar spine contain two separate anatomic elements: a slightly depressed, flat, or slightly concave plateau of a highly specialized, condensed cancellous bone and the ring apophysis that surrounds it. This cancellous bony layer is not very thick, but is extremely strong in normal vertebrae. A rich vascular supply is found underlying the bony endplate. The ring apophysis is likewise composed of a rather thin, but extremely strong, layer of dense, woven bone, and it serves as the attachment site for the anulus fibrosus. This peripheral rim provides more strength than the central regions of the endplate (Fig. 2-5).[5] The configuration of the apophyseal ring can be used to its greatest advantage in a lateral approach surgery, because an implant can be positioned on this dense area, which provides much support.

LIGAMENTS

The six major ligaments of the spine are the anterior longitudinal ligament (ALL), posterior longitudinal ligament (PLL), ligamentum flavum, interspinous ligament, supraspinous ligament, and the intertransverse ligament. The ALL, PLL, and supraspinous ligament are intersegmental, whereas the others are intrasegmental.

The ALL runs along the ventral and ventrolateral surfaces of the vertebral column, from the sacrum to C2. It continues proximally as the atlantooccipital ligament. The ALL has attachments to the vertebral bodies and discs. There are also superficial fibers that span several vertebral segments and deep fibers that run between adjacent vertebrae. The deep fibers blend with the ventral anulus of the disc and reinforce the intervertebral discs. The ALL demonstrates its greatest tensile strength in the lumbar region. In general, the ALL is approximately twice as strong as the PLL. The ALL is usually ventral to the instantaneous axis of rotation and therefore provides resistance to extension.

The XLIF approach to anterior column stabilization preserves the ALL, thereby maintaining significant, inherent spinal stability. Retaining the anterior and posterior anulus and ligaments fosters a stable alignment correction using ligamentotaxis.

CONCLUSION

The XLIF approach to the anterior spinal column has some advantages over traditional anterior or posterior approaches, with respect to avoiding anatomic risks and morbidity and maintaining structural integrity (Box 2-1). A surgeon should attempt to perform a new procedure only after he or she has carefully reviewed the anatomy and appropriate surgical technique; XLIF is no exception. The topics discussed within this chapter offer only an introduction to this important procedure.

BOX 2-1   Advantages of the XLIF Approach

- Disruption of tissues is minimal, resulting in lower blood loss, less postoperative pain, and a shorter recovery time
- Avoids destruction and denervation of the posterior musculature
- Avoids dural retraction and the associated epidural scarring
- Avoids destabilization caused by resection of the posterior arch
- Minimizes the risk of vascular injury, compared with anterior approaches
- Retains all stabilizing ligamentous structures, thus facilitating alignment correction by ligamentotaxis
- Allows access to a large area for disc removal and endplate preparation for fusion
- Allows a spacer with a large surface area to be placed for load distribution
- Maximizes the strongest areas of the endplate with implant placement spanning the ring apophysis, thus supporting axial and coronal alignment restoration

REFERENCES

1. Gray H. Anatomy, Descriptive and Surgical. Special Edition. Birmingham, AL: Leslie B. Adams Jr, 1981, pp 228-236.
2. Moro T, Kikuchi S, Konno S, et al. An anatomic study of the lumbar plexus with respect to retroperitoneal endoscopic surgery. Spine 28:423-428, 2003.
3. Borenstein DG, Wiesel SW, Boden SD. Low Back and Neck Pain: Comprehensive Diagnosis and Management, 2nd ed. Philadelphia: WB Saunders, 1995.
4. Eyo MU, Olofin A, Noronha C, et al. Incidence of lumbosacral transitional vertebrae in low back pain patients. Afr J Radiology 8:1-6, 2001.
5. Grant JP, Oxland TR, Dvorak MF. Mapping the structural properties of the lumbosacral vertebral endplates. Spine 26:889-896, 2001.

3

Biomechanics
of Lateral Arthrodesis

R. Shay Bess ▪ G. Bryan Cornwall ▪ Richard E. Vance
Kent N. Bachus ▪ Darrel S. Brodke

Anterior vertebral column interbody reconstruction provides a superior biomechanical environment for segmental fusion. The anterior column sustains approximately 80% of the axial load in the spine.[1] Interbody reconstruction unloads segmental spine implants in constructs that incorporate structural anterior column support. This creates a load-sharing—rather than load-bearing—environment for segmental implants. Consequently, the amount of unsupported cantilevered load endured by the posterior segmental implants is reduced, and the endurance limit of the construct is increased.[2] Cunningham et al[3] reported on the stiffness and bending strengths of thirteen different pedicle screw spinal constructs without interbody reconstruction. Normal lumbar physiologic loads exceeded the bending strengths of all constructs evaluated. Cunningham and Polly[4] evaluated the biomechanical effects of interbody cage position and variations in posterior rod diameter on spine construct stiffness, posterior rod strain, and interbody cage strain. All interbody cage constructs demonstrated significantly greater construct stiffness than constructs that did not include interbody support. Increased rod diameter did not significantly increase construct stiffness. These findings demonstrate the value of combined anterior and posterior column load sharing, especially when using posterior-based spinal instrumentation. Some authors have postulated that the biomechanical role of posterior implants is less critical in the presence of structural anterior column support, suggesting that the posterior implants may only provide segmental compression and a posterior tension band.[4]

Options for anterior column reconstruction include anterior lumbar interbody fusion (ALIF), posterior lumbar interbody fusion (PLIF), transforaminal lumbar interbody fusion (TLIF), and, more recently, extreme lateral interbody fusion (XLIF®, NuVasive® Inc., San Diego, CA). The clinical benefits of XLIF, compared with ALIF, PLIF, and TLIF, are discussed throughout this book. This chapter focuses on the biomechanics of interbody fusion and recent data on the biomechanics of XLIF constructs.

HISTORICAL DATA FOR LUMBAR INTERBODY FUSION

White and Panjabi[5] evaluated spinal ligamentous tensile strength and demonstrated that the anterior longitudinal ligament (ALL) is the strongest ligament in the spine. Therefore, if form follows function, the ALL may singly provide the greatest stability for the lumbar spine. One of the variables that influences the biomechanics of interbody constructs is the approach taken to the intervertebral space (for example, ALIF, PLIF, TLIF, or XLIF), because it directly relates to which stabilizing structures are preserved or resected and the size and shape of the implant that can be inserted. Therefore the biomechanics of an instrumentation construct are likely reflective of the construct itself and the approach taken to implant the construct. As a result, the biomechanical properties of ALIF constructs reflect the implants and the concomitant damage to the ALL and supporting tissues during anterior placement of the implants, and the strength and stability of PLIF and TLIF constructs reflect both the resection of bony elements and the limited size of the implants that can be inserted from a posterior approach.

Other variables that influence the biomechanics of the interbody constructs, in addition to the size or "footprint" of the interbody device, include the position of the interbody device within the interspace, the composition of the interbody graft (for example, morselized bone graft, femoral ring allograft [FRA], or polymer or titanium cages), and the total construct in which the interbody implant is used (for example, stand-alone device versus interbody graft supplemented with additional fixation).

Phillips et al[6] examined the effects of supplemental fixation to anteriorly placed threaded interbody cages. Eight human lumbar spines from L1 to the sacrum were tested in the intact state and after each of two different treatments—the insertion of two threaded cages at L5-S1 (ALIF), and ALIF supplemented with translaminar facet screws (TLFSs). The specimens were subjected to 0 to 8 Nm torsional flexion moment and a 0 to 6 Nm torsional extension moment. Three compressive preloads of 0 N, 400 N, and 1200 N were applied by the follower load method. The results suggested that the stability created by ALIF was not constant, but instead it varied, depending on the applied compressive load. The supplemental fixation statistically reduced the range of motion (ROM) relative to stand-alone ALIF. In extension, the ALIF cages alone provided relatively little stability when the compressive load was low. The supplemental TLFS provided significant additional stability at lower loads; however, at higher loads, the effect was not as significant.

Beaubien et al[7] compared stand-alone ALIF using freeze-dried FRA allograft as the interbody implant with ALIF supplemented with an anterior plate, pedicle screws, or translaminar screws. The authors evaluated three human lumbar spines from L1 to the sacrum and divided each spine into three individual, functional spine units (L1-2, L3-4, and L5-S1). Each functional level was instrumented, and ROM data were collected. The ROM was measured as the difference between maximal rotations in each physiologic direction—flexion/extension, lateral bending, and axial rotation. All instrumented constructs demonstrated significantly decreased ROM compared with intact spines. ALIF plus an anterior plate significantly reduced the ROM compared with stand-alone ALIF in extension and axial rotation, but did not statistically reduce the ROM in lateral bending. Pedicle screws and TLFSs provided a significantly higher reduction in the ROM than ALIF and ALIF plus an anterior plate in all dimensions.

Slucky et al[8] examined TLIF biomechanics associated with unilateral pedicle screw fixation, bilateral pedicle screw fixation, and unilateral pedicle screw fixation combined with a contralateral facet screw. Seven fresh-frozen human lumbar spines were tested in random construct order in flexion/extension, lateral bending, and axial rotation using $\pm$ 5 Nm of pure moment and 50 N of compressive load; each specimen was tested from L2 to L5 with the operated level at L3-4. Compared with the intact spine, all TLIF constructs with posterior instrumentation resulted in reduced segmental ROM and increased stiffness at the operated level. Bilateral pedicle screw fixation and unilateral pedicle screw fixation combined with a contralateral facet screw reduced the ROM and increased stiffness significantly more than unilateral pedicle screw fixation.

BIOMECHANICS OF LATERAL ARTHRODESIS

Few biomechanical data have been published on interbody reconstruction performed through a lateral approach. Heth et al[9] evaluated the mechanical stability of stand-alone, titanium-threaded interbody fusion cages (TFCs) placed either anteriorly or laterally across the disc space. Fourteen human cadaveric lumbar spines were instrumented at the L4-5 interspace—seven spines were instrumented anteriorly with two adjacent TFCs, and seven spines were instrumented laterally with only one TFC, which was placed transversely across the disc space. Compared with the intact spine, anterior discectomy destabilized the L4-5 motion segment in flexion and axial rotation, whereas lateral discectomy did not significantly increase the angular ROM. Anterior and lateral TFCs restored angular ROM to that of the intact segment; however, the ROM was not significantly less than values obtained for the intact spine. There was no statistical difference in stability imparted by the anterior and laterally placed TFCs.

Tencer et al[10] evaluated the biomechanics of bilateral anterior and single transverse cage placement in the lumbar spine. A single lateral cage performed similar to one or two anterior cages, with the exception that laterally placed cages demonstrated greater stiffness in axial rotation.

Kim et al[11] evaluated the stability of human cadaveric lumbar spine constructs using FRA interbody reconstruction performed via a lateral approach and constructs with FRA interbody placed via a traditional ALIF approach. Specimens were instrumented at the L3-4 and the L4-5 levels and were evaluated in four conditions: (1) intact spine, (2) destabilization by anterior or lateral discectomy, (3) stand-alone interbody reconstruction (anterior or laterally placed FRA), and (4) interbody reconstruction supplemented with additional fixation (lateral interbody reconstruction was supplemented with lateral plate fixation, and ALIF was supplemented with posterior transpedicular fixation). The segmental ROM and the *neutral zone* (NZ; defined as the difference between the original position and the displacement of the spine after the load force is removed) were measured in flexion/extension, lateral bending, and axial rotation. Values were normalized to the intact spine. The ROM and NZ were increased in all dimensions after lateral and anterior discectomy. There was no difference in the ROM or NZ between the lateral and the anteriorly destabilized spine. The stand-alone lateral interbody and ALIF restored the ROM and NZ to intact spine values. There was no significant difference in the ROM or NZ between stand-alone lateral interbody and ALIF. Compared with the intact spine, supplemental instrumentation significantly reduced the ROM and NZ in all loading modes (except for the NZ in lateral bending) in both groups. Lateral interbody reconstruction supplemented with a lateral plate demonstrated significantly reduced ROM in flexion and lateral bending compared with stand-alone lateral interbody. All ALIF/pedicle screw values for the ROM and NZ were significantly lower than the values for stand-alone ALIF. In flexion/extension and lateral bending, the ALIF/pedicle screw constructs also demonstrated lower ROM and NZ values than lateral interbody/lateral plate constructs.

Bess et al[12] used a human cadaver model to compare lumbar spine kinematics of a laterally placed poly-ether-ether-ketone (PEEK) interbody device (CoRoent® XL; NuVasive, Inc.) used as a stand-alone construct with various instrumented constructs. Seven fresh-frozen, human cadaveric lumbar spine specimens were potted at L1 and L5. All specimens underwent nondestructive ROM flexibility testing in three physiologic directions: flexion/extension, lateral bending, and axial rotation. The L3-4 interspace was evaluated in five conditions: (1) intact spine, (2) lateral discectomy and stand-alone lateral interbody device (XLIF), (3) XLIF supplemented by a lateral plate (PLATE), (4) XLIF supplemented by unilateral pedicle screws (UNI, SpheRx® DBR®, NuVasive, Inc.), and (5) XLIF supplemented by bilateral pedicle screws (BILAT, SpheRx DBR) (Fig. 3-1). Testing was performed using a pneumatic seven-axis spine simulator (Fig. 3-2). Intervertebral motion was evaluated using an optoelectronic motion measurement system (OptoTRAK Model 3020; Northern Digital, Waterloo, Ontario, Canada). Intact specimens were precycled with 30 cycles at ± 5 Nm moment in each dimension. All instrumented specimens underwent five ROM cycles in each

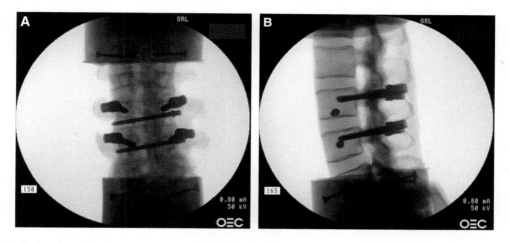

FIG. 3-1 **A** and **B,** Anteroposterior and lateral fluoroscopic images, respectively, of a fresh-frozen, human cadaveric lumbar spine specimen potted at L1 and L5. The L3-4 interspace was evaluated in five conditions: in an intact spine, XLIF, PLATE, UNI, and BILAT.

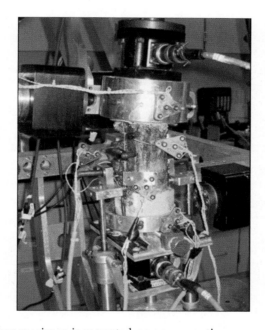

FIG. 3-2 A lumbar specimen is mounted on a pneumatic, seven-axis spine simulator.

axis at ± 5 Nm moment, using position control based on intact specimens. The ROM cycles were performed using 100 N follower load and 50 N axial compression. Data were collected on the fourth and fifth cycles and normalized to the intact specimen. There was no measurable difference between the stiffness and ROM data collected with 100 N follower load and specimens tested with 50 N axial compressive load; consequently, all reported data corresponded to data collected using 100 N follower load.

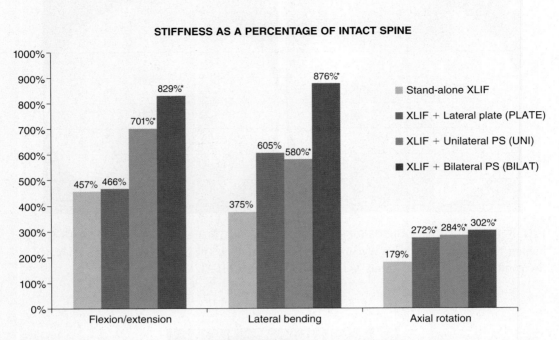

FIG. 3-3 Lumbar stiffness as a function of different XLIF cage constructs. Values are expressed as the percentage of increased stiffness at the L3-4 segment compared with the intact spine. All values are significantly greater than in the intact spine ($p < 0.05$). *, Significantly greater than stand-alone XLIF ($p < 0.05$); *PS*, pedicle screws.

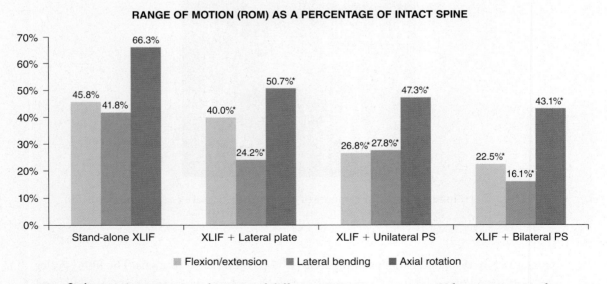

FIG. 3-4 Lumbar ROM as a function of different XLIF cage constructs. Values are expressed as the percentage of increased stiffness at the L3-4 segment compared with the intact spine. All values are significantly lower than in the intact spine ($p < 0.05$). *, Significantly lower than stand-alone XLIF ($p < 0.05$); *PS*, pedicle screws.

XLIF and all supplemented XLIF constructs demonstrated significantly increased stiffness (Fig. 3-3) and deceased ROM (Fig. 3-4) in all dimensions compared with intact specimens. The results for stiffness are presented as normalized values relative to the intact spine (% stiffness) in Fig. 3-3. The results are grouped by applied physiologic motion to facilitate the comparison of the following treatment conditions: stand-alone XLIF, XLIF + lateral plate (PLATE), XLIF + unilateral fixation (UNI), and XLIF + bilateral fixation (BILAT). Compared with the intact spine, stand-alone XLIF increased flexion/extension stiffness by 457%, lateral bending stiffness by 375%, and axial rotation stiffness by 179%. Compared with XLIF alone, supplemental instrumentation using UNI and BILAT constructs significantly increased stiffness in all dimensions, PLATE significantly increased stiffness only in axial rotation.

All XLIF constructs supplemented with instrumentation demonstrated a significantly decreased ROM. Further analysis demonstrated that BILAT constructs had significantly greater stiffness and decreased ROM for flexion/extension and lateral bending compared with XLIF, PLATE, and UNI. In Fig. 3-4, the results are grouped by treatment to facilitate the comparison of applied physiologic motion on the resulting normalized ROM (% ROM) with that of intact spine. The greatest reduction in ROM was observed with lateral bending and flexion/extension in all treatments.

DISCUSSION

When evaluating the biomechanical properties of spinal constructs, the primary clinical concern is whether or not the construct provides adequate segmental rigidity to promote a solid arthrodesis. Numerous studies have reported that stand-alone interbody devices do not sufficiently stabilize a spinal motion segment.[9,13-17] However, Bess et al[12] demonstrated that a laterally placed stand-alone interbody device decreased flexion/extension and lateral bending ROM more than 50% and increased flexion/extension and lateral bending rigidity more than 300% compared with the intact spine. These findings may be because the ALL is preserved with lateral interbody approach and discectomy, but not with a standard ALIF approach. Tencer et al[10] reported that sectioning the ALL in a calf spine model created increased laxity in flexion, extension, and lateral bending. However, other studies have indicated that stabilization in the sagittal plane is primarily generated by the facet joints, whereas the ALL provides an anchor for axial rotation. This may explain why other investigators have reported that a laterally placed lumbar interbody device restores segmental rigidity to the intact spine and is not significantly more stable than stand-alone ALIF.[9-11]

The implants used for study may provide a possible explanation for the differences in the segmental rigidity afforded by lateral interbody fusion, as reported by Bess et al,[12] compared with previous evaluations. All biomechanical studies of lateral interbody instrumentation have evaluated the technique and implants using a cadaveric model. This model does not evaluate fusion. Instead, it is only able to evaluate the immediate stability provided by the implants. The interbody device used by Bess et al[12] has a broad, rectangular shape that is contoured to match the endplates, in addition to machined, serrated edges that contact and interdigitate with the vertebral endplates. The large, rectangular implant is designed to support the anterior column more laterally on the peripheral ring apophysis and may provide greater immediate stability than the smooth FRA interbody placed in the center of the disc space, used by Kim et al.[11] This is consistent with the findings of Hitchcock et al,[18] who reported that interbody implants with serrations imparted greater segmental stability than smooth interbody implants. The interbody implants used by Heth et al[9] were threaded cages. It is possible that the surface serrations on the interbody implants used by Bess et al[12] also increased the resistance to shear forces more effectively than did a threaded cage. To our knowledge, however, the immediate stability provided by threaded cages has not been compared with that of serrated interbody cages.

In addition to preserving the ALL, the lateral approach also preserves the facet joints. Finite element analysis by Zander et al[19] demonstrated that unilateral hemifacetectomy (removal of the left superior articular process of L5 with the corresponding facet capsular ligament) increased intersegmental rotation, and bilateral hemifacetectomy (removal of the left and right superior articular processes of L5 with the corresponding facet capsular ligaments) further increased intersegmental rotation, creating marked segmental instability. This increase in segmental motion is likely a major factor that has lead to the poor clinical results associated with stand-alone PLIF.[20-23] In concordance with the poor clinical results of stand-alone procedures, Ames et al[24] demonstrated that stand-alone PLIF and TLIF do not impart a significant degree of segmental stability after a 1- or 2-level procedure compared with intact spines. Because of these findings, Ames et al recommended pedicle screw supplementation when performing PLIF or TLIF. Similar biomechanical results were reported by Harris et al,[25] who found that stand-alone TLIF did not increase segmental stability, compared with intact spines, and actually destabilized the L4-5 segment in axial rotation. Unlike PLIF and TLIF approaches, the lateral approach to the vertebral disc space spares the facets, retaining much of the native stability of the motion segment. A laterally placed interbody device also benefits from a larger interbody footprint than can be inserted via a PLIF or TLIF approach. The larger interbody device may afford more immediate stability. However, to our knowledge, the stability of lateral interbody devices has not been directly compared with that of PLIF or TLIF devices.

Comparing the XLIF data (Bess et al[12]) with historical values for ALIF (Beaubien et al[7]) and TLIF (Slucky et al[8]), stand-alone XLIF demonstrated greater stability than stand-alone ALIF in flexion/extension and lateral bending. The greatest discrepancy between stand-alone ALIF and stand-alone XLIF was with flexion/extension, because stand-alone XLIF shows greater stability than stand-alone ALIF, possibly for reasons discussed previously. Minimal differences were demonstrated between the groups if supplemental fixation was added to XLIF,

ALIF, or TLIF. Bilateral fixation combined with anterior column support provided the greatest biomechanical reduction in ROM. Finally, comparing the reported changes in axial rotation, TLIF with unilateral pedicle screw fixation provided the least reduction in motion. Bilateral fixation combined with ALIF showed the greatest reduction in ROM, followed by XLIF and bilateral fixation. Some degree of caution is recommended when comparing these studies, because the testing conditions were not entirely the same and the data were obtained at different time points; consequently, an accurate statistical comparison between the values was not performed. These comparisons are intended only to provide relative information.

CONCLUSION

Lateral interbody fusion using the CoRoent XL cage provides immediate segmental stability in the lumbar spine. Compared with historical data, the segmental rigidity provided by the laterally placed CoRoent XL cage exceeds that of stand-alone ALIF, PLIF, and TLIF. Based on results from our study, XLIF significantly increases stiffness and decreases ROM compared with the intact lumbar spine. XLIF supplementation with additional segmental implants further reduces ROM when compared with intact spines and, when compared with stand-alone XLIF, also decreases ROM. Bilateral pedicle screw–supplemented constructs demonstrate the greatest stiffness and decreased ROM. Lumbar biomechanical changes appropriate for fusion constructs are achieved with the XLIF approach for placement of an interbody cage.

REFERENCES

1. Bergmark A. Stability of the lumbar spine. A study in mechanical engineering. Acta Orthop Scand Suppl 230:1-54, 1989.
2. Gaines RW Jr, Carson WL, Satterlee CC, et al. Experimental evaluation of seven different spinal fracture internal fixation devices using nonfailure stability testing. The load-sharing and unstable-mechanism concepts. Spine 16:902-909, 1991.
3. Cunningham BW, Sefter JC, Shono Y, et al. Static and cyclical biomechanical analysis of pedicle screw spinal constructs. Spine 18:1677-1688, 1993.
4. Cunningham BW, Polly DW Jr. The use of interbody cage devices for spinal deformity: a biomechanical perspective. Clin Orthop Relat Res 394:73-83, 2002.
5. White AA, Panjabi MM. Clinical Biomechanics of the Spine, 2nd ed. Philadelphia: Lippincott Williams & Wilkins, 1990.
6. Phillips FM, Cunningham B, Carandang G, et al. Effect of supplemental translaminar facet screw fixation on the stability of stand-alone anterior lumbar interbody fusion cages under physiologic compressive preloads. Spine 29:1731-1736, 2004.
7. Beaubien BP, Derincek A, Lew WD, et al. In vitro, biomechanical comparison of an anterior lumbar interbody fusion with an anteriorly placed, low-profile lumbar plate and posteriorly placed pedicle screws or translaminar screws. Spine 30:1846-1851, 2005.
8. Slucky AV, Brodke DS, Bachus KN, et al. Less invasive posterior fixation method following transforaminal lumbar interbody fusion: a biomechanical analysis. Spine J 6:78-85, 2006.

9. Heth JA, Hitchon PW, Goel VK, et al. A biomechanical comparison between anterior and transverse interbody fusion cages. Spine 26:E261-E267, 2001.

10. Tencer AF, Hampton D, Eddy S. Biomechanical properties of threaded inserts for lumbar interbody spinal fusion. Spine 20:2408-2414, 1995.

11. Kim SM, Lim TJ, Paterno J, et al. Biomechanical comparison: stability of lateral-approach anterior lumbar interbody fusion and lateral fixation compared with anterior-approach anterior lumbar interbody fusion and posterior fixation in the lower lumbar spine. J Neurosurg Spine 2:62-68, 2005.

12. Bess RS, Bacchus K, Vance R, et al. Lumbar biomechanics with extreme lateral interbody fusion (XLIF®) cage construct. Presented at the International Meeting on Advanced Spine Techniques, Paradise Island, Bahamas, July 2007.

13. Tsantrizos A, Andreou A, Aebi M, et al. Biomechanical stability of five stand-alone anterior lumbar interbody fusion constructs. Eur Spine J 9:14-22, 2009.

14. Oxland TR, Hoffer Z, Nydegger T, et al. A comparative biomechanical investigation of anterior lumbar interbody cages: central and bilateral approaches. J Bone Joint Surg Am 82:383-393, 2000.

15. Oxland TR, Lund T. Biomechanics of stand-alone cages and cages in combination with posterior fixation: a literature review. Eur Spine J 9(Suppl 1):S95-S101, 2000.

16. Lavoie S, Lindsey RW, Gugala Z, et al. Load sharing and kinematics of threaded cages for lumbar interbody fusion. Clin Orthop Relat Res 408:174-179, 2003.

17. Vadapalli S, Robon M, Biyani A, et al. Effect of lumbar interbody cage geometry on construct stability: a cadaveric study. Spine 31:2189-2194, 2006.

18. Hitchcock R, Sears W, Gillies RM, et al. In vitro study of shear force on interbody implants. J Spinal Disord Tech 19:32-36, 2006.

19. Zander T, Rohlmann A, Klockner C, et al. Influence of graded facetectomy and laminectomy on spinal biomechanics. Eur Spine J 12:427-434, 2003.

20. Cassinelli EH, Wallach C, Hanscom B, et al. Prospective clinical outcomes of revision fusion surgery in patients with pseudarthrosis after posterior lumbar interbody fusions using stand-alone metallic cages. Spine J 6:428-434, 2006.

21. Elias WJ, Simmons NE, Kaptain GJ, et al. Complications of posterior lumbar interbody fusion when using a titanium threaded cage device. J Neurosurg 93:45-52, 2000.

22. Chen L, Yang H, Tang T. Cage migration in spondylolisthesis treated with posterior lumbar interbody fusion using BAK cages. Spine 30:2171-2175, 2005.

23. Wetzel FT, LaRocca H. The failed posterior lumbar interbody fusion. Spine 16:839-845, 1991.

24. Ames CP, Acosta FL Jr, Chi J, et al. Biomechanical comparison of posterior lumbar interbody fusion and transforaminal lumbar interbody fusion performed at 1 and 2 levels. Spine 30:E562-E566, 2005.

25. Harris BM, Hilibrand AS, Savas PE, et al. Transforaminal lumbar interbody fusion: the effect of various instrumentation techniques on the flexibility of the lumbar spine. Spine 29:E65-E70, 2004.

4

Radiology of Lumbar Degenerative Disease

H. Brad Jones, Jr.

Lumbar degenerative disease is a leading cause of disability, work loss, and medical expenses. With the increase of obesity throughout the world, especially in the United States, degeneration of the spine is increasing in prevalence and is affecting more younger patients than ever before.

An overview of imaging anatomy begins this chapter. It is important to understand normal anatomy first, because this knowledge makes it easier to highlight the progression of findings in lumbar degenerative disease, including disc degeneration, central canal stenosis, lateral encroachment, and degenerative scoliosis. However, the true objective of this chapter is to provide a review of available imaging modalities—information that allows a radiologist to help a clinician with his or her care of a patient. These imaging modalities include plain radiography, myelography, discography, computed tomography (CT), and magnetic resonance imaging (MRI); the advantages and drawbacks of each method are discussed. Also included are the findings of degenerative lumbar disease as they are obtained with both radiography and cross-sectional imaging, an area that has seen significant advancement in recent years. Imaging advances benefit patients, because clinicians can better select the appropriate treatment for each patient's specific problem.

ANATOMY

The lumbar spine is made up of five vertebral bodies; an intervertebral disc exists between each. In some instances, a sixth lumbar vertebra also exists and the terms *six non–rib-bearing vertebrae* and *transitional lumbosacral vertebrae* will be used. In these cases, it is critical that the radiologist and clinician communicate clearly with one another and that they be consistent in the labeling of the disc spaces, especially if an intervention is needed.

Each lumbar vertebra is made up of a body and pedicles, and the bodies are secured by anterior and posterior longitudinal ligaments. The posterior elements include the lamina and spinous processes; an interspinous ligament anchors the spinous process at each level. Bilateral articulating facet joints stabilize the adjacent vertebrae with one another; the ligamentum flavum stabilizes the lamina with the ipsilateral articulating facet.[1]

The intervertebral discs are composed of a peripheral anulus fibrosus and a central nucleus pulposus, which is predominantly made up of water and has a homogeneous high signal on a water-sensitive (T2-weighted) MRI scan. The anulus fibrosus, however, has a low signal in water-sensitive (T2-weighted) MRI scans because of its fibrous content.[2] Because disc degeneration is typically the instigator for lumbar degeneration, it is important to know what normal and abnormal discs look like on cross-sectional imaging (Fig. 4-1).

The conus medullaris of the spinal cord can vary in its termination point. However, it is typically located at the L1 or L2 level. Nerve roots emerge from the distal cord; these travel within the spinal canal to exit through the intervertebral neural foramina at their respective levels. A disease at a specific lumbar level has the potential to affect two separate nerve roots. Because the upper nerve root at a certain level travels under the pedicle and then into the neural foramen, posterolateral and far lateral disc disease or osteophytosis typically affect this nerve root. Central and paracentral disc disease typically affect the lower nerve root.[3] A posterolateral osteophyte or diseased disc at L4-5 often impinges on the ipsilateral L4 nerve root. Central or paracentral osteophytes or a diseased disc at L4-5 often impinge on the L5 nerve root.[1]

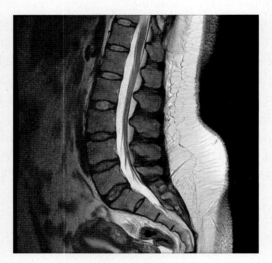

FIG. 4-1   A sagittal T2-weighted image that demonstrates a normal signal in upper lumbar intervertebral discs and water loss with loss of a signal in the lower lumbar intervertebral discs.

DISC DEGENERATION AND IMAGING

Because humans are upright creatures and walk on two legs instead of four, the lumbar spine degenerates as we age. The degeneration process typically begins with the intervertebral discs. The central nucleus pulposus loses its water content and becomes more fibrous. The high signal within the nucleus, seen on T2-weighted images, will start to lower, beginning centrally and then expanding within the disc toward the endplates[2] (see Fig 4-1). The peripheral anulus can also begin to develop cracks along its edge. If these cracks, also known as anular tears, can be visualized on T2-weighted MRI, they have a linear high signal. Anular tears allow nitrogen to enter the central portion of the disc, resulting in continued degeneration. The nitrogen produces air density that can be seen with plain radiography and CT, and it produces a linear low signal within the disc on MRI. These areas of air density are referred to as *vacuum discs* and are signs of advanced degeneration[1] (Fig. 4-2). Disc degeneration and anular tears place the patient at increased risk for symptomatic disc disease. Tears in the anulus, for example, allow the nucleus pulposus to extend outward from its central location.

Although disc morphology can be described in different ways, none is fully correct. The keys for accurately describing disc morphology should be consistent and clearly communicate findings with a surgeon. The location of any abnormal disc morphology is especially crucial. Disc disease can be central, paracentral, posterolateral, or far lateral. As mentioned in the previous section, posterolateral and far lateral disc disease affect the upper nerve roots, whereas central and paracentral disc disease affect the lower nerve roots.[3]

Disc bulges are typically broad-based and extend at least 2 mm beyond the margin of the vertebral body.[2] In addition, they are almost always present with acquired lumbar degenerative disease. Focal disc protrusions or herniations typically occur in central or paracentral

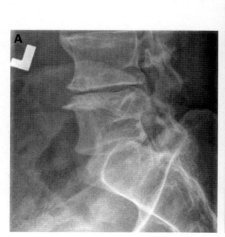
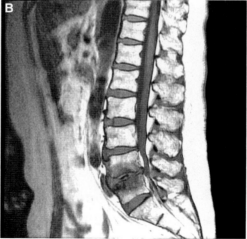

FIG. 4-2   Vacuum discs on **A,** a conventional lateral radiograph and **B,** a sagittal T1 MRI.

locations. Although not always symptomatic, these discs can be quite symptomatic if they occur in certain positions. Posterolateral and foraminal disc protrusions commonly produce root compression and symptoms correlating with the affected level. Far lateral protrusions most commonly affect nerve roots that exit proximal to the disk level involved. Disc extrusions, another type of spinal ailment, have larger anteroposterior dimensions than mediolateral dimensions in axial cross-sectional imaging[2] (Fig. 4-3). Because of the size of these disc extrusions, they often migrate either superiorly or inferiorly behind the adjacent vertebral body. In addition, they are often symptomatic. Another spinal disorder occurs when sequestered disc fragments break away from their parent disc (Fig. 4-4). A sequestered disc fragment shows rim enhancement in postgadolinium MRI scans, and the size and location of a disc fragment determine its clinical significance.

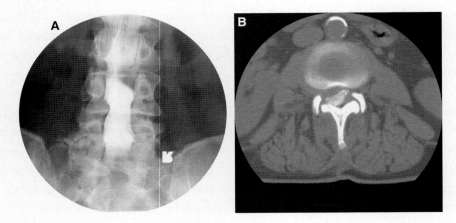

FIG. 4-3   These **A,** myelogram and **B,** postmyelogram CT images both demonstrate a large right paracentral disc extrusion with secondary nerve root impingement.

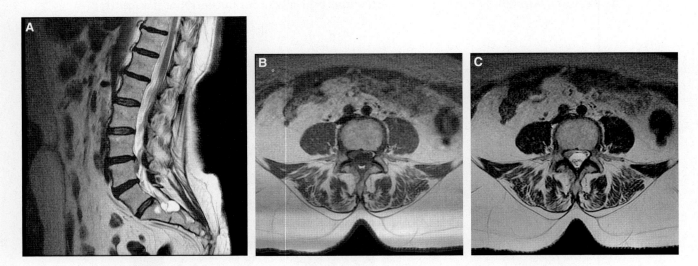

FIG. 4-4   **A,** Sagittal T2, **B,** axial T1, and **C,** axial T2 images demonstrate a right paracentral sequestered disc fragment that originates from the L3-4 disc space and extends inferiorly behind the L4 vertebral body.

CONVENTIONAL RADIOGRAPHY AND DISC DISEASE

Radiographs allow the radiologist and clinician to see preservation of disc height. With progressing disc degeneration, the disc height begins to decrease and endplate degenerative changes occur. This is discussed in more detail in the osseous degeneration section.

MYELOGRAPHY AND COMPUTED TOMOGRAPHY

Although MRI has become the standard, myelography and follow-up CT remain valid and important imaging modalities for disc disease and lumbar degeneration (see Fig. 4-3). These tests are often performed in patients who are unable to undergo MRI, including those individuals with extreme claustrophobia, pacemakers, or spinal stimulators. The obvious disadvantage of myelography is the invasive nature of the procedure—the patient must undergo a lumbar puncture and an injection of contrast into the thecal sac. However, one advantage is that it allows visualization of the individual nerve roots. By visualizing the individual nerve roots, one is able to see their course, as well as specific points of impingement and effacement. Lateral radiographs following myelogram injection allow assessment of central canal preservation or stenosis.

A postmyelogram CT is crucial, because it defines whether a nerve root impingement is related to isolated disc abnormalities and/or osseous degeneration. A CT examination also helps assess the central canal dimensions, as well as lateral recess stenosis and far lateral neuroforaminal stenosis. The facet joints and ligamentum flavum can be well evaluated on CT examinations, and their contributions to acquired central canal, lateral recess, and neuroforanimal stenosis are easily discerned. Today's 16-slice and 64-slice CT scanners allow quick imaging and easy access to three-dimensional reconstructed images. These reconstructed images allow visualization of the individual nerve roots in a coronal plane, as well as easy assessment of degenerative scoliosis in the coronal plane.

MAGNETIC RESONANCE IMAGING

MRI has become the gold standard for evaluating degenerative disc disease. The test has a number of advantages: it is noninvasive, provides results that have great spatial resolution, and avoids any exposure to radiation. In addition, MRI gives exact assessments of the size and locations of disc abnormalities. Broad-based disc bulges, focal disc protrusions or herniations, disc extrusions, and sequestered disc fragments are all easily seen using MRI (see Fig. 4-4). Because of the anatomic detail seen with MRI, an impingement on a specific nerve root can be determined easily. It is also useful for disc degeneration. When a disc loses water or becomes dehydrated, there is a loss of signal on T2-weighted (water-sensitive) images.[2] With further progression, the disc loses height and eventually develops abnormal peripheral morphology.

DISCOGRAPHY

Discography is a provocative procedure that is used to determine the sources and levels of pain in patients with disc degeneration. This invasive procedure is often performed on patients who have not responded to conservative treatments. Needles are placed into multiple discs, then contrast is injected into the disc space. The patient is kept awake throughout the procedure so that he or she can describe the intensity of pain at each disc space level of the spine, thereby confirming a level-specific diagnosis of pain generators.

OSSEOUS DEGENERATION

The preceding sections of this chapter discuss the progression of disc degeneration as it leads to the final stage of lumbar disease—osseous degeneration. With progressive disc degeneration and loss of height, the vertebral endplates come closer to one another, and other changes in the endplates also develop, which are are best seen using MRI. As the endplates change, the facet joints simultaneously begin to lose their articular cartilage. With the loss of these stabilizing elements, abnormal movement occurs in the lumbar spine. Vertebral osteophytes can also form as the disease progresses; these secondarily narrow the central canal and exiting foramina. With loss of cartilage, the facet joints also begin to hypertrophy and become arthropathic. At the same time, the stabilizing ligamentum flavum begins to hypertrophy and bow inward. These factors contribute to progressive central canal, lateral recess, and neuroforaminal stenosis. [2]

Progressive loss of stabilizing elements around the lumbar spine allows continual abnormal motion, which in turn leads to degenerative spondylolisthesis, in the form of either anterolisthesis or retrolisthesis. When an anterolisthesis occurs, the superior vertebral body moves *anterior* to the inferior vertebral body, whereas the superior vertebral body moves *posterior* to the inferior vertebral body in retrolisthesis. Spondylolisthesis in general can be graded in terms of the degree of abnormal movement. A simplistic approach is to divide the vertebral body into quarters. With grade I anterolisthesis, the superior vertebral body moves forward 0% to 25% over the inferior vertebral body. Grade II occurs when the vertebral body moves 25% to 50%, grade III is at 50% to 75%, and grade IV is at more than 75%.[3]

The term *degenerative spondylolisthesis* is used in this section because spondylolisthesis can also be seen with pars interarticularis defects (spondylolysis).[3] Spondylolysis can be recognized with plain radiography or with cross-sectional imaging. It is important for the image interpreter to look for this not-uncommon entity. Degenerative spondylolisthesis can be differentiated from spondylolisthesis secondary to spondylolysis by the central canal diameter. With spondylolysis, the central canal remains patent or widened, whereas degenerative spondylolisthesis leads to a narrowing of the central canal. Both conditions lead to lateral recess and neuroforaminal stenoses (Fig. 4-5).

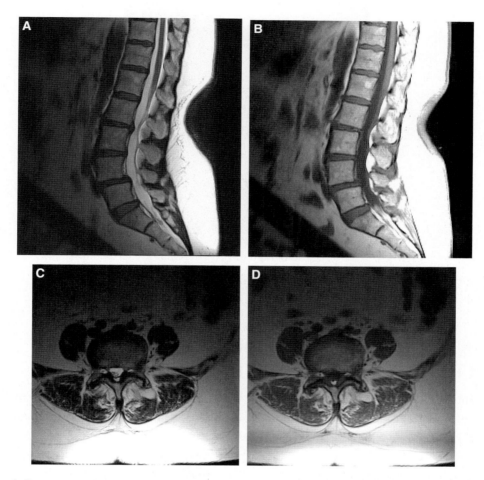

FIG. 4-5   **A,** Sagittal T2 and **B,** sagittal T1 images demonstrate grade I anterolisthesis of L4 on L5. **C,** Axial T2 and **D,** axial T1 images show the central canal stenosis secondary to the spondylolisthesis and facet arthropathy.

With the loss of disc height and facet arthropathy, the lumbar spine begins to collapse. Abnormal lateral curvature with disc and osseous degeneration is termed *degenerative scoliosis.* This condition typically occurs in older patients following years of wear. Degenerative scoliosis also contributes to central canal, lateral recess, and neuroforaminal stenoses. Neuroforaminal stenosis tends to be more severe on the ipsilateral side of the convex portion of the lateral curvature. For example, levoscoliosis centered at the L3-4 level typically causes more severe left-sided neuroforaminal stenosis. Because this contributes to bony canal compromise and progressive facet arthropathy, patients have an increased risk of developing localized pain, lumbar radiculopathy, and neurogenic claudication.

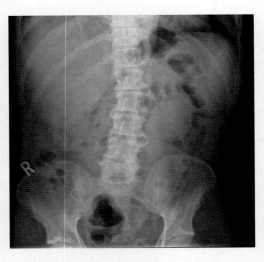

FIG. 4-6   A frontal radiograph displays degenerative levoscoliosis.

CONVENTIONAL RADIOGRAPHY IN OSSEOUS DEGENERATION

Conventional radiographs are often the first imaging modality used when a patient complains of back pain—they are easy to obtain, inexpensive, and provide useful information. Lateral radiographs allow the imager to assess for disc space preservation, vacuum discs, and posterior osteophytes. Lateral radiographs are also excellent for assessing spondylolisthesis. Oblique radiographs are used to exclude spondylolysis as the cause of spondylolisthesis.[4] Frontal radiographs give a quick assessment of disc space preservation. These radiographs are crucial for assessing lateral osteophytosis. Although the lateral recess and neuroforamen cannot be well evaluated with radiographs of the lumbar spine, the presence of lateral osteophytes is usually indicative of foraminal stenosis and encroachment on the exiting nerve roots. Frontal radiographs are also excellent for assessing degenerative scoliosis of the lumbar spine (Fig. 4-6). Large 32-inch cassettes can be used to evaluate the scoliotic curvature of the spine. Anteroposterior and lateral bending radiographs allow the radiologist and clinician to assess the stiffness of a patient's scoliotic curve. The lateral curvature and the presence of lateral osteophytes are seen easily with lumbar radiographs.

COMPUTED TOMOGRAPHY AND MYELOGRAPHY

CT gives an excellent, quick assessment of central canal diameter and neuroforaminal stenoses. Unfortunately, its benefits are limited if an intrathecal contrast medium is not

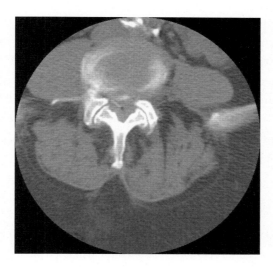

FIG. 4-7   This postmyelogram CT image demonstrates high-grade central canal stenosis and impingement on the thecal sac secondary to posterior spondylosis, facet arthropathy, and ligamentum flavum hypertrophy.

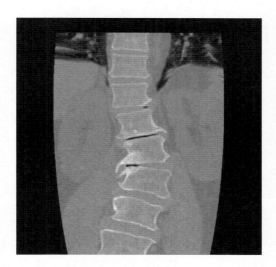

FIG. 4-8   This coronal reformatted CT image demonstrates multilevel disc degeneration, lumbar spondylosis, and secondary degenerative scoliosis.

used. Even though myelography is an invasive procedure, it does allow direct viewing of nerve root effacement. Flexion and extension postmyelogram radiographs also allow assessment of abnormal motion of the lumbar spine. Postmyelogram CT images provide impressive views of the central canal, lateral recess, and neuroforamen. The combination of these studies allows the imager to differentiate nerve root compromise secondary to disc disease from osseous degeneration.

As mentioned in the previous section, posterior osteophytes, facet arthropathy, and ligamentum flavum hypertrophy can all be clearly evaluated with a postmyelogram CT examination (Fig. 4-7). Postprocessing also allows the development of three-dimensional sequences. Sagittal sequences allow excellent assessment of degenerative spondylolisthesis, whereas coronal sequences allow assessment of degenerative scoliosis (Fig. 4-8) and secondary lateral recess and neuroforaminal compromise. With intrathecal contrast, the nerve roots are directly visualized. Therefore impingement of the nerves secondary to osseous degeneration is easily assessed.

MAGNETIC RESONANCE IMAGING

MRI is also the standard for assessing osseous degeneration. Vertebral body endplate changes following disc degeneration are visualized earlier with MRI than they are with any other modality. These changes, first described by Modic et al,[5] are as follows: type 1 changes produce a low signal along the endplates on T1-weighted images and a high signal on T2-

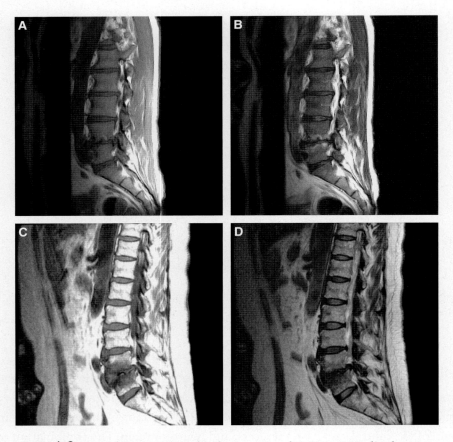

FIG. 4-9   **A** and **B,** Type 2 Modic changes. **C** and **D,** Type 3 Modic changes.

weighted images, type 2 changes produce a high signal along the endplates on both T1- and T2-weighted images, and type 3 changes produce a low signal along the endplates on both T1- and T2-weighted images. Conventional radiographs allow visualization of only the type 3 changes because of the sclerosis along the endplates. Sclerosis produces a low signal with MRI (Fig. 4-9).

With disc degeneration and endplate degenerative changes, abnormal movement begins in the lumbar spine. Facet joints begin to have abnormal motion, which leads to a progressive loss of the articular cartilage. The facets begin to become hypertrophic and arthropathic. Simultaneously, the ligamentum flavum begins to hypertrophy and encroach on the central lumbar spinal canal and the lateral recess. MRI gives a multiplane view of these acquired degenerative changes[6] (Fig. 4-10).

Sagittal MRIs provide a clear look at degenerative spondylolisthesis (see Fig. 4-5). Comparing axial images with sagittal images allows assessment of central canal stenosis and exclusion of pars interarticularis defects. With degenerative spondylolisthesis, the central canal becomes narrowed and compromised. Weight-bearing MRI scanners have been introduced into modern imaging technology. Although not yet widely available, these scanners have been reported to be superior in assessing spinal cord and nerve root impingement.

Degenerative scoliosis is the final stage of lumbar degeneration. Coronal and axial MRI allow assessment of abnormal lateral curvature. Degenerative scoliosis leads to further osseous encroachment of the lateral recess and neuroforamen—findings that are also seen clearly with MRI.

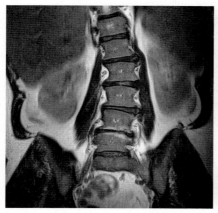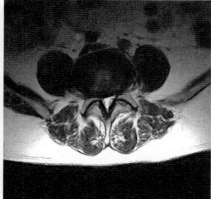

FIG. 4-10   This multiplane T2-weighted MRI demonstrates multilevel disc degeneration with secondary central canal and lateral recess stenoses. The advanced disc and osseous degeneration has led to secondary degenerative scoliosis.

Lumbar degeneration proceeds in a stepwise fashion. Disc degeneration allows disc collapse, abnormal motion, and misalignment of the lumbar spine. Abnormal motion leads to posterior and lateral osteophytes. Facet arthropathy and cartilage loss allow an additional increase in abnormal motions of the lumbar spine. Further progression of lumbar degeneration leads to spondylolisthesis and degenerative scoliosis. The combination of disc degeneration and osseous degeneration leads to central canal, lateral recess, and neuroforaminal stenoses (see Fig. 4-10).

CONCLUSION

Although conventional radiographs remain beneficial for assessing lumbar degenerative disease, advancements in cross-sectional imaging, including multiplane MRI and three-dimensional CT, have provided improved assessment of disc spaces and the osseous lumbar spinal canal. This enhanced assessment improves the ability to localize a patient's symptoms. As assessment and diagnosis accuracy improves, treatments and clinical outcomes for lumbar degeneration will also continue to improve.

REFERENCES

1. Grossman RI, Yousem DM, eds. Anatomy and degenerative diseases of the spine. In Neuroradiology: The Requisites. St Louis, MO: Mosby–Year Book, 1994, pp 447-476.
2. Kaplan PA, Dussault R, Helms CA, et al, eds. Spine. In Musculoskeletal MRI. Philadelphia: Saunders, 2001, pp 279-331.
3. Helms CA. Lumbar spine: disc disease and stenosis. Brant WE, Helms CA, eds. Fundamentals of Diagnostic Radiology. St Louis, MO: Mosby–Year Book, 1994, pp 316-325.
4. Greenspan A. Orthopedic Radiology: A Practical Approach, 3rd ed. Philadelphia: Lippincott Williams & Wilkins, 2000.
5. Modic MT, Steinberg PM, Ross JS, et al. Degenerative disc disease: assessment of changes in vertebral body marrow with MRI imaging. Radiology 166:194-199, 1988.
6. Stoller D. The spine. In Magnetic Resonance Imaging in Orthopedics and Sports Medicine, 2nd ed. Philadelphia: Lippincott Williams & Wilkins, 1997, pp 1097-1111.

5

Clinical Evaluation of Low Back and Leg Pain

Robert A. McGuire

When a patient presents with complaints of back and leg pain, the surgeon must consider many causes. To successfully treat the problem, of course, the correct diagnosis must first be made. The mode of onset of the problem is important, because injury mechanisms can give insight into the structures that serve as pain generators. It is extremely important to determine whether the pain is predominantly axial or radicular in nature, because the causes of each type of pain can be quite different. This chapter discusses the importance of a patient's history, the differential diagnosis, and the physical examination when evaluating patients with back and leg pain.

HISTORY AND DIFFERENTIAL DIAGNOSIS

When evaluating patients with back pain, it is paramount for the surgeon to determine whether the problem is predominantly axial or radicular (Box 5-1). Structures in the lower back that cause pain are muscular, ligamentous, and fascial. The intervertebral disc anulus can be painful, because it is highly innervated circumferentially in the peripheral portion of the structure. Kuslich et al[1] has elegantly shown that torn anular fibers can also result in radicular symptoms from irritation of the nerve and dorsal root ganglion as they pass near the inflamed structure. Bone and facet joints can also be a source of pain, and as the degenerative cascade progresses, degenerative by-products such as cytokines can produce centralized axial back pain. Compression of the neural structures, on the other hand, predominantly leads to either radicular or claudication symptoms.

When evaluating a patient's complaints of pain, it is important to assess—in detail—the patient's medical and surgical history, the onset and duration of the pain; exacerbating factors such as standing, sitting, coughing, sneezing, or other Valsalva maneuvers; and the quality of

BOX 5-1   History: Questions to Ask Patients Who Present With Low Back Pain
(With or Without Leg Pain)

- What is the onset of pain (acute or gradual)?
- Is the pain episodic or continuous and progressive?
- What factors precipitate the pain or alleviate the symptoms? Does the pain occur with activity? Is the pain alleviated with recumbency?
- Are there any constitutional symptoms (fever, chills, or weight loss)?
- Is there a history of bowel, bladder, or gait disturbance?
- Does the pain radiate? If so, to what locations (for example, buttock, thigh, or below knee to foot; unilateral or bilateral)?
- Is there a history of smoking? How much and for how long?
- Is there a medical history?
  - Hypertension
  - Diabetes
  - Other medical condition for which medications or therapy has been prescribed
  - Allergies

the pain. This information can assist the surgeon in determining the dermatomal pattern and locations of specific root involvement.[2] The history should include questions about exercise and social habits, such as tobacco and alcohol use.[3] Recent unexplained weight loss, chronic pain that has not responded to conservative management, a history of smoking, and being older than 50 can indicate a possible neoplastic process, which should be thoroughly evaluated. Previous surgeries, especially spinal procedures, should also be considered. Likewise, medical conditions that can cause neuropathy, such as diabetes, should be addressed, as should vascular conditions that can lead to either aneurysms or vascular occlusions, which, in turn, can result in back and leg symptoms.

Paresthesias (abnormal neurologic sensations that can include numbness, tingling, burning, and prickling), hyperalgesias (increased sensitivity), hypalgesias (decreased sensitivity), deep aching, or loss of sensation point to compression of a specific root. Nociceptive fibers to muscles, joints, and fascia are fewer in number and, when irritated, can result in a vague ache instead of specific radicular symptoms. Activities that aggravate or improve the problem should be explored. Hyperextension maneuvers of the spine that aggravate the symptoms suggest abnormalities of the facet joint or stenosis that is located either centrally or in the lateral recess. Pain that is aggravated by standing or active flexion or extension movements, but is relieved with recumbency, suggests mechanical instabilities.

Changes in neurologic function are of immediate concern. Any difficulties with bowel or bladder control, perineal anesthesia, and severe leg pain suggest a possible cauda equina syndrome, which should be evaluated as an immediate priority. Progressive weakness in spite of conservative management indicates a need for urgent surgical consideration. Symptoms of myelopathy occur more commonly in the cervical and thoracic levels with involvement of the spinal cord, so abnormalities of gait with spasticity or lower extremity weakness, either unilaterally or bilaterally, suggest the need to evaluate the more cephalad upper motor neuron condition in greater detail.

A patient's psychological history is also important, because depression can manifest as low-back somatization complaints. Finally, it is important to find out whether a patient with leg or back pain is actively involved in a worker's compensation claim or litigation. Studies have shown that patients who are involved in such claims or litigation often exhibit exaggeration or somatization of their symptom complex.[4,5]

The quality of the pain is very important when evaluating back and leg pain symptoms. When looking specifically at low back pain, one must also consider the structures in the pelvis and the abdomen as potential pain generators. A deep ache in the lower back can be a result of abnormalities of the kidneys, ureters, or pancreas, and a thorough evaluation of the aorta must be performed to rule out a potential aneurysm. In addition to the soft tissues and vascular structures, the sacroiliac and hip joints can be a source of the deep ache from the bony structures of the pelvis.

Pain that extends into the lower extremities can also result from structures within the pelvis.[6] If the sacroiliac joint is inflamed, for example, the sciatic nerve can be irritated, resulting in radiating leg pain. Vascular claudication can result in leg pain that is classically described as a dull ache beginning in the calf region; this is aggravated by ambulation and is usually relieved with rest or by stopping the activity.

Inflammatory arthritic conditions such as rheumatoid arthritis and ankylosing spondylitis can also cause a deep ache in the lower back. Serology consisting of antinuclear antibodies (ANAs), sedimentation rate, rheumatoid factors, and genetic markers such as HLAB 27 can assist in the diagnosis of these conditions.

Neoplasia and infection should be considered as possible diagnoses in patients with low back and leg pain. Patients with primary bone tumors like myeloma often present with spinal pain; these patients can be evaluated using both serum electrophoresis, to check for monoclonal elevations, and urine studies, to evaluate for elevated Bence Jones proteins. Discitis and osteomyelitis can both initially result in intense local back pain; if allowed to progress, these conditions can result in radicular complaints as the nerve itself becomes compromised from the abscess—directly or indirectly—which occurs after disc space or vertebral body collapse. The nerve can also experience potential vascular compromise locally.

The patient's age can assist in the diagnosis of specific degenerative problems. Disc herniations, which result in both back and leg pain, usually occur in the third and fourth decades of life. Instability symptoms usually occur in the late fourth or fifth decade, whereas stenosis and degenerative spondylolisthesis usually manifest in the latter fifth, sixth, or seventh decades.

PHYSICAL EXAMINATION

After a thorough history has been obtained, a physical examination completes the evaluation (Fig. 5-1).[7] Visual analog pain scales can be helpful in assessing the intensity of the patient's pain; such a tool can be reliable and valid. Pain drawings provide information that can assist surgeons as they diagnose low back and radicular problems, although there are conflicting data about the success of predicting surgical outcomes using these tools.[8] These drawings can provide valuable insights into a patient's complaints as they relate to either radicular or sclerodermal symptoms or to psychological overlay (Fig. 5-2). These tools also yield relatively high, repeatable results. They are good for evaluating pain intensity, and, if nonanatomic in presentation, they can steer the care provider to focus more on the psychological profile instead of on the specific problem of nerve compression. Functional studies such as the Oswestry Disability Index and SF-36 give a self-rated assessment of impairment of daily activities as a result of the spinal problem. These tests are easy to administer and have high validity and responsiveness.[9,10]

Attention should be paid to the patient's demeanor in the examination room, which provides the surgeon with insights about whether the patient might have an anxious personality or significant psychosocial overlays.[11] The patient's gait should also be evaluated, as should the manner in which the patient sits, stands, and transitions from sitting to standing. Furthermore, the surgeon should conduct a thorough vascular examination to assess the patient's femoral, popliteal, dorsalis pedis, and posterior tibial pulses. The patient should also be questioned about whether he or she has experienced trophic skin changes such as loss of hair, dystrophic nails, and rubor; these are warning signs of poor circulation.

Sensory testing is performed in all dermatomes of the lower extremity, and the ability to detect differences in light touch, pain, and temperature should be checked during the examination. If differences are found in nonanatomic or stocking distributions, one should consider metabolic neuropathy, such as that caused by diabetes, as the potential cause. Dermatomal deficits, on the other hand, are usually the result of root compression from herniated nucleus pulposus, lateral recessed stenosis, or spondylolisthesis. Also, a strength evaluation confirms radicular symptoms, because muscle groups are innervated by specific nerve roots; the muscles may be weak if the corresponding innervating root is compromised. Reflexes also should be thoroughly evaluated as part of the physical examination. A decreased response indicates a compromise of the lower motor neuron or root level, and, again, if the nerve root is compromised, this indicates potential radiculopathy. A hyperactive response is present if there is upper motor compromise; if present, lesions of the brain or the cervical or thoracic cord must be considered.

Once the physical examination is complete, any necessary radiographic studies should be performed. These results can assist the surgeon in verifying the clinical findings and in deciding on an appropriate treatment.

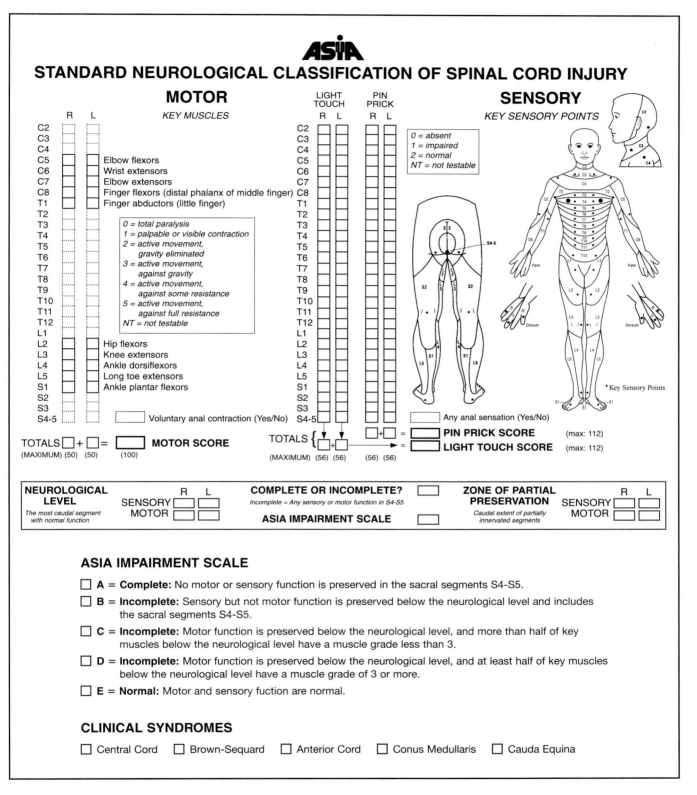

FIG. 5-1 Physical examination, based on American Spinal Injury Association (ASIA) classification. (Reproduced with permission from ASIA.)

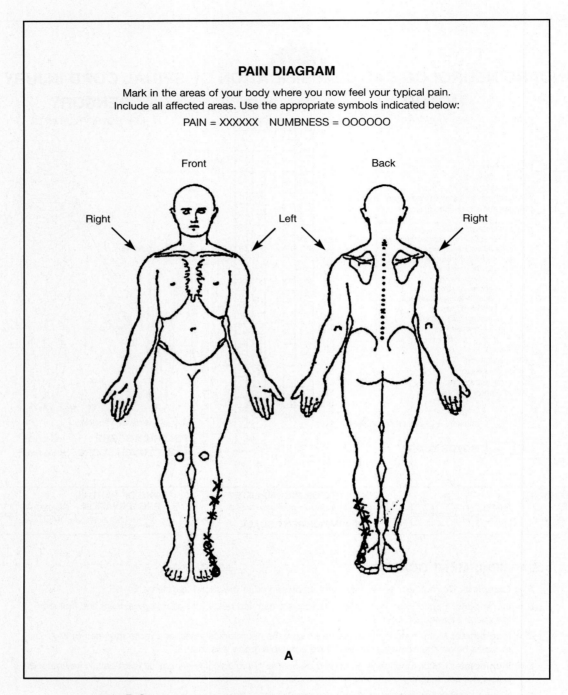

FIG. 5-2 **A,** Classic radiculopathy with pain in a dermatomal pattern.

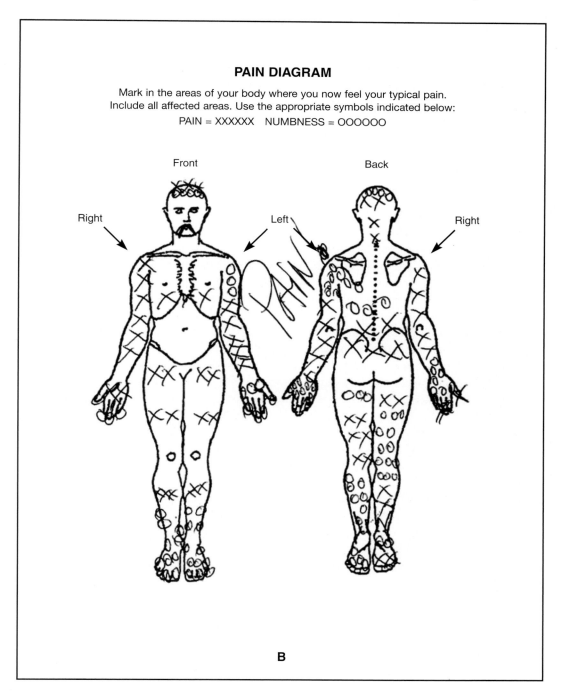

FIG. 5-2, cont'd   B, The nonorganic presentation of pain in a patient with chronic pain who had two previous spinal procedures and a compensation claim pending.

CONCLUSION

A thorough history and physical examination in a patient with back and leg pain often provide an understanding of the patient's complaints, aggravating factors, and the specific areas of involvement. In addition, they can help facilitate the diagnosis and treatment planning.

REFERENCES

1. Kuslich SD, Ulstrom CL, Michael CJ. The tissue origin of low back pain and sciatica: a report of pain response to tissue stimulation during operations on the lumbar spine using local anesthesia. Orthop Clin North Am 22:181-187, 1991.
2. Marks R. Distribution of pain provoked from lumbar facet joints and related structures during diagnostic spinal infiltration. Pain 39:37-40, 1989.
3. Deyo RA, Rainville J, Kent DL. What can the history and physical examination tell us about low back pain? JAMA 268:760-765, 1992.
4. Fransen M, Woodward M, Norton R, et al. Risk factors associated with the transition from acute to chronic occupational back pain. Spine 27:92-98, 2002.
5. DeBerard MS, Masters KS, Colledge AL, et al. Outcomes of posterolateral lumbar fusion in Utah patients receiving workers' compensation: a retrospective cohort study. Spine 26:738-747, 2001.
6. Dreyfuss P, Michaelsen M, Pauza K, et al. The value of medical history and physical examination in diagnosing sacroiliac joint pain. Spine 21:2594-2602, 1996.
7. Bradley WG, Daroff RB, Fenichel GM, et al. Neurology in Clinical Practice: Principle of Diagnosis and Management, 3rd ed. Boston: Butterworth-Heinemann, 2000.
8. Ohnmeiss DD. Repeatability of pain drawings in a low back pain population. Spine 25:980-988, 2000.
9. Fairbank JC, Couper J, Davies JB, et al. The Oswestry low back pain disability questionnaire. Physiotherapy 66:271-273, 1980.
10. Millard RW. A critical review of questionnaires for assessing pain-related disability. J Occup Rehabil 1:289-302, 1991.
11. Waddell G, McCulloch JA, Kummel E, et al. Nonorganic physical signs in low-back pain. Spine 5:117-125, 1980.

6

Principles of Direct and Indirect Decompression With XLIF®

Mark D. Peterson ▪ Kelli M. Howell

The extreme lateral interbody fusion (XLIF, NuVasive®, Inc., San Diego, CA) procedure has been presented as an alternative approach to anterior column stabilization in conditions resulting from degenerative processes, deformity, and traumatic injury of the thoracolumbar spine. Perhaps because it was first presented in comparison to anterior lumbar interbody fusion (ALIF),[1] early indications focused on such conditions as degenerative disc disease without significant stenosis. Successful application of the procedure in more complicated conditions, such as degenerative spondylolisthesis and scoliosis, broadened its usage as a minimally invasive treatment for conditions requiring anterior column stabilization of the thoracolumbar spine. Discussion continues regarding the use of XLIF alone to treat leg pain versus back pain, with a not uncommon assumption that leg symptoms require additional direct decompression. However, many patients have had resolution of radicular symptoms without direct posterior decompression.

In this chapter, we summarize the causes of radicular leg symptoms in lumbar degenerative conditions, review the literature on indirect decompression, and discuss what can reasonably be expected to be clinically affected by the indirect decompression afforded by XLIF.

PATHOPHYSIOLOGY

The earliest description of stenosis in the literature is attributed to Verbiest,[2] who described the anatomic changes of hypertrophic articular processes causing spinal canal stenosis. However, stenosis may be defined as occurring in the central, lateral recess, or foraminal areas; we may also categorize stenosis as caused by soft tissue or hard tissue encroachment and/or spinal malalignment. Central stenosis occurs in the central part of the spinal canal, usually by redundant ligamentum flavum or by anterior constriction of the disc as a consequence of disc narrowing and bulging (that is, soft tissue encroachment). When degeneration causes significant reduction of disc height, the interlaminar space is also reduced, and the ligamentum flavum, which may have become thickened, buckles anteriorly into the spinal canal. The posterior anulus and/or posterior longitudinal ligament may also bulge into the canal. Bony encroachment may also play a factor. The facets may become hypertrophied, with the medial margins of both facet joints approaching midline. Together, these contribute to the hourglass deformity of the dural sac, which can be seen in coronal, sagittal, and transverse magnetic resonance imaging (MRI) views. Hypertrophy primarily affects the superior facet of the inferior vertebra so that the superior articular process subluxes cranially toward the inferior margin of the pedicle of the superior vertebra, which progressively narrows the lateral recess and intervertebral foramina, usually bilaterally.[3] Osteophyte formation on the posterior or posterolateral margins of the vertebral endplate or on the lamina or articular processes may also contribute to the stenosis.

Degenerative spondylolisthesis or retrolisthesis often leads to concomitant stenosis. Subluxation and osteoarthritic changes of facet joints as a consequence of disc degeneration result in segmental instability, causing the cranial vertebra to be displaced anteriorly and the motion segment to become kyphotic. This displacement, accompanied by disc space narrowing, ligamentum flavum redundancy, and osteophyte formation, contributes to the existence of spinal stenosis involving the central canal, lateral recess, and neuroforamina.[4-7] Isthmic spondylolisthesis produces the same results, and the presence of Gill's nodules can contribute to narrowing of the foramen.[8]

CLINICAL PRESENTATION

Patients with nerve root compression demonstrate a radicular syndrome; the clinical presentation is characterized by pain in one or both buttocks and legs, often in a radicular pattern. Stenosis of the neural foramina and/or lateral recess is the most frequent cause of radiculopathy in patients over 50 years of age. Central stenosis may not present in a radicular pattern, but instead be heralded by intermittent claudication, demonstrated by generalized buttock and/or leg pain and difficulty with walking. Patients seek relief for neurogenic claudication or leg pain by sitting or assuming a more flexed or rounded posture as they walk, often supported by a cane, walker, or shopping cart. Frequently, the stenotic spine segment is limited to one or two levels, and it is not necessary to flex the entire spine forward or to round the whole back. If the one or two involved levels of stenosis are flexed forward, the symptoms can be relieved. Such postural relief is a positive sign for the potential to achieve indirect decompression.

The clinical evaluation should include determining the proportion of axial to radicular symptoms; the extent, nature, and location of neural compression (that is, central, subarticular, foraminal, extraforaminal, or a combined compression); the number of levels and degree of involvement; whether the compression is static or dynamic; whether the cause is hard or soft tissue; and the stability of the involved motion segments and the potential instability after decompression.

Although many surgeons use MRI as the preferred preoperative diagnostic tool to determine central stenosis, computed tomography (CT) has been reported to be better than MRI at enabling the surgeon to see the degenerative changes of the posterior elements and displaying lateral recess morphology.[9] CT may also help to identify calcification of any posterior anular ligamentous bulges. Foraminal stenosis is clear from lateral radiographs, with the foramen appearing flattened rather than oval, although surgical decision-making regarding the foramen should be based on MRI or CT, rather than on lateral radiographs. The foraminal morphology and effect on the exiting nerve are well appreciated on parasagittal MRI views.[9]

MECHANISMS OF TREATMENT

The surgical management of lumbar spine pathology presenting with radicular symptoms is well established in clinical practice and the literature. Compressive lesions in a stable spine are traditionally treated with direct decompression (Box 6-1). "Direct" decompression in this context refers to posterior excisional procedures: laminectomy, partial facetectomy, and/or foraminotomy are the typical surgical methods of choice, with or without fusion, depending on the presence and severity of instability. Complications associated with direct lumbar decompressive surgery are well documented and include bleeding, epidural hematoma, deep vein thrombosis, dural tear, infection, nerve root injury, iatrogenic instability, and recurrence of symptoms.

BOX 6-1   Decompression Guidelines

Conditions Amenable to Indirect Decompression
- Disc bulge, as in contained disc herniation (recurrent)
- Collapsed disc with loss of foraminal height and/or soft tissue encroachment (such as posterior anulus, PLL, or ligamentum flavum) of the canal
- Lateral listhesis, retrolisthesis, or spondylolisthesis, with narrowing of the central and intervertebral foramina because of malalignment
- Degenerative scoliosis with unilateral central or foraminal stenosis caused by the malalignment

Conditions That May Require Direct Decompression
- Congenital stenosis/congenitally short pedicles
- Uncontained disc herniation
- Significant facet arthropathy/osteophyte formation coupled with calcified disc, posterior longitudinal ligament, or osteophytes arising from the posterior endplates, with complete or near-complete compromise of the lateral recess
- Synovial cysts
- Radicular symptoms that do not improve with flexion

When instability is present with radicular symptoms, decompression (usually direct) with fusion is traditionally preferred. Indications include unstable spondylolisthesis, significant scoliosis or kyphosis, a second surgery for stenosis at the same segment, iatrogenic instability, or when radical discectomy is performed. Degenerative instability, in fact, has been shown to play a role in the cause of spinal stenosis,[10,11] and stabilizing the motion segment by fusion may therefore be beneficial to its treatment. In point of fact, fusion without decompression has been shown to be effective in alleviating radicular symptoms in the management of lytic spondylolisthesis. De Loubresse et al[12] compared the clinical results of posterolateral fusion only with posterolateral fusion with decompression in isthmic spondylolisthesis patients with radicular pain. They concluded that there was no significant statistical difference between the two groups and that resection of the loose lamina and direct decompression are not mandatory.

INDIRECT DECOMPRESSION

The principle of providing indirect neural decompression by restoration of disc height and foraminal volume by interbody fusion is well established. Indeed, in the cervical spine this approach is routinely used to treat foraminal stenosis from osteophytes or disc material. Research has shown that interbody distraction augments the space available for the spinal cord.[13] This treatment philosophy has been less studied in the lumbar spine, although one area of recent research has concerned the advent of spinous process spacing devices. Recent work with these devices suggests that claudicant or radicular symptoms caused by spinal stenosis and degenerative spondylolisthesis may be improved with indirect decompression. Interspinous process spacers have been specifically designed to distract the stenotic segment, stretching the soft tissues such as ligamentum flavum and/or disc encroaching on the canal, resulting in an increase in the dimensions of the canal and an alleviation of symptoms. Cadaveric[14] and clinical[15] studies of interspinous process distraction have shown a significant increase in the dural sac and exit foraminal area at the implanted level. A prospective, randomized, multicenter clinical study further showed significantly improved clinical outcome at 1 year postoperatively compared with patients whose condition was managed nonoperatively.[16]

Lumbar interbody distraction can produce the same decompressive effect. Vamivanij et al[17] performed a cadaveric study examining increases in the canal and foraminal cross-sectional area after placement of an interbody device in the lumbar spine. A 33% increase in the cross-sectional canal area and a 41% increase in the foraminal area were observed when a threaded distraction plug was placed from a lateral approach. A clinical study of anteriorly placed femoral ring allograft found effective indirect neuroforaminal decompression via the distractive effect of placing the graft.[18] Interbody grafting also has a lordosing effect on anterior column reconstruction. A comparison between posterolateral fusion and posterior interbody fusion showed better maintenance of disc space height and correction of sagittal alignment.[19] Further, anterior approaches to interbody fusion have been shown to more effectively restore disc height, foraminal volume, and lumbar lordosis compared with posterior approach.[20]

Much of the literature on the subject of indirect decompression through interbody fusion focuses on spondylolisthesis correction. In a study by Kim et al,[21] changes in the spinal canal were measured after anterior interbody fusion in both spondylolisthesis and disc herniation. It was shown that anterior interbody fusion corrects malalignment of the lumbar spine, reduces anterior slippage, restores disc height, and resolves nerve compression indirectly by increasing volume of the stenotic canal. The effect of stabilization also appears to assist in alleviating radicular symptoms. The authors concluded that it is possible to obtain satisfactory clinical results by anterior interbody fusion without instrumentation or direct decompression, especially in patients with radicular pain.[21]

Inoue et al[5] compared the preoperative and postoperative myelograms performed in patients with intervertebral disc herniation treated by anterior interbody fusion. Their study showed normalization of the radicular sheath in 60% of patients, normalization of the large hourglass defect and total block of the dural sac in the anteroposterior view in 82%, and normalization of the dural sac indentation in the lateral view in 70%. Inoue et al[22] reported another comparison of myelograms performed before and after anterior interbody fusion in patients with spondylolisthesis. There was normalization of the dural sac in the anteroposterior view in 44% and in the lateral view in 58%. The authors suggested that good clinical results might be attributed to the normalization of the myelographic pattern obtained by restoration of disc height and correction of the spinal malalignment after anterior interbody fusion.[22]

In the treatment of degenerative spondylolisthesis, comparable clinical outcomes have been observed between anterior interbody fusion without direct posterior decompression and posterolateral fusion with decompressive laminectomies.[7,21-25] Anterior interbody fusion reverses the pathogenesis of these features by distraction and restoration of the disc height, reduction of facet subluxation, and stabilization of the motion segment.[21,22,25]

In a long-term study of 39 patients who underwent anterior decompression and interbody fusion for degenerative spondylolisthesis, Takahashi et al[7] reported that 76% of their patients had satisfactory results for 10 years, 60% for 20 years, and 52% for 30 years. Neurogenic claudication resolved in 28 of the 32 patients who had the symptoms before surgery.

In a CT analysis, Kim and Kim[23] showed an increase in anteroposterior diameter of the dural sac and a decrease in the amount of disc bulging after anterior lumbar interbody fusion in patients with spondylolisthesis or intervertebral disc herniation. Other reports showed uniform satisfactory outcomes.[7,21,24,25] These results were similar to those for a laminectomy and posterolateral instrumentation.[24]

Indeed, as a treatment option for spondylolisthesis in particular, anterior column fusion appears to have some advantages over posterior approaches in that a stiffer arthrodesis is obtained and the posterior spinal musculature and other stabilizing structures are preserved. Minimally invasive procedures appear to have even greater advantages. Lee et al[26] found that a mini-ALIF followed by percutaneous pedicle screw fixation is an effective alternative for low-grade isthmic spondylolisthesis, and posterior decompression is not necessary to relieve leg symptoms. This minimally invasive combined procedure offers many advantages, such as preservation of the posterior arch, no neural retraction, less blood loss, excellent cosmetic results, a high fusion rate, and early patient discharge.

The preference among surgeons at this time is to treat grades I and II isthmic spondylolisthesis with normal adjacent discs with an anterior fusion. This procedure allows indirect foraminal decompression by restoring the disc height, decreasing the slip angle, and reducing the magnitude of the slip, as demonstrated by Kim and Lee.[27] Other studies support this, finding that anterior interbody fusion alone, without decompression, is more effective than decompression alone for the treatment of degenerative spondylolisthesis with associated stenosis.[23,25]

Further along the disease process, osteophytes form on the anterior and posterior surfaces of the superior articular processes of the lower vertebra, and the inferior articular processes of the upper vertebra continue to slip. Lateral recess and foraminal stenosis are mainly created by osteophyte formation. Low back pain is usually diminished or absent, and leg pain persists at rest. Anterior distraction and fusion may not adequately decompress lateral and foraminal stenosis in this stage, because the osteophytes on the posterior surface of superior articular processes block the reduction of the slippage, and anterior osteophytes still impinge on the neural elements.

Kuslich[28] recommended performing anterior interbody fusion without concomitant decompression when:
- The symptoms are a balanced combination of back and leg symptoms
- The segment is mildly unstable (for example, grade 1 spondylolisthesis)
- The stenosis is mild to moderate and subarticular or "up-down" as a result of the descent of the pedicle
- The stenosis involves only one or two motion segments
- The anterior approach is feasible

Kuslich determined these criteria when he found that "the case procedure can distract the disc sufficiently to open the foramen and reduce and/or eliminate the subarticular compression by preventing sagittal plane instability. If the stenotic symptoms are not relieved, a simple but complete posterior decompression can be done later without concerns of iatrogenic instability."[28]

XLIF FOR INDIRECT DECOMPRESSION

Clinical experience with XLIF suggests fusion without direct decompression is effective in treating neurologic symptoms in an unstable, scoliotic, and degenerative lumbar spine. Unlike anterior or posterior approaches, the lateral approach is ligament sparing and allows a

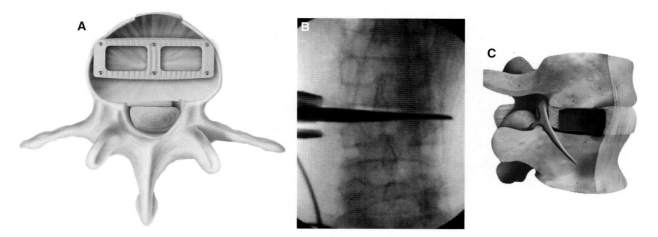

FIG. 6-1 **A,** The relative size of the XLIF implant and its placement across the disc space so that it rests on the ring apophysis bilaterally. **B,** Intraoperative fluoroscopic image showing intentional release of the contralateral anulus, an important step in reconstructing the height and alignment of the segment. **C,** The mechanism of disc space height and alignment restoration by implant placement and ligamentotaxis.

large, intrinsically stable implant to be placed completely across the interspace, resulting in a very stable interbody construct (Fig. 6-1, *A*). Proper surgical technique includes aggressive disc removal and the release of contralateral anulus (Fig. 6-1, *B*). This process not only ensures a proper graft bed but also allows interbody distraction that restores disc height and facilitates the reduction of the deformity through ligamentotaxis (Fig. 6-1, *C*). The supplemental use of lateral or posterior hardware increases construct stability (and possibly fusion rates) but is not necessary to achieve indirect decompression of the neural elements.

A staged approach is recommended; the surgeon should counsel the patient that an additional microdecompression might be required if symptoms persist. Severe central spinal stenosis is a relative contraindication if the patient is unwilling to accept the possibility of a second operation (direct decompression) if neurologic symptoms persist postoperatively. The second procedure is unnecessary in the vast majority of cases and spares the patient undue morbidity and risk of neural injury or scarring from direct posterior surgery.

CASE EXAMPLE

A 54-year-old nurse, previously very active (hiking, tennis, and basketball), presented with a history of 2 years of progressive low back pain and bilateral leg pain that worsened with standing and walking and improved when she sat. Symptoms persisted despite the use of NSAIDs, epidural injections, physical therapy, and giving up all recreational activities. Having difficulty with simple activities of daily living and work, she wanted surgical treatment. Preoperative imaging showed degenerative changes at L3-4 and L4-5, with spondylolisthesis at L3-4 and central, lateral recess, and foraminal stenosis at both levels (Fig. 6-2, *A* through *F*). The treatment plan included two-level XLIF from a left-sided approach using lordotic implants, then percutaneous pedicle screw fixation (SpheRx® DBR®, NuVasive, Inc.) from L3 to L5 (Fig. 6-2, *G* through *M*). No posterior (direct) decompression was performed. She tolerated the surgery very well and had no exposure-related thigh pain or numbness. The length of her hospital stay was 1 day, and she returned to part-time work at 4 weeks postoperatively and full-time at 8 weeks. At 8 weeks, she still had mild low back pain (a VAS of 3 compared with 8.5 preoperatively), with no leg pain. At 14 weeks, MRI demonstrated significant improvements in the central, lateral recess, and foraminal areas (Fig. 6-2, *N* through *X*); she had very minimal low back pain (a VAS of 0.5) and no leg pain. One year postoperatively, her radiographs showed improved disc height at L3-4 and L4-5, and her VAS was 0.0 (Fig. 6-2, *Y* through *AA*). She has returned to full work and recreational activities.

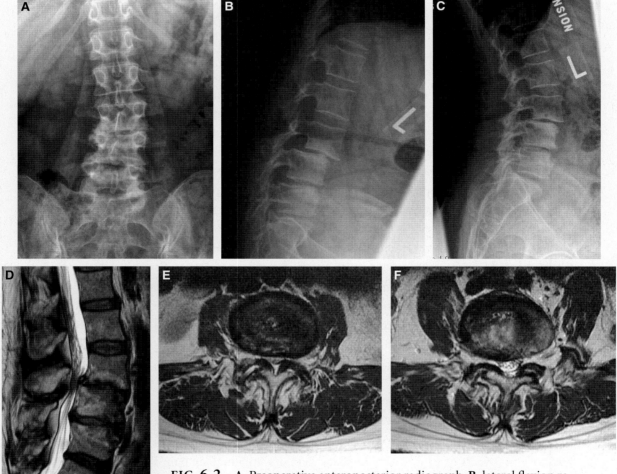

FIG. 6-2   A, Preoperative anteroposterior radiograph, **B,** lateral flexion radiograph, and **C,** lateral extension radiograph showing disc collapse at L3-4 and L4-5, with L3-4 spondylolisthesis. **D,** Preoperative sagittal MRI and **E** and **F,** axial MRI showing stenosis at the L3-4 and L4-5 levels, respectively.

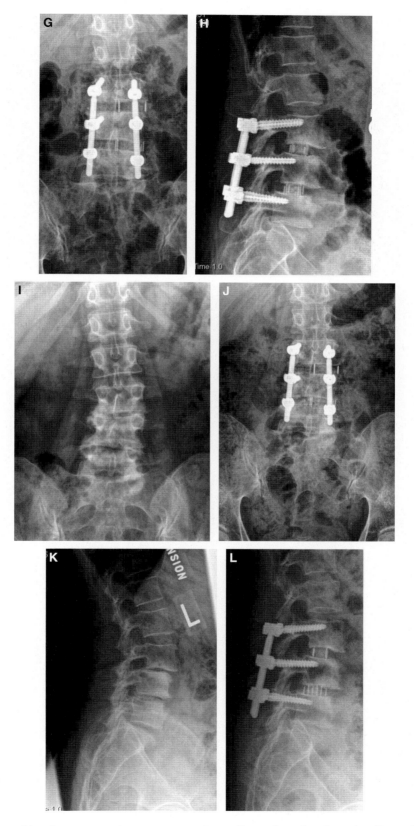

FIG. 6-2, cont'd   G, Postoperative anteroposterior radiograph and **H,** lateral radiograph showing an L3-5 XLIF with percutaneous pedicle screw fixation. Notice restoration of disc height and **I** and **J,** correction of coronal and **K** and **L,** sagittal alignment.   *Continued*

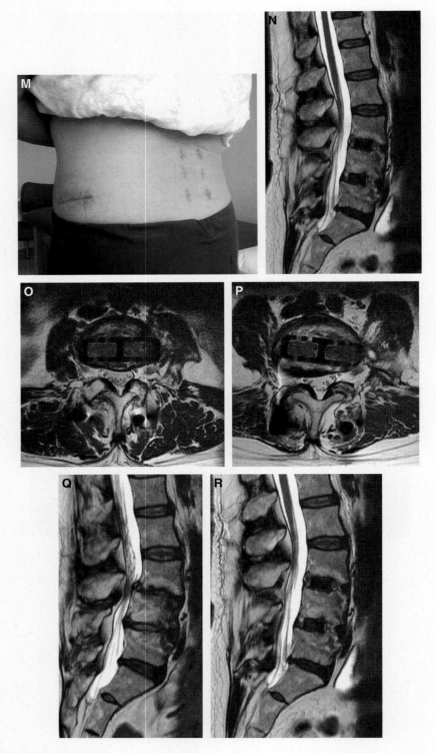

FIG. 6-2, cont'd   M, The patient's incisional scars are seen, laterally from two-level XLIF and posteriorly from two-level bilateral placement of percutaneous pedicle screws/rods. **N,** Postoperative sagittal and **O** and **P,** axial MRI showing restoration of canal dimensions. Comparison of canal dimensions **Q,** preoperatively with **R,** postoperatively in midsagittal MRI section.

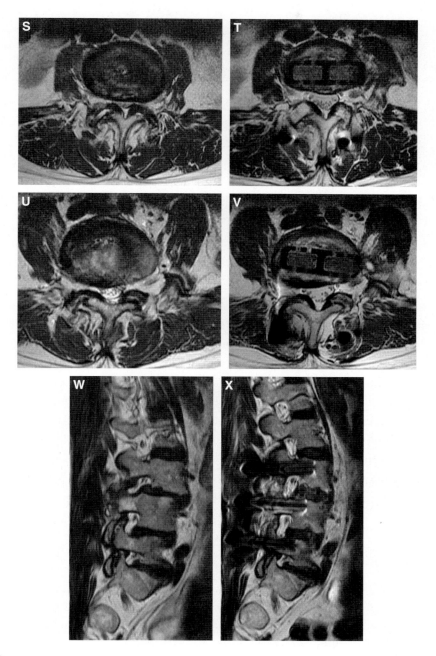

FIG. 6-2, cont'd   Comparison of central and lateral recesses in axial MRI at **S** and **T,** L3-4; **U** and **V,** L4-5; and foraminal dimensions in **W** and **X,** left parasagittal MRI section.   *Continued*

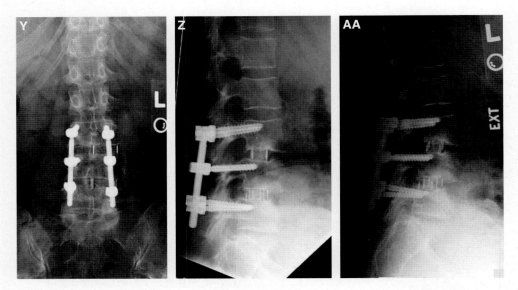

FIG. 6-2, cont'd   Y, One-year postoperative anteroposterior radiograph. **Z,** Flexion radiograph showing improved disc height at L3-4 and L4-5. **AA,** Lateral extension radiograph.

CONCLUSION

There is support in the literature for the practice of fusion with indirect decompression for spinal pathologies presenting with neurologic symptoms. Clinical experience suggests XLIF offers a mechanism for achieving indirect decompression through interbody distraction for several common lumbar disorders. XLIF avoids many of the potential complications of traditional surgery, including those associated with direct decompression. Adequate disc clearance and anular release are essential steps in achieving interbody distraction. Interbody distraction and stability are maintained through the use of an intrinsically stable interbody device that spans the vertebral body and rests on the apophyseal ring. Supplemental hardware is not necessary to achieve indirect decompression. Posterior or lateral hardware will increase construct stiffness and may protect the indirect decompression.

REFERENCES

1. Ozgur BM, Aryan HE, Pimenta L, et al. Extreme Lateral Interbody Fusion (XLIF): a novel surgical technique for anterior lumbar interbody fusion. Spine J 6:435-443, 2006.
2. Verbiest H. A radicular syndrome from developmental narrowing of the lumbar vertebral canal. J Bone Joint Surg Br 36:230-237, 1954.
3. Crock HV, Crock MC. Congenital versus acquired lumbar canal stenosis. In Gunzberg R, Szpalski M, eds. Lumbar Spinal Stenosis. Philadelphia: Lippincott Williams & Wilkins, 2000, pp 43-47.
4. Crock HV. Normal and pathological anatomy of the lumbar spinal canal nerve root canal. J Bone Joint Surg Br 63:487-490, 1981.
5. Inoue S, Watanabe T, Hirose A, et al. Anterior discectomy and interbody fusion for lumbar disc herniation. A review of 350 cases. Clin Orthop Relat Res 183:22-31, 1984.

6. Newman PH. Stenosis of the lumbar spine in spondylolisthesis. Clin Orthop Relat Res 115:116-121, 1976.

7. Takahashi K, Kitahara H, Yamagata M, et al. Long-term results of anterior interbody fusion for treatment of degenerative spondylolisthesis. Spine 15:1211-1215, 1990.

8. Crock HV. Anterior lumbar interbody fusion: indications for its use and notes on surgical technique. Clin Orthop 165:157-163, 1982.

9. Widelec J, Bacq C, Peetrons P. Conventional x-rays and computed tomographic scan in lumbar spinal stenosis. In Gunzberg R, Szpalski M, eds. Lumbar Spinal Stenosis. Philadelphia: Lippincott Williams & Wilkins, 2000, pp 91-96.

10. Kirkaldy-Willis WH, Farfan HF. Instability of the lumbar spine. Clin Orthop 165:110-113, 1982.

11. Kirkaldy-Willis WH, Wedge JH, Yong-Hing K, et al. Lumbar spinal nerve lateral entrapment. Clin Orthop 169:171-178, 1982.

12. De Loubresse CG, Bon T, Deburge A, et al. Posterolateral fusion for radicular pain in isthmic spondylolisthesis. Clin Orthop 323:194-201, 1996.

13. Bayley JC, Yoo JU, Kruger DM, et al. The role of distraction in improving the space available for the cord in cervical spondylosis. Spine 20:771-775, 1995.

14. Richards JC, Majumdar S, Lindsey DP, et al. The treatment mechanism of an interspinous process implant for lumbar neurogenic intermittent claudication. Spine 30:744-749, 2005.

15. Siddiqui M, Karadimas E, Nicol M, et al. Influence of X Stop on neural foramina and spinal canal area in spinal stenosis. Spine 31:2958-2962, 2006.

16. Zucherman JF, Hsu KY, Hartjen CA, et al. A prospective randomized multicenter study for the treatment of lumbar spinal stenosis with the X Stop interspinous implant: 1-year results. Eur Spine J 13:22-31, 2004.

17. Vamivanij V, Ferrara LA, Hai Y, et al. Quantitative changes in spinal canal dimensions using interbody distraction for spondylolisthesis. Spine 26:E13-E18, 2001.

18. Kozak JA, Heilman AE, O'Brien JP. Anterior lumbar fusion options. Technique and graft materials. Clin Orthop Relat Res 300:45-51, 1994.

19. Kim KT, Lee SH, Lee YH, et al. Clinical outcomes of three fusion methods through the posterior approach in the lumbar spine. Spine 31:1351-1357, 2006.

20. Hsieh PC, Koski TR, O'Shaughnessy BA, et al. Anterior lumbar interbody fusion in comparison with transforaminal lumbar interbody fusion: implications for the restoration of foraminal height, local disc angle, lumbar lordosis, and sagittal balance. J Neurosurg Spine 7:379-386, 2007.

21. Kim NH, Kim HK, Suh JS. A computed tomographic analysis of changes in the spinal canal after anterior lumbar fusion. Clin Orthop 286:180-191, 1993.

22. Inoue S, Watanabe T, Goto S, et al. Degenerative spondylolisthesis: pathophysiology and results of anterior interbody fusion. Clin Orthop 227:90-98, 1988.

23. Kim NH, Kim DJ. Anterior interbody fusion for spondylolisthesis. Orthopedics 14:1069-1076, 1991.

24. Mardjetko SM, Connolly PJ, Shott S. Degenerative lumbar spondylolisthesis: a meta-analysis of literature 1970-1993. Spine 19(20 Suppl):S2256-S2265, 1994.

25. Satomi K, Hirabayahi K, Toyama Y, et al. A clinical study of degenerative spondylolisthesis: radiographic analysis and choice of treatment. Spine 17:1329-1336, 1992.

26. Lee SH, Choi WG, Lim SR, et al. Minimally invasive anterior lumbar interbody fusion followed by percutaneous pedicle screw fixation for isthmic spondylolisthesis. Spine J 4:644-649, 2004.

27. Kim NH, Lee JW. Anterior interbody fusion versus posterolateral fusion with transpedicular fixation for isthmic spondylolisthesis in adults: a comparison of clinical results. Spine 24:812-817, 1999.

28. Kuslich SD. The utility of interbody arthrodesis using BAK cages in treatment. In Gunzberg R, Szpalski M, eds. Lumbar Spinal Stenosis. Philadelphia: Lippincott Williams & Wilkins, 2000, pp 287-301.

7

Bone Grafting Options for Lumbar Spine Fusions

Jonathan A. Tuttle ▪ Norman B. Chutkan

The number of spine fusions performed annually has increased dramatically since the early 1990s.[1-4] More than 400,000 spine fusions are done in the United States and Europe, combined, every year.[5,6] As the rate of spine fusions increases, so does the economic impact. According to Medicare's own statistics, lumbar fusions in the United States made up 14% of the agency's spinal surgery payments in 1992; this increased to 50% by 2003.[4]

The goal of spine fusion is to achieve a bony union across the vertebral segments. Common indications for surgery include instability, deformity, and discogenic pain. *Nonunion,* or *pseudarthrosis,* is the failure of a bony union to occur. One way to increase the rate of bony fusion is to use instrumentation; however, nonunions can still approach 15% for instrumented single-level anterior lumbar fusions.[6-9] Reported nonunion rates have varied in the literature, depending on the study and the type of lumbar fusion performed. Unfortunately, nonunion rates are still higher for multilevel fusions and posterolateral intertransverse fusions when compared with single-level fusions and anterior lumbar interbody fusions, respectively.[10,11]

Nonunions often lead to increased morbidity and require additional surgeries to achieve an arthrodesis. Bone grafting techniques increase the percentage of successful bony fusions. Available grafting options include autogenous iliac crest bone graft, bone marrow aspirate, allograft, ceramics, and recombinant human bone morphogenic proteins (BMPs) (Table 7-1).

Fusion Model

Urist[12] and Urist et al[13] described the concept of osteoinduction and were the first to identify a bone morphogenic protein. Osteoinduction, osteoconduction, and osteogenicity make up

TABLE 7-1   Properties of Clinically Available Bone Grafting Options

	Osteoinductive	Osteoconductive	Osteogenic
Autograft	++	+++	+++
Allograft	Weakly +	+	
Ceramic		+++	
Bone morphogenic proteins (for example, INFUSE, OP-1)	+++		

the three desired properties of bone grafts used for spine fusion. *Osteoinduction* refers to the maturation of primitive mesenchymal cells into osteoblasts, whereas *osteoconduction* is the scaffold that allows an ingrowth of osteoprogenitor cells in an environment that also allows vascular support.[14] *Osteogenicity* refers to the availability of osteoblasts, osteoclasts, and osteocytes—cells that are capable of depositing, resorbing, and remodeling bone, respectively.

Each bone graft material is evaluated in terms of its osteoinductivity, osteoconductivity, and osetogenicity, and the clinical utility of materials as graft enhancers, graft extenders, or graft substitutes should also reflect this.[6] Graft enhancers increase the rate of fusion when compared with autologous graft alone, whereas graft extenders decrease the amount of autologous graft needed to achieve the same fusion. Extenders also allow for additional segmental fusion levels that would not have been possible because of limited autograft. Graft substitutes completely replace autologous bone graft and have similar fusion rates.

AUTOGRAFT

Autogenous iliac crest bone graft has been the standard for bone grafting, because it is inherently osteoinductive, osteoconductive, and osteogenic. Compared with allograft, autograft has a higher rate of fusion, fewer incidences of interbody graft subsidence and pseudarthrosis, and no potential for disease transmission or immunologic rejection. Autograft is used in the form of cortical or cancellous bone, bone marrow aspirate, or vascularized graft but is only available in limited quantities. In revision surgeries, the previous harvesting of iliac crest autograft may limit its availability. The morbidities associated with autograft include chronic donor-site pain, increased operative time, increased blood loss, a necessity for additional surgical sites, infection, hematoma, abdominal herniation, nerve or vascular injury, cosmetic deformity, or iliac wing fracture.[15-22] By far, the most common problem is chronic donor-site pain, which is commonly reported to be around 8% but can be as high as 30%.[22,23] This is especially frustrating for a patient—and his or her surgeon—if back pain resolves but iliac crest pain persists.

It is preferable to use autograft whenever possible. Because iliac crest bone grafting is associated with increased morbidity, bone marrow aspiration is routine, with rare morbidity. Recently, transpedicular aspiration of the vertebral body and iliac crest aspirate have been shown to have a similar amount of osteogenic cells.[24] For anterior lumbar interbody grafting, a 2 mm bone marrow aspiration provides the ideal concentration of osteoblast progenitor cells; larger volumes are diluted with peripheral blood.[25] For posterolateral intertransverse fusions after decompression, laminar autograft may be sufficient; if not, it may be mixed with a combination of bone marrow aspirate and bone graft extender, such as allograft or tricalcium phosphate.

ALLOGRAFT

Allograft, traditionally the first choice for autograft replacement, has advantages and disadvantages compared with autograft. Allograft is osteoconductive and mildly osteoinductive, and it can be used as a graft substitute or a graft extender. Allograft is available in greater supply—albeit not unlimited—and there is no need for an additional incision or increased surgical time as with autograft. However, fusion rates are slightly lower, and allograft use carries a risk of disease transmission and immunologic rejection.[26,27]

The risk of disease transmission is linked to the method of allograft preservation. Allograft is often preserved at cadaveric harvest, but it can also be fresh frozen or freeze dried. Freeze-dried, or lyophilized, grafts are less immunogenic, but the freeze-drying process also decreases the mechanical strength and osteoinductivity more than fresh-frozen preservation. In addition, there has never been a documented case of HIV transmission with the use of freeze-dried allograft; four infections resulted from two fresh-frozen allograft donors.[28] However, these infections predated current HIV testing; no infections have been discovered since the mid-1980s.[29-31]

Conducting extensive medical and social history reviews of potential donors can prevent viral transmission, as can allograft sterilization, which is accomplished with ethylene oxide gas or gamma irradiation. However, chemical sterilization is ineffective against HIV.[32-35] Gamma irradiation is the preferred method for sterilizing intraarticular grafts; high failure rates are reported with ethylene oxide. The exception is when ethylene oxide is used to sterilize lumbar interbody grafts; Ma[36] evaluated this method and reported an 89% fusion rate.

As noted previously, the mechanical properties of allograft vary according to the preservation technique. Fresh-frozen allograft retains torsional, bending, and compressive strength compared with fresh allograft. Fresh allograft is ideal for a kidney donation, for example, but fresh allograft bone is not used for spine surgeries because of its immunogenicity and potential for disease transmission. The freeze-drying preservation technique maintains the compressive strength of fresh or fresh-frozen allograft; however, it only retains 55% to 90% of its bending strength and 39% of its torsional strength.[37,38]

Another type of allograft is demineralized bone matrix (DBM), a ground cadaveric corticocancellous bone that contains variable amounts of proteins and growth factors.[39,40] The Food and Drug Administration (FDA) requires that each lot of DBM come from a single donor, but donor characteristics are not standardized, nor are assays used to ensure that the DBM meets minimal quality standards. Most DBM contains 93% collagen carrier, 5% soluble proteins, and 2% mineral matrix.[41] However, multiple formulations of DBM exist, and the fillers and carrier materials vary, depending on the manufacturer. Each formulation has different handling characteristics, allowing a surgeon to select a DBM based on his or her preference. DBM is both a graft enhancer and a graft extender.

CERAMICS

Osteoconductive ceramic materials that are commonly available for spine surgeries include calcium sulfate, tricalcium phosphate (TCP), and hydroxyapatite (HA).[42] Calcium sulfate is a salt that dissolves if it enters a joint space, and it remains in place for only a short time after implantation. TCP and HA persist longer, with HA remaining in place the longest.[43] When HA/TCP are mixed together, they are referred to as *biphasic calcium phosphate.* The HA component of the compound has the benefit of long-term osteoconductivity, and the TCP is rapidly replaced with new bone. When assembled within a collagen matrix (such as FormaGraft®, NuVasive®, Inc., San Diego, CA [Fig. 7-1]), the material possesses superb handling properties and the ability to absorb osteogenetic cells and osteoinductive factors from bone marrow aspirate (Table 7-1). As such, the composite of FormaGraft and bone marrow aspirate closely mimics the composition and biology of normal human bone.

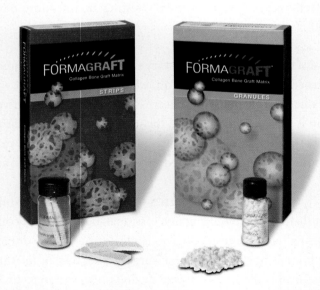

FIG. 7-1   FormaGraft strips and granules (Courtesy NuVasive, Inc.).

Biphasic calcium phosphate has been studied as a carrier for BMP-2 in posterolateral inter-transverse lumbar fusions and appears to provide comparable fusion rates to autograft.[10,44] Other studies show that when biphasic calcium phosphate is mixed with local bone, the fusion rate is similar to that of iliac crest autograft.[45-47]

BONE MORPHOGENIC PROTEINS

Bone morphogenic proteins belong to the transforming growth factor beta superfamily.[48,49] Originally discovered by Urist,[12,13] BMP has been further delineated to include designations from BMP-1 to BMP-16. BMP-2 through BMP-7 and BMP-9 are capable of de novo bone formation; however, clinical use centers around BMP-2 (INFUSE Bone Graft, Medtronic Sofamor Danek, Memphis, TN [Fig. 7-2]) and BMP-7, also known as osteogenic protein one, or OP-1 (Stryker Biotech, Hopkinton, MA).[50-56] At this time, INFUSE has been approved for lumbar fusions, and it is currently being evaluated for use in poly-ether-ether-ketone (PEEK) cervical cages for cervical fusions, whereas OP-1 has FDA humanitarian device exemption for long bone nonunions.[57]

Burkus et al[58] published the controlled study that resulted in FDA approval for recombinant human BMP-2 (rhBMP-2) use in single-level anterior lumbar fusions, with a threaded LT CAGE, for degenerative disc disease at L4-S1 in skeletally mature patients. Additional studies have indicated that fusion rates are superior to autograft for single-level anterior lumbar or transforaminal interbody fusions—without the morbidity, increased operative time, and blood loss associated with autograft.[47,59-62]

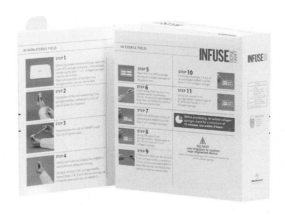

FIG. 7-2 INFUSE Bone Graft (Courtesy Medtronic, Inc., Memphis, TN).

The benefits of INFUSE and OP-1 for posterolateral fusions have been evaluated in several studies.[6,40,63-70] The bovine type-1 absorbable collagen sponge carrier appears to have a higher fusion rate when used with interbody grafts than with posterolateral fusions. Also, the amount of BMP-2 required is greater in posterolateral fusions.[10,44,65] Preliminary data appear positive when biphasic calcium phosphates are used as carriers, because of their osteoconductive and compression-resistance qualities.[64]

CONCLUSION

The use of bone-grafting technologies in spine fusion surgeries continues to evolve. Although autografts remain the current standard, it is likely that BMPs will soon take over that role. As the availability and variety of these proteins increase, so will the indications for their use. In addition, future spine fusion technologies will likely involve tissue modulation, which has the potential to render the use of autograft and allograft obsolete.

REFERENCES

1. Deyo RA, Gray DT, Kreuter W, et al. United States trends in lumbar fusion surgery for degenerative conditions. Spine 30:1441-1445, 2005.
2. Gray DT, Deyo RA, Kreuter W, et al. Population-based trends in volumes and rates of ambulatory lumbar spine surgery. Spine 31:1957-1963, 2006.
3. Taylor VM, Deyo RA, Cherkin DC, et al. Low back pain hospitalization. Recent United States trends and regional variations. Spine 19:1207-1212, 1994.
4. Weinstein JN, Lurie JD, Olson PR, et al. United States' trends and regional variations in lumbar spine surgery: 1992-2003. Spine 31:2707-2714, 2006.
5. Becker S, Maissen O, Ponomarev I, et al. Osteopromotion by a beta-tricalcium phosphate/bone marrow hybrid implant for use in spine surgery. Spine 31:11-17, 2006.
6. Boden SD. Overview of the biology of lumbar spine fusion and principles for selecting a bone graft substitute. Spine 27(16 Suppl 1):S26-S31, 2002.
7. Boden SD, Schimandle JH. Biologic enhancement of spinal fusion. Spine 20(Suppl 24):113S-123S, 1995.
8. Boden SD, Titus L, Hair G, et al. Lumbar spine fusion by local gene therapy with a cDNA encoding a novel osteoinductive protein (LMP-1). Spine 23:2486-2492, 1998.
9. Peterson B, Whang PG, Iglesias R, et al. Osteoinductivity of commercially available demineralized bone matrix: preparations in a spine fusion model. J Bone Joint Surg Am 86:2243-2250, 2004.
10. Glassman SD, Carreon L, Djurasovic M, et al. Posterolateral lumbar spine fusion with INFUSE bone graft. Spine J 7:44-49, 2007.
11. Steinmann JC, Herkowitz HN. Pseudarthrosis of the spine. Clin Orthop Relat Res 284:80-90, 1992.
12. Urist MR. Bone: formation by autoinduction. Science 150:893-899, 1965.
13. Urist MR, Silverman BF, Büring K, et al. The bone induction principle. Clin Orthop Relat Res 53:243-283, 1967.
14. Carlisle E, Fischgrund JS. Bone morphogenetic proteins for spinal fusion. Spine J 5(Suppl 6):S240-S249, 2005.

15. Arrington ED, Smith WJ, Chambers HG, et al. Complications of iliac crest bone graft harvesting. Clin Orthop Relat Res 329:300-309, 1996.

16. Banwart JC, Asher MA, Hassanein RS. Iliac crest bone graft harvest donor site morbidity: a statistical evaluation. Spine 20:1055-1060, 1995.

17. Fernyhough JC, Schimandle JJ, Weigel MC, et al. Chronic donor site pain complicating bone graft harvesting from the posterior iliac crest for spinal fusion. Spine 17:1474-1480, 1992.

18. Kurz LT, Garfin SR, Booth RE Jr. Harvesting autogenous iliac bone grafts: a review of complications and techniques. Spine 14:1324-1331, 1989.

19. Robertson PA, Wray AC. Natural history of posterior iliac crest bone graft donation for spinal surgery: a prospective analysis of morbidity. Spine 26:1473-1476, 2001.

20. Sasso RC, Williams JI, Dimasi N, et al. Postoperative drains at the donor sites of iliac-crest bone grafts. A prospective, randomized study of morbidity at the donor site in patients who had a traumatic injury of the spine. J Bone Joint Surg Am 80:631-635, 1998.

21. Summers BN, Eisenstein SM. Donor site pain from the ilium. A complication of lumbar spine fusion. J Bone Joint Surg Br 71:677-680, 1989.

22. Younger EM, Chapman MW. Morbidity at bone graft donor sites. J Orthop Trauma 3:192-195, 1989.

23. Laurie SW, Kaban LB, Mulliken JB, et al. Donor-site morbidity after harvesting rib and iliac bone. Plast Reconstr Surg 73:933-938, 1984.

24. McLain RF, Fleming JE, Boehm CA, et al. Aspiration of osteoprogenitor cells for augmenting spinal fusion: comparison of progenitor cell concentrations from the vertebral body and iliac crest. J Bone Joint Surg Am 87:2655-2661, 2005.

25. Muschler GF, Boehm C, Easley K. Aspiration to obtain osteoblast progenitor cells from human bone marrow: the influence of aspiration volume. J Bone Joint Surg Am 79:1699-1709, 1997.

26. Smith RA, Ingels J, Lochemes JJ, et al. Gamma irradiation of HIV-1. J Orthop Res 19:815-819, 2001.

27. Tomford WW. Transmission of disease through transplantation of musculoskeletal allografts. J Bone Joint Surg Am 77:1742-1754, 1995.

28. Asselmeier MA, Casperi RB, Bottenfield S. A review of allograft processing and sterilization techniques and their role in transmission of the human immunodeficiency virus. Am J Sports Med 21:170-175, 1993.

29. Buck BE, Malinin TI, Brown MD. Bone transplantation and human immunodeficiency virus. An estimate of risk of acquired immunodeficiency syndrome (AIDS). Clin Orthop Relat Res 240:129-136, 1989.

30. Buck BE, Resnick L, Shah SM, et al. Human immunodeficiency virus cultured from bone. Implications for transplantation. Clin Orthop Relat Res 251:249-253, 1990.

31. Centers for Disease Control (CDC). Transmission of HIV through bone transplantation: case report and public health recommendations. MMWR Morb Mortal Wkly Rep 37:597-599, 1988.

32. Bujía J, Wilmes E, Kastenbauer E, et al. Influence of chemical allograft preservation procedures on the human immunodeficiency virus. Laryngoscope 106:645-647, 1996.

33. Conway B, Tomford WW, Hirsch MS, et al. Effects of gamma irradiation on HIV-1 in a bone allograft model. Trans Orthop Res Soc 15:225-230, 1990.

34. Czitrom A. Principles and techniques of tissue banking. In Heckam JD, ed. AAOS Instructional Course Lectures, 42nd ed. Rosemont, IL: American Academy of Orthopaedic Surgeons, 1993, pp 359-362.

35. Fideler BM, Vangsness CT Jr, Moore T, et al. Effects of gamma irradiation on the human immunodeficiency virus. A study in frozen human bone-patellar ligament-bone grafts obtained from infected cadavera. J Bone Joint Surg Am 76:1032-1035, 1994.

36. Ma GW. Posterior lumbar interbody fusion with specialized instruments. Clin Orthop Relat Res 193:57-63, 1985.

37. Pelker RR, Friedlaender GE, Markham TC. Biomechanical properties of bone allografts. Clin Orthop Relat Res 174:54-57, 1983.

38. Triantafyllou N, Sotiropoulos E, Triantafyllou J. The mechanical properties of the lyophylized and irradiated bone grafts. Acta Orthop Belg 41(Suppl 1):S35-S39, 1975.

39. Bae HW, Zhao L, Kanim LE, et al. Intervariability and intravariability of bone morphogenetic proteins in commercially available demineralized bone matrix products. Spine 31:1299-1306, 2006.

40. Martin GJ Jr, Boden SD, Marone MA, et al. Posterolateral intertransverse process spinal fusion arthrodesis with rhBMP-2 in a nonhuman primate: important lessons learned regarding dose, carrier, and safety. J Spinal Disord 12:179-186, 1999.

41. Lee KJ, Roper JG, Wang JC. Demineralized bone matrix and spinal arthrodesis. Spine J 5(6 Suppl):S217-S223, 2005.

42. Kelly CM, Wilkins RM, Gitelis S, et al. The use of a surgical grade calcium sulfate as a bone graft substitute: results of a multicenter trial. Clin Orthop Relat Res 382:42-50, 2001.

43. Jarcho M. Calcium phosphate ceramics as hard tissue prosthetics. Clin Orthop Relat Res 157:259-278, 1981.

44. Glassman SD, Dimar JR III, Burkus K, et al. The efficacy of rhBMP-2 for posterolateral lumbar fusion in smokers. Spine 32:1693-1698, 2007.

45. Epstein NE. A preliminary study of the efficacy of Beta Tricalcium Phosphate as a bone expander for instrumented posterolateral lumbar fusions. J Spinal Disord Tech 19:424-429, 2006.

46. Fujibayashi S, Shikata J, Tanaka C, et al. Lumbar posterolateral fusion with biphasic calcium phosphate ceramic. J Spinal Disord 14:214-221, 2001.

47. Resnick DK, Choudhri TF, Dailey AT, et al. American Association of Neurological Surgeons/Congress of Neurological Surgeons, et al. Guidelines for the performance of fusion procedures for degenerative disease of the lumbar spine. Part 16: Bone graft extenders and substitutes. J Neurosurg Spine 2:733-736, 2005.

48. Cheng H, Jiang W, Phillips FM, et al. Osteogenic activity of the fourteen types of human bone morphogenetic proteins (BMPs). J Bone Joint Surg Am 85:1544-1552, 2003.

49. Termaat MF, Den Boer FC, Bakker FC, et al. Bone morphogenetic proteins. Development and clinical efficacy in the treatment of fractures and bone defects. J Bone Joint Surg Am 87:1367-1378, 2005.

50. Chen P, Carrington JL, Hammonds RG, et al. Stimulation of chondrogenesis in limb bud mesoderm cells by recombinant human bone morphogenetic protein 2B (BMP-2B) and modulation by transforming growth factor beta 1 and beta 2. Exp Cell Res 195:509-515, 1995.

51. Chen TL, Bates RL, Dudley A, et al. Bone morphogenetic protein-2b stimulation of growth and osteogenic phenotypes in rat osteoblast-like cells: comparison with TGF-beta 1. J Bone Miner Res 6:1387-1393, 1991.

52. Gitelman SE, Kobrin MS, Ye JQ, et al. Recombinant Vgr-1/BMP-6-expressing tumors induce fibrosis and endochondral bone formation in vivo. J Cell Biol 126:1595-1609, 1994.

53. Mayer H, Scutt AM, Ankenbauer T. Subtle differences in the mitogenic effects of recombinant human bone morphogenetic proteins-2 to -7 on DNA synthesis on primary bone-forming cells and identification of BMP-2/4 receptor. Calcif Tissue Int 58:249-255, 1996.

54. Thies RS, Bauduy M, Ashton BA, et al. Recombinant human bone morphogenetic protein-2 induces osteoblastic differentiation in W-20-17 stromal cells. Endocrinology 130:1318-1324, 1992.

55. Vukicevic S, Luyten FP, Reddi AH. Stimulation of the expression of osteogenic and chondrogenic phenotypes in vitro by osteogenin. Proc Natl Acad Sci USA 86:8793-8797, 1989.

56. Vukicevic S, Luyten FP, Reddi AH. Osteogenin inhibits proliferation and stimulates differentiation in mouse osteoblast-like cells (MC3T3-E1). Biochem Biophys Res Commun 166:750-756, 1990.

57. Brown A, Stock G, Patel AA, et al. Osteogenic protein-1: a review of its utility in spinal applications. BioDrugs 20:243-251, 2006.

58. Burkus JK, Gornet MF, Dickman CA, et al. Anterior lumbar interbody fusion using rhBMP-2 with tapered interbody cages. J Spinal Disord Tech 15:337-349, 2002.

59. Burkus JK, Heim SE, Gornet MF, et al. Is INFUSE bone graft superior to autograft bone? An integrated analysis of clinical trials using the LT-CAGE lumbar tapered fusion device. J Spinal Disord Tech 16:113-122, 2003.

60. Burkus JK. Bone morphogenetic proteins in anterior lumbar interbody fusion: old techniques and new technologies. Invited submission from the Joint Section Meeting on Disorders of the Spine and Peripheral Nerves, March 2004. J Neurosurg Spine 1:254-260, 2004.

61. Burkus JK, Transfeldt EE, Kitchel SH, et al. Clinical and radiographic outcomes of anterior lumbar interbody fusion using recombinant human bone morphogenetic protein-2. Spine 27: 2396-2408, 2002.

62. Mummaneni PV, Pan J, Haid RW, et al. Contribution of recombinant human bone morphogenetic protein-2 to the rapid creation of interbody fusion when used in transforaminal lumbar interbody fusion: a preliminary report. Invited submission from the Joint Section Meeting on Disorders of the Spine and Peripheral Nerves, March 2004. J Neurosurg Spine 1:19-23, 2004.

63. Akamaru T, Suh D, Boden SD, et al. Simple carrier matrix modifications can enhance delivery of recombinant human bone morphogenetic protein-2 for posterolateral spine fusion. Spine 28:429-434, 2003.

64. Barnes B, Boden SD, Louis-Ugbo J, et al. Lower dose of rhBMP-2 achieves spine fusion when combined with an osteoconductive bulking agent in non-human primates. Spine 30:1127-1133, 2005.

65. Boden SD, Kang J, Sandhu H, et al. Use of recombinant human bone morphogenetic protein-2 to achieve posterolateral lumbar spine fusion in humans: a prospective, randomized clinical pilot trial. Spine 23:2662-2673, 2002.

66. Johnsson R, Strümqvist B, Aspenberg P. Randomized radiostereometric study comparing osteogenic protein-1 (BMP-7) and autograft bone in human noninstrumented posterolateral lumbar fusion: 2002 Volvo Award in clinical studies. Spine 27:2654-2661, 2002.

67. Kanayama M, Hashimoto T, Shigenobu K, et al. A prospective randomized study of posterolateral lumbar fusion using osteogenic protein-1 (OP-1) versus local autograft with ceramic bone substitute: emphasis of surgical exploration and histologic assessment. Spine 31:1067-1074, 2006.

68. Patel TC, Erulker JS, Grauer JN, et al. Osteogenic protein-1 overcomes the inhibitory effect of nicotine on posterolateral lumbar fusion. Spine 26:1656-1661, 2001.

69. Vaccaro AR, Patel T, Fischgrund J, et al. A pilot study evaluating the safety and efficacy of OP-1 Putty (rhBMP-7) as a replacement for iliac crest autograft in posterolateral lumbar arthrodesis for degenerative spondylolisthesis. Spine 29:1885-1892, 2004.

70. White AP, Maak TG, Prince D, et al. Osteogenic protein-1 induced gene expression: evaluation in a posterolateral spinal pseudarthrosis model. Spine 31:2550-2555, 2006.

Part II

Surgical Techniques and Clinical Applications

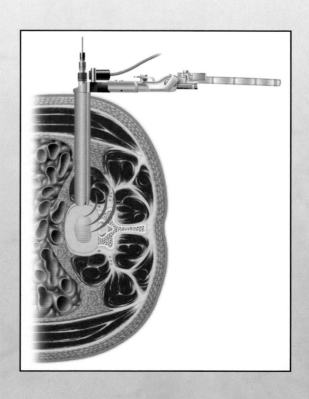

PART II

Surgical Techniques and Clinical Applications

8

Surgical Technique: eXtreme Lateral Interbody Fusion

Luiz Pimenta ▪ Thomas D. Schaffa

Attention to detail and accurate surgical technique are of the utmost importance for surgeons learning the extreme lateral interbody fusion (XLIF®, NuVasive®, Inc., San Diego, CA) surgical procedure. The XLIF procedure can be broken down into five key steps, which, if adhered to meticulously, produce safe and reproducible results (Box 8-1). By following the guidelines in this chapter, we have had continued success with lateral access surgery for many patients and for multiple surgical indications. Indications include any pathology requiring anterior column stabilization in the thoracolumbar spine above L5. Relative contraindications include pathologies at the L5-S1 level (because of limitations of access around the iliac crest) and high-grade spondylolisthesis (≥grade 3). Prior retroperitoneal surgery need not preclude secondary access via XLIF, although caution is required when approaching the upper lumbar levels in patients who have undergone bilateral renal surgery. In this chapter, we focus on the steps of the technique, with particular attention to the nuances that contribute to a successful outcome.

BOX 8-1   Five Key Steps for Performing the XLIF Procedure

---

1. Appropriate patient positioning
2. Retroperitoneal access
3. Transpsoas access
4. Disc space preparation
5. Implant insertion

SURGICAL CONSIDERATIONS

The XLIF procedure allows access to the spine via a direct lateral retroperitoneal approach. The anatomic landmarks the surgeon should consider when preparing for this technique include the iliac crest, the twelfth rib, and the lateral border of the erector spinae muscles. Two small incisions are made during this procedure. The first incision, located near the lateral border of the erector spinae muscles, is used to access the retroperitoneal space and safely guide the initial NeuroVision® Dilator (NuVasive, Inc.) to the psoas muscle. The second incision, located in a direct lateral position, is used to place the Dilators and Retractor and provides disc space access. This two-incision technique was specifically developed to offer simple and efficient access to the spine and to minimize the potential for peritoneal injury. If cosmesis is a concern, an advanced technique using a single skin incision with two fascial incisions can be used to the same effect.

To successfully complete the XLIF technique, the following equipment is required:
- Radiolucent, bendable surgical table
- C-arm
- Light source
- MaXcess® III Access System (NuVasive, Inc.)
- MaXcess Articulating Arm
- MaXcess Disposable Kit
- XLIF Instruments
- Anterior/lateral general instruments
- NeuroVision® JJB System
- NeuroVision XLIF Disposable Module

STEP ONE: PATIENT POSITIONING AND OPERATING ROOM SETUP

The patient is placed on a bendable surgical table in a direct lateral decubitus position, with the greater trochanter directly over the table break. A true lateral (90-degree) position is critical to the safety and reproducibility of lateral access surgery. In a lateral decubitus position the abdominal contents fall forward, away from the approach to the disc space. This simplifies the approach in even the heaviest patients. A true lateral position allows the surgeon to work directly perpendicular to the floor to ensure a safe trajectory across the disc space and to avoid anterior or posterior structures. After initial positioning, the patient is secured with tape (Fig. 8-1).

This configuration ensures that the pelvis tilts away from the spine, allowing access to all lumbar levels, particularly L4-5.

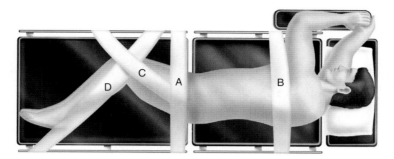

FIG. 8-1   The patient is positioned in a direct lateral decubitus position and secured with tape just below the iliac crest *(A)*, over the thoracic region *(B)*, from the iliac crest to the knee and to the table *(C)*, and from the table to the knee, past the ankle, and to the table *(D)*.

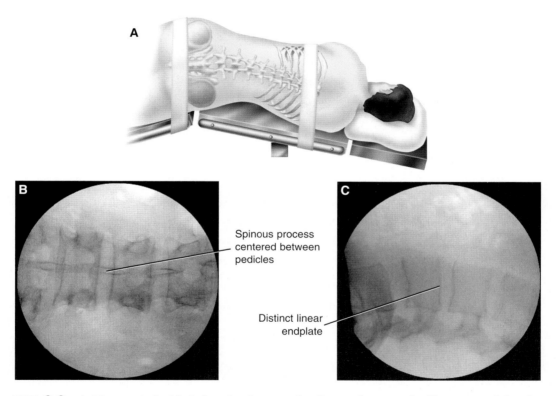

Spinous process
centered between
pedicles

Distinct linear
endplate

FIG. 8-2   **A,** The surgical table is flexed to increase the distance between the iliac crest and the ribs to gain direct access to the disc. **B** and **C,** True anteroposterior and true lateral fluoroscopic images confirm patient positioning.

Using fluoroscopy to verify the location, the surgical table should be flexed to increase the distance between the iliac crest and the ribs and to allow direct access to the disc (Fig. 8-2, *A*). Once the patient has been secured with tape, the table can be adjusted so that the C-arm provides true anteroposterior and true lateral images (Fig. 8-2, *B* and *C*). The table should be readjusted as the surgeon accesses each level to maintain this relationship, particularly in cases of rotational deformity. Careful attention to imaging ensures that the patient is in a

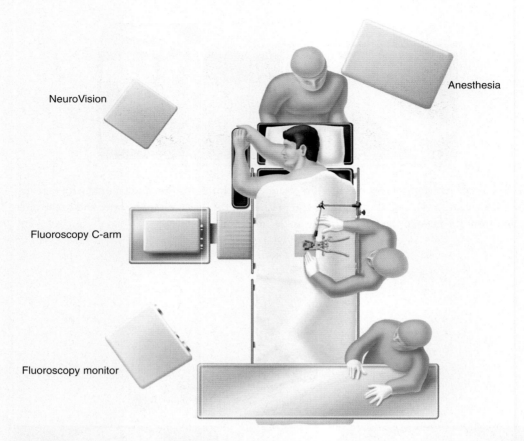

FIG. 8-3   Operating room setup, with the fluoroscopy monitor and the NeuroVision Control Unit placed opposite the surgeon for an unobstructed view.

true lateral position, which is achieved by rotating the table rather than the C-arm. The NeuroVision Control Unit should be placed opposite the surgeon to provide an unobstructed view (Fig. 8-3).

ANATOMIC LANDMARK IDENTIFICATION AND INITIAL INCISIONS

After preparing the patient aseptically, the disc space is localized using lateral fluoroscopy. This is accomplished by crossing two K-Wires over the pathologic level and centering them over the indicated disc space (Fig. 8-4, *A* and *B*). A mark on the skin is made at the intersection of the K-Wires to serve as the location of the skin incision for the operative corridor. Another mark is made on the skin at a posterolateral location, approximately midway between the ilium and the rib cage. Typically, this mark is a finger length's distance from the lateral incision and just lateral to the erector spinae muscles (Fig. 8-4, *C*). The retroperitoneal space is accessed through this incision with blunt scissors and finger dissection.

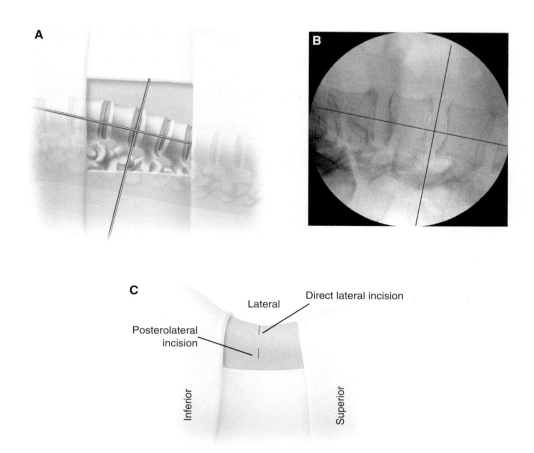

FIG. 8-4 **A** and **B,** Using lateral fluoroscopy, the disc space is localized by crossing two K-Wires over the pathologic level and centering them over the indicated disc space. **C,** A mark on the skin is made at the intersection of the K-Wires to serve as the location of the skin incision for the operative corridor (direct lateral incision). Another mark is made between the ilium and the rib cage (posterolateral incision), indicating the access to the retroperitoneal space.

STEP TWO: RETROPERITONEAL ACCESS

Through the posterolateral incision, the subcutaneous tissue layers are dissected using alternating blunt scissors and finger dissection (Fig. 8-5, *A*). The blunt scissors are used to carefully spread the muscle fibers, and subsequent finger advancement allows the surgeon to determine whether resistance by the muscle tissue is present. Typically, a loss of resistance by the muscle tissue indicates that the retroperitoneal space has been reached. Care should be taken to avoid abrupt advancement, which could cause perforation of the peritoneum. Once the index finger is inside the retroperitoneal space, a gentle sweeping motion is used to release the peritoneum anteriorly and to ensure that the abdominal contents have

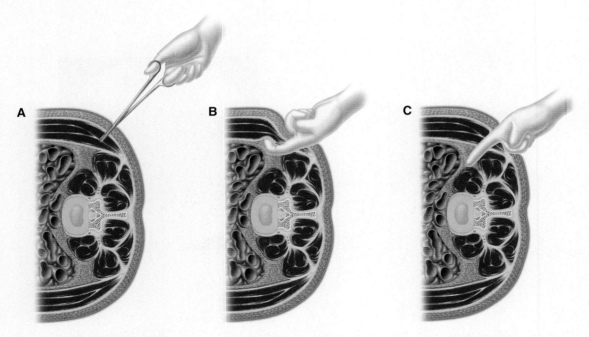

FIG. 8-5 **A,** The subcutaneous tissue layers are dissected using blunt scissors and alternating them with finger dissection. **B,** Using a gentle sweeping motion, the index finger releases the peritoneum anteriorly and ensures that the abdominal contents have fallen forward. **C,** After the peritoneum is released, the finger palpates the psoas muscle, or anterior tip of the transverse process, for landmark identification.

fallen forward, creating a safe space through which the Dilators and Retractor will pass (Fig. 8-5, *B*). When the peritoneum is released, the finger is used to palpate the psoas muscle or anterior tip of the transverse process (Fig. 8-5, *C*) for landmark identification.

POSTEROLATERAL INCISION

Once the psoas muscle is located through the posterolateral incision, the index finger is swept up to the inside abdominal wall, underneath the direct lateral skin mark (Fig. 8-6, *A*). This step ensures that a safe pathway is present between the abdominal wall and the psoas muscle. An incision is made at this location (Fig. 8-6, *B*), and the initial NeuroVision Dilator (black) is introduced (Fig. 8-6, *C*). The Dilator is passed through the oblique muscle layers to meet the index finger that is just inside the retroperitoneal space. This finger is used to guide the initial Dilator safely past the peritoneum, down to the surface of the psoas muscle (Fig. 8-6, *D*).

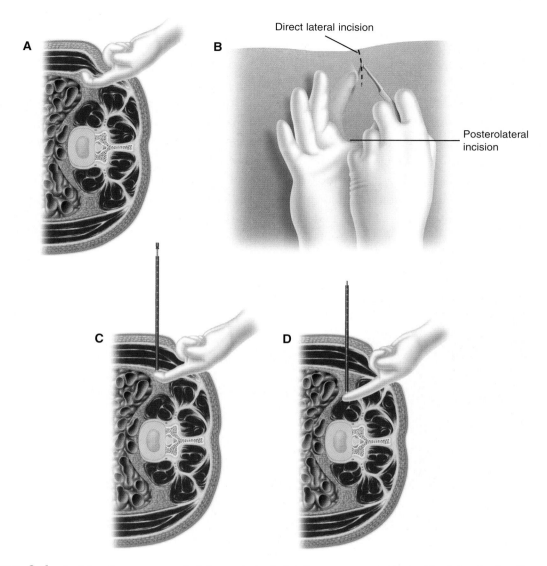

FIG. 8-6 **A,** After the psoas muscle is located, the index finger sweeps to the inside abdominal wall underneath the direct lateral skin mark to ensure a safe pathway between the abdominal wall and the psoas muscle. **B,** An incision is made at this location. **C,** The initial NeuroVision Dilator (black) is introduced and meets the index finger just inside the retroperitoneal space. **D,** The finger guides the Dilator to the surface of the psoas muscle.

STEP THREE: TRANSPSOAS APPROACH

When the NeuroVision Dilator contacts the surface of the psoas muscle, the location is verified with a lateral fluoroscopic image. The ideal location is approximately at the center (or just posterior to the center) of the disc space (Fig. 8-7). NeuroVision EMG stimulation is connected to the Dilator. The Large NeuroVision Dynamic Stimulation Clip is attached to the proximal end of the initial Dilator, and the system is activated in Detection mode (Fig. 8-8, *A* and *B*). The fibers of the psoas muscle are split using blunt dissection with the initial

Dilator, which is slowly advanced while NeuroVision remains active in the Detection mode (Fig. 8-8, *C*). As the Dilator is advanced through the psoas, NeuroVision's dynamically stimulated discrete EMG guidance is used to identify and avoid the nerves of the lumbar plexus (Fig. 8-8, *D*). A direct lateral trajectory, targeting approximately the middle of the disc, minimizes the chance of encountering a nerve and ensures that the anterior vessels remain well anterior to the access corridor. If the Dilator approaches too close to a nerve, it is slowly rotated 360 degrees to determine the location of the nerve. A line on the proximal end of the Dilator corresponds to an electrode on the side of the distal tip. NeuroVision indicates a higher stimulation threshold value when the electrode faces away from the nerve. In this case, the Dilator is removed from the psoas, moved slightly in this direction, and a new path through the psoas muscle is attempted (see Fig. 8-7). The NeuroVision Twitch Test is used to determine the level of muscle relaxants in the patient (Fig. 8-8, *E*).

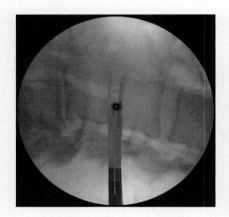

FIG. 8-7   After the initial NeuroVision Dilator reaches the surface of the psoas muscle, the location is verified with a lateral fluoroscopic image. The ideal location is approximately at the center (or just posterior to the center) of the disc space.

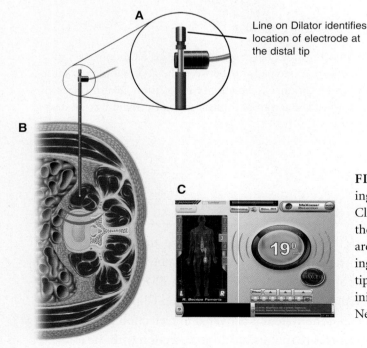

FIG. 8-8   NeuroVision EMG Monitoring. **A,** The Large Dynamic Stimulation Clip is attached to the proximal end of the NeuroVision Dilator. **B,** The Dilators are insulated to minimize current shunting, and an isolated electrode at the distal tip acts as the stimulation source. **C,** The initial Dilator is slowly advanced while NeuroVision is active in Detection mode.

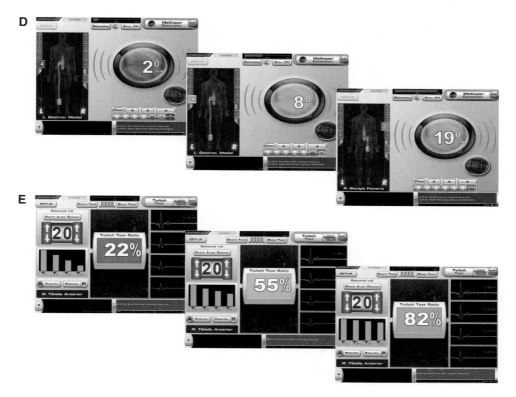

FIG. 8-8, cont'd **D,** The descending nerves of the lumbar plexus tend to lie in the posterior one third of the psoas muscle. The NeuroVision System assists with safe passage past these nerves and/or confirmation of their posterior location via evoked EMG monitoring. In Detection mode, the NeuroVision System continuously searches for the stimulus threshold that elicits an EMG response on the myotomes being monitored and audibly and visually reports the thresholds. As the Dilator is advanced through the psoas muscle, the stimulus necessary to elicit an EMG response varies with the distance from the nerve. For example, as the stimulus source moves closer to the nerve, less stimulus intensity is required to elicit a response, resulting in a lower threshold, which provides an indication of the relative proximity of the Dilator to the nerves. Literature reports suggest that stimulation thresholds of less than 5 mA may indicate direct nerve stimulation,[1-3] and other experience has suggested that threshold values greater than 10 mA indicate a distance that allows both continued nerve safety and ample working space.[4] **E,** The Twitch Test can be performed either in peripheral stimulation mode (the stimulation is directed through an electrode at the popliteal fossa) or direct stimulation mode (the stimulation is directed through instruments in the surgical wound). The system stimulates with four pulses and displays the results of each twitch as a percentage of the first one. A fourth twitch with at least 75% of the strength of the first is required to ensure accurately quantifiable EMG readings.

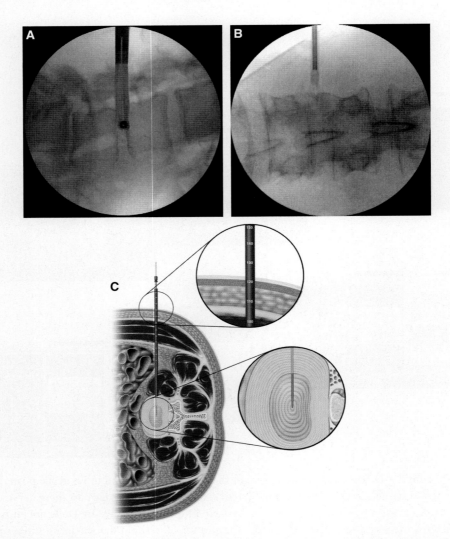

FIG. 8-9 **A,** After the initial Dilator is on the disc, a lateral radiograph confirms that the Dilator is approximately centered on, and parallel with, the disc. **B,** A cross-table anteroposterior image confirms that the Dilator is in the plane of, and flush with, the disc space. **C,** A K-Wire is introduced about halfway into the disc space to secure the position.

Once the initial Dilator is on the disc, fluoroscopy is used to confirm its position. A lateral image should confirm that the Dilator is approximately centered on and parallel with the disc (Fig. 8-9, *A*). If the Dilator is not at the optimal position, NeuroVision's Detection mode may be reactivated and the Dilator's position adjusted. A cross-table anteroposterior image should confirm that the Dilator is in the plane of and flush with the disc space (Fig. 8-9, *B*). After confirming the position, a K-Wire is introduced approximately halfway into the disc space to secure the position (Fig. 8-9, *C*). Subsequent dilation and muscle-splitting retraction are used to establish the operative corridor. Depth markings on the Dilator indi-

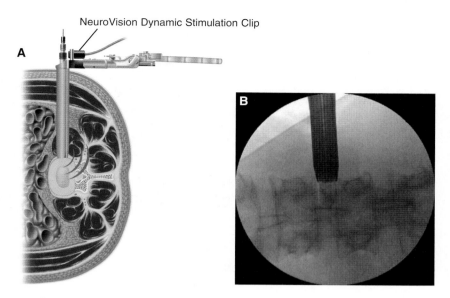

FIG. 8-10   A, The NeuroVision Dynamic Stimulation Clip is attached to the post on top of the center Blade to stimulate an electrode on the distal end of the Blade. **B,** A cross-table anteroposterior fluoroscopic image is used to confirm the correct position of the Access Driver Blades on the spine and to ensure that the Blades are parallel with the disc space.

cate the appropriate length of the Blade to be loaded onto to the MaXcess Access Driver. The Blades are tightened via set screws.

The next two NeuroVision Dilators (magenta and blue) are subsequently introduced over the initial Dilator using a twisting motion. As with the previous Dilator, NeuroVision's dynamically stimulated EMG guidance is used to minimize potential nerve contact. The Access Driver is introduced over the third Dilator, with the handles pointing posteriorly. The NeuroVision Dynamic Stimulation Clip may be attached to the post on top of the center Blade to stimulate an electrode on the distal end of the Blade (Fig. 8-10, *A*). Cross-table anteroposterior fluoroscopy is used to confirm that the position of the Access Driver Blades on the spine is correct and that the Blades are parallel with the disc space (Fig. 8-10, *B*).

The MaXcess Retractor is stabilized to the table by attaching an Articulating Arm from the bedrail to the Access Driver (Fig. 8-11, *A*). The Access Driver allows two different points of attachment: (1) attachment on the center Blade, which ensures that the exposure opens only anteriorly from that position, avoiding pressure on the nerves posterior to the center Blade and (2) attachment closer to the handles of the Retractor, which results in the center Blade moving posteriorly when opened and having more posterior exposure. However, in this scenario, extra care must be taken to avoid compression of neural elements against the transverse processes behind the center Blade.

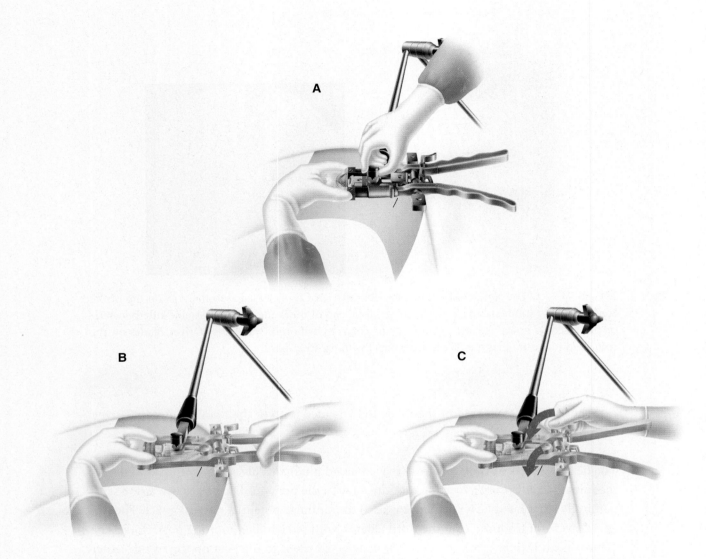

FIG. 8-11   A, The MaXcess Retractor is stabilized to the table by attaching an Articulating Arm from the bedrail to the Access Driver. **B,** The Retractor is gently opened by squeezing the handles on the Access Driver until the Blades are expanded in a superior/inferior direction by approximately three "clicks." **C,** Anterior/posterior exposure is achieved by turning the knobs on the sides of the Access Driver forward.

While holding the Access Driver in position and using downward pressure, the Retractor is gently opened by squeezing the handles on the Access Driver so that the Blades are expanded approximately three "clicks" in a superior/inferior direction (Fig. 8-11, *B*). Anterior/posterior exposure is achieved by turning the knobs on the sides of the Access Driver forward (Fig. 8-11, *C*).

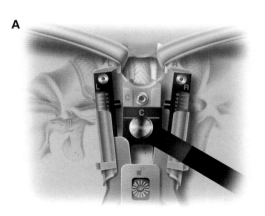
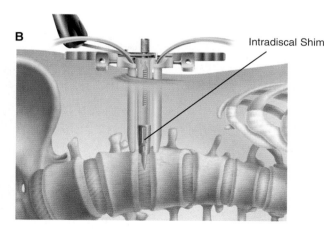

Intradiscal Shim

FIG. 8-12   A, Direct, illuminated visualization is achieved by passing the two ends of the bifurcated Light Cable about halfway down the left and right Blades of the Access Driver. The two ends of the Light Cable are bent flush to the surface of the Access Driver. **B,** An Intradiscal Shim may be placed into the disc space to further stabilize the Retractor to the patient.

Direct, illuminated visualization is achieved by passing the two ends of the bifurcated Light Cable about halfway down the left and right Blades of the Access Driver. The two ends of the Light Cable are bent flush to the surface of the Access Driver (Fig. 8-12, *A*). The proper anterior/posterior position should be verified using lateral fluoroscopy. Any residual tissue at the bottom of the exposure should be thoroughly explored. The NeuroVision Pedicle Probe is used to confirm that nerves are not within the exposure. Shims are available in various sizes to either effectively widen or lengthen the Blades to keep tissue out of the exposure. An Intradiscal Shim may be placed into the disc space to further stabilize the Retractor to the patient (Fig. 8-12, *B*).

The XLIF instrument set contains tools such as Penfields, Nerve Retractors, and Psoas Retractors, which can be used to tuck residual tissue behind the Shims. If electrocautery is necessary for further visualization of the disc, bipolar—not monopolar—cautery should be used sparingly to avoid thermal injury to the nearby nerves and unnecessary trauma to the psoas muscle.

The distal part of the exposure can be widened without enlarging the skin incision by rotating either one or both of the Blades using the Blade Rotation Wrenches or Blade Rotation Spreader. This may be helpful to preferentially adjust the exposure in either direction (for example, inferiorly at L4-5 under the iliac crest) to gain optimal access to the disc space, but care should be taken to avoid expanding the Blades to the midvertebral body to minimize psoas trauma and the risk of segmental vessel injury. Exposure need only be as wide as the disc space. Blade rotation locks automatically slide toward the Blades on the left and right arm of the Access Driver to secure the Blades' position.

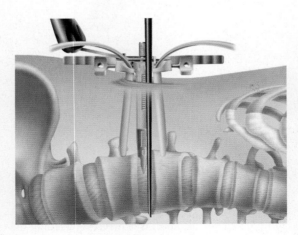

FIG. 8-13   Contralateral anular release is performed by passing the Cobb Elevator along both endplates and completely through the contralateral anulus.

STEP FOUR: DISC SPACE PREPARATION

With the operative corridor in place and disc exposure achieved, the disc space can be prepared in a conventional manner using intradiscal instruments, such as the Rongeurs, Curettes, and Rasps found in the XLIF instrument set. The anulotomy must be at least 18 mm long (anterior to posterior) to accommodate the XLIF implant. A number of XLIF instruments can be used to measure this space and thoroughly evacuate the disc and to prepare the endplates for fusion. Contralateral anular release is critical to the parallel distraction of the disc space and proper coronal alignment. This release can safely be performed by passing the Cobb Elevator along both endplates and completely through the contralateral anulus (Fig. 8-13). The contralateral anular release ensures symmetrical disc space preparation, parallel disc distraction, and the ability to place a large implant on the dense ring apophysis bilaterally.

STEP FIVE: IMPLANT SIZING AND PLACEMENT

One of the biggest advantages of a lateral approach to the spine is the ability to place a large implant that makes use of the densest areas of endplate support. For this reason, the implant length should allow the lateral margins of the implant to span the ring apophysis, aligning with the lateral borders of the endplate on an anteroposterior image. The implant height should allow adequate disc height restoration without excessive strain on the endplates or anterior longitudinal ligament. Sagittal alignment can be restored through the anterior

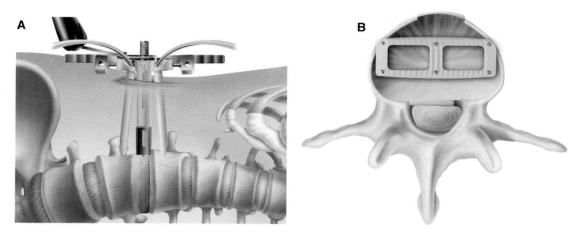

FIG. 8-14 **A** and **B,** The implant is ideally centered across the disc space from a medial/lateral perspective and placed between the anterior third and middle third of the disc space from an anterior/posterior perspective.

placement of a nonlordotic implant or through a more central placement of a 10-degree lordotic implant. Indirect decompression can be expected from corrections in the disc height, sagittal and coronal alignment, and anterior and lateral listheses.

The XLIF Distractor and Sizers are used to distract the disc space and to gauge the appropriately sized Trial, which is gently impacted into the disc space under anteroposterior fluoroscopy until it is centered. The proper anterior/posterior position should be verified using lateral fluoroscopy. The corresponding implant, filled with graft material, is gently impacted into the disc space under anteroposterior fluoroscopy and NeuroVision Free-Run EMG monitoring. Ideally, the implant is centered across the disc space from a medial/lateral perspective (Fig. 8-14, *A*) and placed between the anterior third and middle third of the disc space from an anterior/posterior perspective (Fig. 8-14, *B*).

LATERAL PLATING: XLP™

Supplemental instrumentation may include lateral or posterior fixation systems. If lateral plating (XLP, NuVasive, Inc.) is chosen, the pilot hole is prepared and the Bolt is inserted through XLP Guides (NuVasive, Inc.). A Guide of the appropriate length is introduced through the XLIF exposure and centered over the disc space. With the Guide properly positioned, the spikes are inserted into both vertebral bodies to secure them in place. Several instruments are available in the XLP set to create pilot holes, including Taps, Drills, and Awls. The selected instruments are inserted through the XLP Guide, and a pilot hole is created to the desired depth and trajectory (Fig. 8-15, *A*).

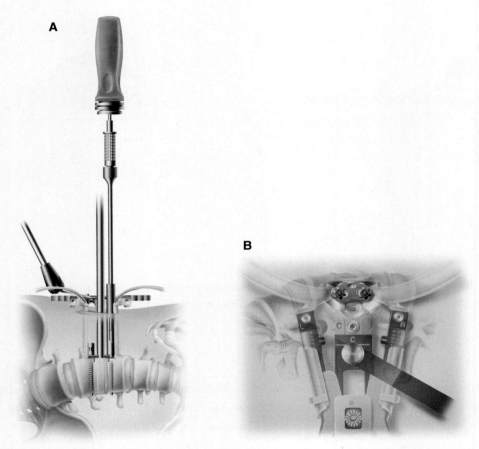

FIG. 8-15 **A,** A pilot hole is created to the desired depth and trajectory. **B,** The Plate is fully seated, and Lock Nuts are inserted onto both Bolts and tightened.

After the pilot hole is prepared, a Bolt is introduced through the Guide barrel and inserted to depth. The Bolt insertion procedure is repeated on the adjacent level. With the Bolts in place, the Plate is inserted over both Bolts, ensuring that the heads are properly exposed above the Plate for Lock Nut insertion. The Plate is confirmed to be fully seated by direct visualization, and Lock Nuts are inserted onto both Bolts and tightened (Fig. 8-15, *B*).

CLOSURE

After the procedure is completed, the Access Driver is removed, and direct visualization is used to verify the absence of significant bleeding in the disc space or psoas muscle. The skin is closed using standard subcuticular suture. Supplemental posterior instrumentation is added as warranted.

POSTOPERATIVE MANAGEMENT AND EXPECTATIONS

Patients should be encouraged to walk within hours of the surgery to aid their recovery and muscle function. Postoperative pain from the lateral incision tends to be minimal, and, depending on the supplemental procedures performed and any preexisting comorbidities, patients may be discharged after only an overnight hospital stay.

Postoperative tenderness with hip flexion on the operative side is common and resolves spontaneously within the first 2 weeks after surgery as the psoas muscle heals. Less commonly, sensory disturbances in the operative side leg may occur; these can also be expected to resolve within the first weeks after surgery. Painful dysesthesias are rare, and most cases resolve within 6 weeks. Motor disturbances in the operative side leg are exceedingly rare, but possible. In these situations, it is recommended to obtain a postoperative CT scan to rule out a psoas hematoma. If a hematoma is found, draining it improves symptoms. Continued mobilization, physical therapy, and treatment with gabapentin (Neurontin), pregabalin (Lyrica), levetiracetam (Keppra), or other anticonvulsant/nerve stabilizing agents are recommended. To date, there have been no known cases of permanent motor deficit.

All of these side effects can be minimized through gentle muscle manipulation and care during the approach, with the stringent use of EMG guidance and careful nerve retraction when necessary.

Technical Tips

- Placing the patient in a true lateral position is critical to the safety and reproducibility of lateral access surgery. The time spent properly positioning the patient facilitates the ease with which the procedure then proceeds.
- Careful attention to properly positioning the patient over the break in the table and flexing the table ensures access to the L4-5 disc space in all cases by moving the pelvis away from the spine.
- Finger dissection and guidance of the initial Dilator through the retroperitoneal space adds safety and reproducibility by preventing visceral injury.
- Dynamic EMG stimulation with discrete threshold monitoring allows the directional identification of nerves and their avoidance during the transpsoas approach.
- Disc space preparation must include the contralateral release of the anulus to ensure parallel distraction, the placement of a large implant across the ring apophysis, and alignment correction.

REFERENCES

1. Calancie B, Madsen P, Lebwohl N. Stimulus-evoked EMG monitoring during transpedicular lumbosacral spine instrumentation: initial clinical results. Spine 19:2780-2786, 1994.
2. Holland NR, Lukaczyk TA, Riley LH, et al. Higher electrical stimulus intensities are required to activate chronically compressed nerve roots. Spine 23:224-227, 1998.
3. Maguire J, Wallace S, Madiga R, et al. Evaluation of intrapedicular screw position using intraoperative evoked electromyography. Spine 20:1068-1074, 1995.
4. Peloza J. Validation of neurophysiological monitoring of posterolateral approach to the spine via discogram procedure. Poster presented at the Ninth International Meeting on Advanced Spine Techniques, Montreux, Switzerland, May 2002.

9

Safety of XLIF® Afforded by Automated Neurophysiology Monitoring With NeuroVision®

W. Blake Rodgers ▪ G. Bryan Cornwall
Kelli M. Howell ▪ Bernard Allan Cohen

The innovative spinal surgery technique of extreme lateral interbody fusion, or XLIF, (NuVasive®, Inc., San Diego, CA) is a novel, minimally disruptive spine procedure that is directed laterally, or 90 degrees, off midline. The technique is described in more detail in Chapter 8. This chapter focuses on the safety of the procedure. XLIF provides the biomechanical benefit of preserving the anterior and posterior longitudinal ligaments. In addition, a large graft is placed, providing indirect decompression with excellent height restoration.[1-3] Historically, lateral approach surgery is not new[4-9]; however, a lateral approach surgery that is minimally invasive, safe, and reproducible in the hands of many surgeons *is* new. In a recent series by Bergey et al,[4] the authors reported positive results with a lateral approach, but with a significant complication rate. It is important to note that intraoperative neurophysiologic monitoring was not used during the transpsoas approach in that series.

The XLIF technique is unique in that the automated, surgeon-driven neurophysiologic guidance using the NeuroVision JJB System (NuVasive, Inc.) helps to ensure safety by avoiding neural injury. The safety and reproducibility of the XLIF procedure have been replicated in many centers.[1-3,10-13] The evolution of the surgical technique and experience has demonstrated that the following five cardinal principles are essential to making XLIF a safe, simple, and efficacious procedure:

1. Careful patient positioning
2. Gentle retroperitoneal dissection
3. Meticulous psoas traverse using NeuroVision
4. Complete disc removal, with release of the contralateral anulus and preparation of the fusion site
5. Appropriate-sized interbody implant placement

In this chapter, we discuss the third step—meticulous psoas traverse using NeuroVision, an automated neurophysiologic monitoring technology based on stimulated electromyography (EMG). Without reliable neurologic monitoring in real time, the lateral approach is fraught with risk.

BASIC NEUROANATOMY

Intraoperative neurophysiologic monitoring has been a part of spinal reconstruction surgeries since the early 1970s. Some of the earliest spinal cord monitoring in humans was done by Nash et al[14] during surgeries to treat patients with scoliosis and other spinal deformities. They monitored spinal cord function during spinal instrumentation procedures to minimize the chances of postoperative neurologic deficits. This early work evaluated only the sensory pathways by using somatosensory evoked potential (SSEP) monitoring. One clear drawback of this single-modality neurophysiologic monitoring was the likelihood of missing motor abnormalities during the procedure. The desire to monitor both the motor pathways in general and the nerve root–level characteristics led to the development of new neurophysiology monitoring modalities, such as stimulated EMG monitoring[15] and motor evoked potential (MEP) monitoring.[16-17]

TYPES OF INTRAOPERATIVE NEUROMONITORING

Fig. 9-1 presents the four main types of neuromonitoring—EMG, transcranial motor evoked potentials (TcMEPs), SSEPs, and dermatomal somatosensory evoked potentials (DSEPs). These are described as follows:

1. **EMG** assesses nerve root function by recording muscle activity during the surgical procedure. The general process involves locating the specific muscles or myotomes related to the root entry levels involved in the surgical procedure. Recording elicited myotome responses allows real-time assessment of nerve root irritation caused by electrical stimulation or triggered electromyography (trEMG), or mechanical irritation caused by spontaneous, free-run electromyography (SFrEMG). For trEMG, the amount of current required to depolarize the nerve root and elicit the peripherally innervated muscle to contract is recorded. Studies have indicated that direct, triggered stimulation of a healthy nerve root elicits a muscular response at approximately 2 mA.[18,19] One hallmark of trEMG is the ability to track a motor pathway to ensure continuous conduction, thus providing information concerning the integrity of the pathway.

2. **TcMEPs** generally allow tracking of the motor pathways along the anterior columns of the spinal cord to the peripheral muscles as a result of electrical or magnetic stimulation over the motor cortex. Magnetic stimulation is used under certain circumstances in the clinical laboratory, and electrical stimulation is generally used in the surgical environment. Responses can be recorded from the same muscle groupings as those in conjunction with trEMG or SFrEMG.

3. **SSEPs** are recorded from afferent fibers and long tract, dorsal column pathways. The earliest reported cases of surgical monitoring involved SSEPs.[14] Studies of this pathway have been widely reported. However, SSEP monitoring offers no information concerning individual nerve root function, and SSEP data are not a real-time measurement, because there is a delay while the response is averaged.[20]

4. **DSEPs** are methodologically identical to the previously discussed SSEPs, except that the stimulation site, rather than being a peripheral nerve, is a peripheral dermatomal patch on an extremity or other part of the body.[20] The information obtained is a sensory indication of conduction characteristics related to specific dermatomal regions rather than to large mixed nerves, as in SSEP recordings. Although a broad cross section of literature is available on SSEPs, this is not true for dermatomal responses. Generally speaking, dermatomal responses are smaller in amplitude and somewhat more difficult to obtain, particularly in patients who are obese or edematous.

The most appropriate type of monitoring for the XLIF procedure is stimulated EMG monitoring, which provides neurophysiologic information concerning the nerve roots and plexus during the transpsoas approach to the anterolateral lumbar disc.

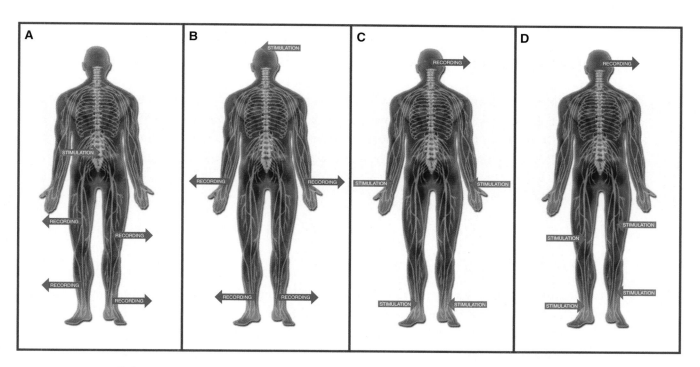

FIG. 9-1 Stimulation and recording for four types of monitoring. **A,** EMG. **B,** TcMEPs. **C,** SSEPs. **D,** DSEPs.

ANATOMIC CONSIDERATIONS

The use of neurophysiologic guidance is particularly important when traversing the psoas muscle to avoid injury to the lumbar plexus and exiting nerve roots. Moro et al[21] conducted an anatomic study to assess the relationship between the position of the lumbar plexus and nerve roots relative to the lumbar vertebral body and the relationship between the genitofemoral nerve and the psoas muscle. In their study, 30 cadavers were examined. Six lumbar spine specimens were analyzed by sectioning the spine from L1 to the sacrum; the positions where the genitofemoral nerve emerged on the abdominal surface of the psoas major muscle were analyzed using the remaining 24 cadavers. Cuts were made parallel to the lumbar disc and then at the cranial third and caudal third of the vertebral body. Analyzing the relationship between the lumbar plexus and nerves involved defining the transverse section view in terms of six zones: zone A was anterior to the anterior margin of the vertebral body, and zone P was posterior to the posterior margin of the vertebral body. The area between the anterior and posterior borders of the vertebral body was divided into four zones: zone 1 was the anteriormost part, and zone 4 was the posteriormost part. For level L2-3 and above, all parts of the lumbar plexus and the nerves were located in the posterior fourth of the vertebral body or more dorsally. For L3-4 and L4-5, the lumbar plexus and the nerves were located in the posterior half of the vertebral body or more dorsally. The genitofemoral nerve was found to descend obliquely forward through the psoas muscle, emerging to its surface between L3 and L4. This anatomic study clearly demonstrates the importance of using neurophysiologic guidance to avoid motor injury when performing a transpsoas approach.

Bergey et al[4] reported on their clinical series, in which they used a lateral approach without neurophysiologic assessment. They reported a 30% complication rate associated with the approach. In contrast, several large reports[10-13] have shown that the XLIF technique is extremely safe when NeuroVision is used to guide the surgeon through a safe path in the psoas muscle.

SAFETY PROVIDED BY AUTOMATED NEUROPHYSIOLOGY

The NeuroVision JJB System provides validated EMG information. In a recent study, Youssef and Salas[22] directly compared the automated NeuroVision system with a conventional system (Axon Epoch XP, Axon Systems, Inc., Hauppauge, NY) for testing pedicle screws. Clinical and numeric agreement between the two systems was high, and the authors commented that the key differentiating feature between the two systems was the manner in which the information was presented to the surgeon, with the automated system providing direct feedback to the surgeon. They concluded: "EMG testing has been shown in other studies to be a useful tool to help identify misplaced pedicle screws. Automated EMG systems may widen the availability of this technology."[22]

In addition, the NeuroVision JJB System provides capabilities that conventional neurophysiologic assessment does not, including a dynamic Detection mode to provide real-time information concerning proximity to nerves. The NeuroVision system uses a patented hunting algorithm that provides 5 pulses per second of increasing amplitude current until the appropriate myotome has responded (Fig. 9-2). Once the maximum current level to elicit a response is achieved, the current output is maintained at that level. The Detection mode uses evoked EMG to test the proximity of neural structures to prevent postoperative radicular irritation or injury from surgical instruments and implanted instrumentation. Obser-

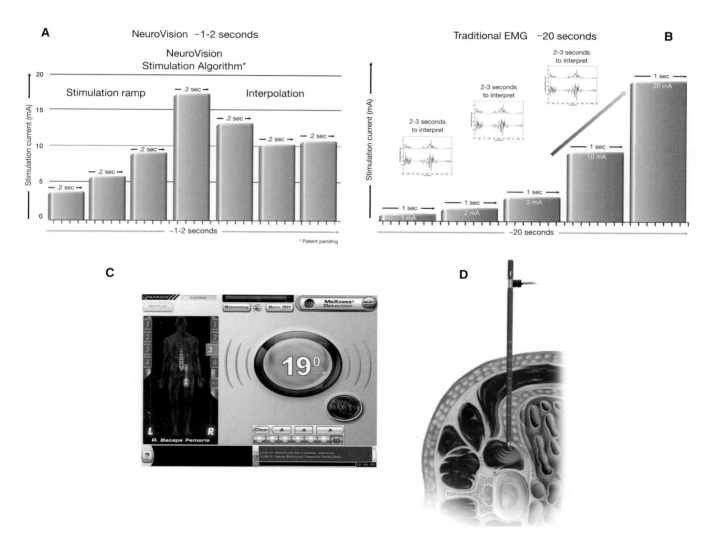

FIG. 9-2 A and **B,** Comparison of the NeuroVision hunting algorithm with traditional EMG monitoring. The NeuroVision system applies stimulation in a nonlinear fashion to quickly (1 to 2 seconds) determine the EMG threshold for nerve roots in proximity of the surgical instrument. Automation of this process allows real-time results to be delivered directly to the surgeon precisely when needed. **C** and **D,** XLIF Nerve Detection. NeuroVision provides directional nerve proximity information, true trajectory of the nerve with directed stimulation values, and safe and reproducible passage through the psoas muscle.

NUMERIC READING	COLOR CORRESPONDENCE		INTERPRETATION
11 mA or Greater	GREEN	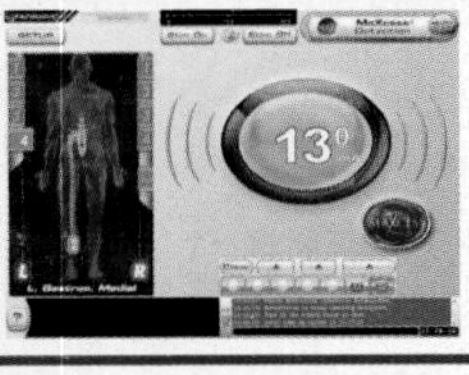	Acceptable
5-10 mA	YELLOW	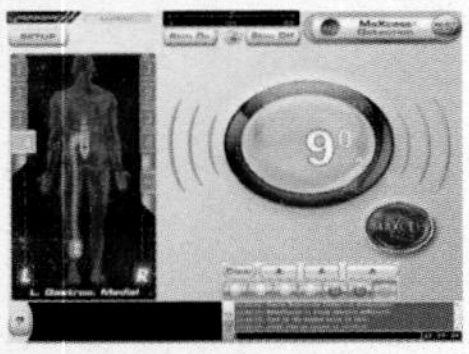	Caution
Less than 5 mA	RED	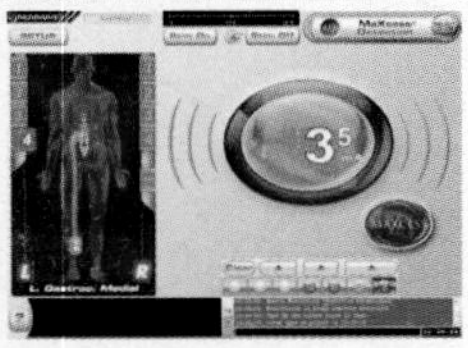	Alert

FIG. 9-3 Interpretation of color-coded results for NeuroVision's Detection mode, which is essential for safe and reproducible passage through the psoas muscle.

vations made from direct nerve stimulation during instrumentation procedures indicate that clinically normal nerves elicit an EMG response under an applied stimulus ranging from 1 to 5 mA, with an average of approximately 2 mA.[18,19] Therefore the closer the proximity of the nerve, the closer the threshold is to 2 mA. Experience with lateral approach procedures has shown that thresholds are divided into the following three groupings (Fig. 9-3):
1. Acceptable (green) thresholds are those greater than 10 mA.
2. Caution (yellow) thresholds are those between 5 and 10 mA.
3. Alert (red) thresholds are those less than 5 mA.

In the Detection mode of the NeuroVision JJB System, the stimulus is applied with the Dynamic Stimulation Clip to the MaXcess® Dilators (NuVasive, Inc.). The Dilators are insulated, except for a triangular-shaped electrode at the distal tip. This tip continuously emits the stimulus while the EMG electrodes are monitored for a myotome response. Insulating the Dilators is important to concentrate the electrical current at the desired location. The closer that tip electrode is to a nerve, the lower the resulting EMG threshold will be. Also, by judiciously rotating the tip of the exposed electrode portion in different directions, the surgeon can determine the general anatomic relationship between the Dilator and the adjacent nerves. With this feedback, the Dilator can be advanced and/or repositioned to avoid nerve contact and to determine proximity.

The NeuroVision JJB System displays the stimulus responses on a color-coded, numeric, graphical user interface, or GUI. The responses are accompanied by an audio feature where-

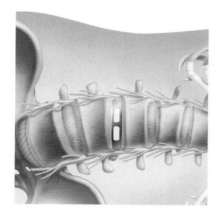 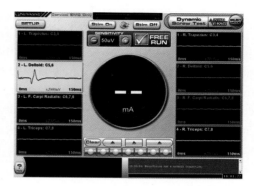

FIG. 9-4 Free-run EMG. Continuous monitoring of multiple spinal nerves warns the surgeon of neurologic insult from mechanical stimuli, such as when the disc space is distracted. NeuroVision provides both visual and audio alerts to free-run activity.

by changes in tone indicate the change in color coding, allowing the surgeon the freedom to focus on the surgical site instead of the screen (see Fig. 9-3). This feature provides near instantaneous feedback in real time and allows neural protection.

In addition to the safety provided by the electrophysiologic monitoring while in the Detection mode, the NeuroVision JJB System can be set to display free-run events, which are typically associated with mechanical stimulation of the cauda equina or exiting nerve roots.[20] Free-run monitoring is especially helpful while restoring disc height, because of the neural stretch that is inherent with height restoration (Fig. 9-4).

METICULOUS PSOAS TRAVERSE USING NEUROVISION

It is impossible to overemphasize the importance of reliable, timely monitoring of the neural elements while the surgeon traverses the psoas. Visual identification of the lumbar plexus is challenging, even with an extensive surgical exposure, and is essentially impossible in any minimally disruptive procedure. Thus it is essential that the plexus be protected by using an automated electrophysiology technology. The NeuroVision System, in Detection mode, provides information concerning the direction of the neural structures, because the stimulating electrode can be oriented to direct the current. By rotating the electrode 360 degrees, different current values corresponding to the recording myotome are displayed, providing information about the spatial orientation of the neural structures. Once the maximum current level required to elicit a response is achieved, the current output stabilizes.

ANESTHESIA REQUIREMENTS

Effective and accurate intraoperative neurophysiologic monitoring requires careful collaboration with the anesthesia personnel. The wide varieties of available anesthetic agents have differing effects on the neuromonitoring modalities. In general, if EMG monitoring is used, all muscle relaxants must be cleared from the patient's system before traversing the psoas muscle. One of the best ways to evaluate the muscle relaxant clearance is the so-called Twitch Test, which is more accurately known as the "train of four" neuromuscular junction transmission testing (Fig. 9-5). This test is used to assess the residual effect of paralytic agents used during intubation by electrically stimulating the temporalis muscle. If such stimulation evokes four muscle twitches in response, the paralytic agents have been cleared from the patient's system and it is safe to proceed.

It is acceptable to use small quantities of rapidly cleared relaxants during intubation, but it is imperative that the patient be tested to ensure that the "train of four" twitches have returned before proceeding. In our experience, psoas traversal begins less than 1 minute after the skin incision is made, thus it is our practice to ask the anesthesia provider to confirm the return of twitches before we incise the skin. No further muscle relaxants are permitted. It is important to emphasize this rule with each anesthesia provider during an XLIF procedure. In addition, TcMEP has been used for XLIF in the thoracic region, and it is important to note that testing for relaxants in the upper body may not be indicative of their effect in the lower limbs.

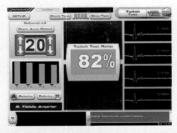

COLOR	RESULT	COMMENT
RED	0%-30%	Little or no muscle response
YELLOW	30%-75%	Marginal muscle response
GREEN	75%-100%	Good muscle response

FIG. 9-5   NeuroVision Twitch Test (also known as the "train of four") provides real-time information about the patient's muscle relaxants with out reliance on anesthesia.

EXPERIENCE WITH NEUROVISION

Since the NeuroVision JJB System was introduced to spine surgeons in 2002, this automated, neurophysiology technology has been used in over 70,000 spine surgery procedures. The applications range from pedicle screw testing to the dynamic monitoring of pedicle screw pilot holes, spinal cord monitoring using TcMEP, and the dynamic monitoring of the transpsoas approach during XLIF.

The records of 903 XLIF surgeries were reviewed to determine how often nerve identification occurred during the lateral approach through the psoas muscle (these records, obtained from cases performed between January and June 2007, contained no patient or other case-related information). The number of times an EMG threshold value fell within an "Alert" range category was documented. The time during which NeuroVision Nerve Detection dynamic-evoked EMG was active was also documented. From these numbers, the frequency of positive nerve proximity feedback was determined (Table 9-1).

Of the 903 cases evaluated, positive nerve proximity (that is, a myotome response was found at a value below the maximum stimulus intensity, usually set at a default of 20 mA) was identified in 758/903 (84%). "Acceptable" responses (green) occurred in 80% of all cases, 60% of all cases had "Caution" responses (yellow), and "Alert" responses (red) were detected in 50% of all cases.

TABLE 9-1   Intraoperative Data from 903 XLIF Surgeries Using the NeuroVision JJB System Monitoring

	Alert Range Category			
	Red	**Yellow**	**Green**	**Any**
	Alert	Caution	Acceptable	
	0.5 to 4.5	5 to 10	11 to 20	
	mA	mA	mA	
Percentage of all cases with nerves detected	49.8%	60.2%	80.4%	83.9%
Average number of detections per surgery	2.76	5.26	17.26	25.28
Average number of detections per hour of monitoring	4.57	6.90	21.60	33.06

SIGNIFICANCE OF FINDINGS

The XLIF approach offers the surgeon a safe pathway through the psoas muscle, because it is performed anterior to the nerves that tend to lie in the posterior third of the muscle.[21] However, it is clear from the values reported in Table 9-1 that nerve proximity during the approach is not only variable—and detectable—in the vast majority of cases (84%), but has been detected at values that should cause at least caution in more than half of the cases (60%). "Caution" responses (yellow) should encourage careful examination during the approach. It is generally recommended, however, that the path of the approach through the psoas muscle be redirected if the responses fall within the "Alert" (red) range, based on the direct nerve-stimulation values of 1 to 5 mA reported in the literature.[19,21,22] The findings from the data presented in Table 9-1 imply that pathway redirection may be necessary in as many as 50% of cases to avoid nerve injury. The low incidence of neural complications attributable to the monitored XLIF approach underscores the safety that NeuroVision Nerve Detection brings to this procedure. It is the only system that can provide real-time neurophysiologic information.

CONCLUSION

The utility of XLIF for multiple indications is becoming increasingly recognized. However, the safety of minimally invasive lateral spine surgery remains a point of discussion. It is incumbent on surgeons to ensure that the procedure is performed proficiently and with a minimal level of risk of neural or visceral injury. By following the five cardinal principles, safe and successful completion of the procedure is ensured. Of the five principles, the reliance on real-time neurologic monitoring has most often been neglected in previously reported series. It is not surprising that blind passage through the psoas results in neural injury. In our own series of more than 250 XLIF procedures using NeuroVision guidance, we have noted only two transient neurapraxias (0.7%).[11] Similar results are seen in other series using NeuroVision monitoring.[1,10,12,13] XLIF is a safe technique when it is carried out properly. NeuroVision neurophysiologic monitoring is a required part of the procedure.

REFERENCES

1. Heim SE, Pimenta L. Surgical anatomy and approaches to the anterior lumbar and lumbosacral spine. In Kim DH, Vaccaro AR, Fessler RG, eds. Spinal Instrumentation: Surgical Techniques. New York: Thieme, 2005, pp 706-711.
2. Ozgur BM, Aryan HE, Pimenta L, et al. Extreme Lateral Interbody Fusion (XLIF): a novel surgical technique for anterior lumbar interbody fusion. Spine J 6:435-443, 2006.
3. Pimenta L, Diaz RC, Guerrero LG. Charité lumbar artificial disc retrieval: use of a lateral minimally invasive technique. Technical note. J Neurosurg Spine 5:556-561, 2006.
4. Bergey DL, Villavicencio AT, Goldstein T, et al. Endoscopic lateral transpsoas approach to the lumbar spine. Spine 29:1681-1688, 2004.

5. Dezawa A, Yamane T, Mikami H, et al. Retroperitoneal laparoscopic lateral approach to the lumbar spine: a new approach, technique, and clinical trial. J Spinal Disord 13:138-143, 2000.

6. Hovorka I, de Peretti F, Damon F, et al. Five years' experience of retroperitoneal lumbar and thoracolumbar surgery. Eur Spine J 9(Suppl 1):S30-S34, 2000.

7. Le Huec JC, Liu M, Skalli W, et al. Lumbar lateral interbody cage with plate augmentation: in vitro biomechanical analysis. Eur Spine J 11:130-136, 2002.

8. Mayer HM. A new microsurgical technique for minimally invasive anterior lumbar interbody fusion. Spine 22:691-700, 1997.

9. McAfee PC, Regan JJ, Geis WP, et al. Minimally invasive anterior retroperitoneal approach to the lumbar spine: emphasis on the lateral BAK. Spine 23:1476-1484, 1998.

10. Diaz RC, Phillips F, Pimenta L, et al. XLIF® for lumbar degenerative scoliosis: outcomes of minimally invasive surgical treatment out to 3 years postoperatively. Spine J 6:75S, 2006.

11. Rodgers WB, Cox CS, Gerber EJ. Experience and early results with a minimally invasive technique for anterior column support through eXtreme Lateral Interbody Fusion (XLIF®). US Musculoskeletal Review 1:28-32, 2007.

12. Smith W. XLIF: one surgeon's interbody fusion technique of choice. Presented at the Ninth Joint Annual Meeting of the American Association of Neurological Surgeons/Congress of Neurological Surgeons, Orlando, FL, Feb 2006.

13. Wright N. XLIF: the United States experience 2003-4. Presented at the Twelfth International Meeting on Advanced Spine Techniques, Banff, Alberta, Canada, July 2005.

14. Nash CL Jr, Lorig RA, Schatzinger RA, et al. Spinal cord monitoring during operative treatment of the spine. Clin Orthop Related Res 126:100-105, 1977.

15. Calancie B, Madsen P, Lebwohl N. Stimulus-evoked EMG monitoring during transpedicular lumbosacral spine instrumentation. Initial clinical results. Spine 19:2780-2786, 1994.

16. Calancie B, Harris W, Broton JG, et al. "Threshold-level" multipulse transcranial electrical stimulation of motor cortex for intraoperative monitoring of spinal motor tracts: description of method and comparison to somatosensory evoked potential monitoring. J Neurosurg 88:457-470, 1998.

17. Calancie B, Harris W, Brindle GF, et al. Threshold-level repetitive transcranial electrical stimulation for intraoperative monitoring of central motor conduction. J Neurosurg 95:161-168, 2001.

18. Holland NR, Lukaczyk TA, Riley LH, et al. Higher electrical stimulus intensities are required to activate chronically compressed nerve roots. Spine 23:224-227, 1998.

19. Maguire J, Wallace S, Madiga R, et al. Evaluation of intrapedicular screw position using intraoperative evoked electromyography. Spine 20:1068-1074, 1995.

20. Devlin VJ, Schwartz DM. Intraoperative neurophysiologic monitoring during spinal surgery. J Am Acad Orthop Surg 15:549-560, 2007.

21. Moro T, Kikuchi S, Konno S, et al. An anatomic study of the lumbar plexus with respect to retroperitoneal endoscopic surgery. Spine 28:423-428, 2003.

22. Youssef JA, Salas VM. Surgeon-interpreted intra-operative electromyography (EMG) versus conventional EMG pedicle screw testing—a prospective comparison. US Musculoskeletal Review 1:37-40, 2007.

10

Potential Complications of eXtreme Lateral Interbody Fusion (XLIF®)

Eli M. Baron ▪ Neel Anand
Alexander R. Vaccaro

Extreme lateral interbody fusion (XLIF, NuVasive®, Inc., San Diego, CA) is a novel, minimally invasive technique for the performance of anterior lumbar interbody fusion (ALIF).[1] Advantages of anterior lumbar interbody over posterior approaches include the potential for a more complete and thorough discectomy, sparing of the posterior elements, and avoidance of scarring adjacent to the neural elements by avoiding entry into the spinal canal.[2-4] Theoretically, interbody fusion also provides a higher fusion rate, because the graft is placed under compression rather than in tension such as following a posterolateral fusion. Anterior interbody fusion also results in greater lordosis than is achievable with posterior surgical methods.[5-8] ALIF, however, is associated with several serious complications, more so than the posterior approach; these include a higher potential for ureteral injury,[9] vascular injury,[10,11] bowel injury, and sexual dysfunction.[11]

Minimally invasive methods have been developed, including mini-open, laparoscopic, and endoscopic techniques.[12-16] These require a significant learning curve, and the potential for the aforementioned serious complications still remains.[1] By using a transpsoas approach, many of the complications of ALIF theoretically may be avoided. Nevertheless, the XLIF approach does not entirely avoid the risk of complications. In this chapter, we review the relevant surgical anatomy—specifically with regard to the potential operative complications that are associated with XLIF—and make recommendations on how to minimize these maloccurrences.

COMPLICATIONS ASSOCIATED WITH ALIF AND POSTERIOR METHODS OF INTERBODY FUSION

XLIF is a novel method of performing conventional anterior column reconstruction; therefore a review of the complications associated with the traditional ALIF approach is useful. Complication rates range from 2.8% to 80% following ALIF.[17,18] Rajaraman et al[11] noted an overall surgical complication rate of 40% associated with the surgical exposure. Vascular injury occurred in 6.6% of patients, and somatic neurologic injury (i.e., injury of the ilioinguinal and/or iliohypogastric nerves) occurred in 5.0% of patients.[11] Vascular injuries have been reported, with a range of 0.5% to 15.6% in patients undergoing the ALIF procedure.[10,17] However, a frequency of 6.66% is more consistent with the literature, especially when one considers the higher rates of injury seen with threaded cage placement.[11] Deep venous thrombosis may also occur in association with ALIF and has been reported at a rate of 7% to 8% following surgery that was adjacent to major pelvic vasculature.[19]

Another serious complication of ALIF is sexual dysfunction. The recorded incidence of sexual dysfunction following ALIF has been reported at 0.42% to 20%.[20-23] Retrograde ejaculation has been reported to occur in 5% to 22% of patients, with partial resolution of the symptoms over 1 to 2 years.[23,24] This is believed to be caused by injury to bilateral sympathetic chains contributing to the superior hypogastric plexus.[11]

Ureteral injury is a less frequently reported serious complication associated with ALIF (0.4%).[17,25] Bowel injury has a reported incidence of 1.6%.[11] Postoperative ileus is more commonly encountered, occurring in 0.6% to 6% of patients undergoing the anterior retroperitoneal approach.[12,26] Lumbar sympathetic dysfunction usually has no long-term sequelae and presents in a variety of ways. Often the leg on the side of surgical approach feels warmer than the other leg. However, there may be dysesthetic pain or a change in limb coloration,[11] which has been reported in 6% of patients postoperatively.[11] Wound dehiscence and hernias may also be a problem following ALIF; these reportedly occur in 0.4% to 3.3% of patients.[11,17]

Complication rates from posterior approaches (posterior and transforaminal lumbar interbody fusion) are generally considerably lower than those of ALIF procedures. Complications associated with posterior approaches include dural tears and postoperative radiculopathy, possibly caused by intracanal scarring. Elias et al[27] reported on a series of 67 patients who underwent posterior lumbar interbody fusion (PLIF). Of these patients, 15% experienced dural tears, and 15% experienced the new onset of postoperative radiculopathy. There were no visceral or vascular injuries. One death was reported in a patient who was morbidly obese. In another study of 33 patients who underwent transforaminal lumbar interbody fusion (TLIF), Houten et al[28] reported that one patient (3%) had severe postoperative radiculopathy. Very low complication rates have been reported in several contemporary series of patients who have undergone TLIF.[5,29-31] Nevertheless, traditional midline approaches to the spine have been associated with muscular damage and dysfunction, which may lead to chronic muscle fatigue and, possibly, failed back syndrome.[32-38]

Villavicencio et al[39] compared patients who had received ALIF and posterior spinal fusion with patients who had TLIF. The total rate of complications was 76.7% for those patients who had anteroposterior reconstruction; 62.8% had major complications, and 13.9% had minor ones. Patients who had transforaminal lumbar interbody fusion had an overall complication rate of 30.1%; 21.9% had minor complications, and 8.2% had major ones.

Hee et al[40] reported surgical results of 164 patients—53 had anterior/posterior fusion, and 111 had TLIF. The overall complication rate was considerably higher in patients who had received anteroposterior fusion (51% and 28%, respectively). The most common perioperative surgical complications in those who had the anteroposterior procedure (excluding screw malposition) were wound infection (11%) and radiculopathy (9%). The most common complications in the TLIF group were radiculopathy (8%), wound infection (8%), and dural tear (5%). Scaduto et al[26] reported a considerably higher complication rate in patients who received PLIF compared with those who had anterior lumbar interbody fusion; this discrepancy can be explained by the aggressive neurologic manipulation that is necessary for PLIF. The relative risk of having a major postoperative complication was 6.8 times higher for the PLIF group than for the ALIF group. Anterior complications included visceral complications (ileus, 6%) and vascular complications (deep venous thrombosis, 2%). In the posterior group, patients experienced neural- and dura-related complications (pseudomeningocele, 16%; epidural hematoma, 3%); these occurred most frequently in patients who had previous posterior lumbar surgery (31% of these patients had major complications).

XLIF: POSSIBLE COMPLICATIONS RELATED TO APPROACH

PATIENT SELECTION

XLIF is a minimally invasive, alternative approach for achieving anterior interbody fusion. Exposure is limited, however, by the superior edge of the iliac crest. Thus for lumbar interbody fusion, XLIF is limited to segments above L5.[1] Additionally, the approach is strictly retroperitoneal, one in which the surgeon's finger "escorts" an initial Dilator to the psoas muscle. Therefore bilateral scarring of the retroperitoneal space is a relative contraindication to XLIF.

NEURAL ANATOMY

Given the transpsoas approach to the disc space, complications may involve the neural structures that are close to this muscle. These structures include the lumbar nerve roots and the lumbosacral plexus, particularly the genitofemoral nerve. The lumbosacral neural plexus forms from the ventral primary rami of the T12-S4 nerve roots and courses through the psoas muscle. The rami enter posteromedially into the psoas and then pass anterolaterally. These fibers often pass very close to the lateral border of the disc space. Anatomic anomalies are seen in the configuration of the lumbosacral plexus as often as 20% of the time.[41] Moro et al[42] studied the configuration of the lumbosacral plexus and genitofemoral nerve in cadavers to assess the theoretical safety of the endoscopic transpsoas approach. They identified the anterior and posterior borders of the vertebral bodies and divided the distance into 4 zones; zone I was located anteriorly, and zone IV was located adjacent to the posterior margin of the vertebral body. They discovered that at L2-3 and above, the lumbar plexus and lumbar nerves were found in zone IV, or posterior to the vertebral body. If the genitofemoral nerve was excluded, however, these results changed; starting at L4-5, the most anterior nerve location was zone III. Thus they concluded that, "if the possibility of damaging the genitofemoral nerve is not considered, the safety zone (for performing an endoscopic transpsoas approach) should be at L4-5 and above."[42]

The genitofemoral nerve typically consists of branches from the L1 and L2 nerve roots, although variations exist with potential contributions from T12-L3.[43] Most commonly, the nerve pierces the psoas muscle and emerges on its surface near the L3-4 vertebral levels.[42] Thus injury to the genitofemoral nerve—with resultant transient postoperative groin paresthesias—has been reported as a complication of the transpsoas approach.[44] Based on the more anterior location of neural structures at L3-4 and L4-5, a neural injury is more likely when performing the transpsoas approach at these levels as opposed to performing the approach at more proximal lumbar segments.

VISCERAL AND VASCULAR ANATOMY

The kidneys and ureter lie anterior to the psoas muscles. The aorta and vena cava lie anterior to the vertebral bodies with the aortic bifurcation, which is typically anterior to the L4-5 disc space; the iliac veins join just below and to the left of this point.[41] Therefore, a transpsoas approach to the disc space is associated with a substantially reduced risk of vascular injury compared with a standard ALIF approach. Nevertheless, vascular injury still may occur, especially if there are vascular anomalies, if instruments are improperly placed, or if the anterior longitudinal ligament is penetrated anteriorly.

OBSERVED COMPLICATIONS

Few studies have reported XLIF outcomes. Nevertheless, safety and feasibility data do exist. Wright[45] reviewed the initial outcomes of the 145 cases of XLIF performed in the United States. No vascular complications or abdominal complications were noted. Five patients (3.4%) had hip flexor weakness, and one patient (0.07%) had a foot drop; these complications resolved. Another patient (0.07%) had transient dermatomal numbness. Other, smaller series have noted no complications.[1,46]

At Cedars-Sinai Medical Center, located in Los Angeles, California, more than 50 XLIF procedures have been performed to date. The incidence of hip flexor weakness in this series has been approximately 10%, with a large percentage of these patients complaining of transient groin pain. This is invariably transient and resolves completely. The majority of patients were able to ambulate by postoperative day 2 or 3. The symptoms described are thought to be related mainly to psoas muscle manipulation and possibly the presence of psoas hematoma. Three cases (6%) of transient quadriceps weakness have also been encountered, and each of these patients has completely recovered within 3 months; two patients recovered within 6 weeks. All three of these patients had XLIF at L4-5. This deficit is thought to be lumbosacral plexus neuropraxia. A single case (2%) of iliac vein injury was noted. No visceral injuries were noted. In accessing the L1-2 disc space, pleural space penetration has occurred with subsequent pneumothorax, caused by the necessary entry through the T11-12 rib space. In some instances, these patients were treated with chest tube management. For other patients, a simple aspiration of the pneumothorax with a syringe/red rubber catheter was performed. A single case of posterior graft malposition with subsequent nerve root irritation occurred; this patient underwent a successful posterior revision.

COMPLICATION AVOIDANCE

The keys to performing XLIF successfully and with minimal complications are careful patient selection, proper positioning, and meticulous surgical technique. Patients are positioned in the lateral decubitus position, with the break of the table at roughly the level of the iliac crest. An axillary roll is used to minimize the risk of axillary nerve neuropraxia.

To prevent lumbosacral plexus injury, intraoperative monitoring is used. This includes both free-run EMG and discrete dynamic triggered EMG using the NeuroVision® JJB EMG monitoring system (NuVasive, Inc.). This system seamlessly couples the stimulation and recording with direct attachment to the access instrumentation to provide real-time nerve proximity measurements, which are critical for avoiding nerve injury during the transpsoas approach.

Fluoroscopy is mandatory for real-time spine viewing. Clear anteroposterior and lateral projections must be obtained before the procedure can be performed. The disc space of interest is marked on the lateral fluoroscopy view. It is important at all times to maintain the fluoroscope at 90 degrees to the patient, while also rotating or tilting the table to obtain a true lateral view of the disc. This helps to maintain a straight, up-down orientation and trajectory of all instruments being passed in and out of the disc. Failure to maintain a strict up-down orientation can result in serious vascular or neurologic injuries caused by inappropriate trajectory. For the direct lateral incision, one may use an oblique incision running parallel to the fibers of the external abdominal oblique musculature. A second posterior incision is used lateral to the border of the erector spinae musculature to introduce a finger bluntly into the retroperitoneal space, open the space, and guide the initial Dilators safely to the surface of the psoas muscle. The NeuroVision system is attached to the initial Dilator that is placed into the lateral incision. As the Dilator is introduced toward the psoas muscle, it is escorted by the surgeon's finger (which is placed through the posterior incision) to ensure the absence of viscera or vasculature in the path to the psoas. This ensures appropriate passage of the Dilators in the retroperitoneal space, and we believe that this is an important aspect of preventing any inadvertent bowel injuries. The location of the Dilator is confirmed with lateral fluoroscopy before the placement of a K-Wire into the disc space. Before the dissection through the psoas musculature with a Penfield dissector, a triggered EMG Probe is used to stimulate the area to identify any traversing neural elements. The Dilator should be placed between the anterior and the middle third of the vertebral body to minimize risk to neural structures, as discussed earlier in this section. Frequent use of fluoroscopy is imperative when placing the Dilators and the MaXcess® Retractor (NuVasive, Inc.).

The NeuroVision system is used with all Dilators that are passed through the psoas muscle (Fig. 10-1). Threshold values greater than 10 mA likely indicate a safe distance from neural structures.[1] Even after the MaXcess Retractors are placed, a nerve may occasionally be seen in the field, despite safe readings from other monitors. If a nerve is seen in the field, it may be gently moved using a Penfield dissector to position it posteriorly behind the MaXcess Retractor Blades. Shims or Retractor Blade extenders may be attached to the Retractor Blades to keep soft tissues from migrating into the path of surgery.

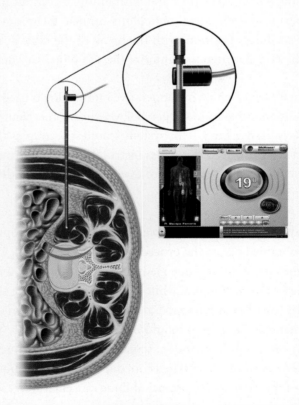

FIG. 10-1 NuVasive NeuroVision JJB EMG monitoring system (NuVasive, Inc.). The system is used intraoperatively to monitor the Dilator's passage and proximity to neural structures, reducing the likelihood of neural injury.

Once the MaXcess Retractors are placed, a lateral fluoroscopic image is obtained to ensure that the Retractor is in the proper AP location. If the Retractor is still anterior, the Retractor arm is loosened and the Retractor itself is repositioned posteriorly. It is critical that the working zone is not too anterior; it should lie between the anterior and the middle third of the lateral disc space. Once the Retractor is opened, the location of the anterior vertebral body is defined. In this manner, the locations of the anterior fibers of the anterior longitudinal ligament are identified. These should not be violated during the discectomy and graft placement; this will help minimize the risks of vascular injury and of anterior graft placement or dislodgment. It is important to continue to reassess the location of the anterior longitudinal ligament during the discectomy procedure (Fig. 10-2).

Before performing the discectomy, the disc space is clearly identified. This is done by gently splitting fibers of the psoas muscle posteriorly and anteriorly as needed using a bayoneted Penfield dissector. Monopolar cautery is avoided at all times. Likewise, bipolar cautery is used only if there is bleeding. Cautery is used sparingly to minimize the risk of neural injury.

The discectomy is performed using a semicircumferential anular release. Controlled passing of a Cobb Elevator is performed across the disc space beyond the contralateral anulus under fluoroscopic guidance. This is done by gently tapping the Cobb across the disc space under fluoroscopic observation. The Cobb is then rotated after it passes through the opposite anulus. In this manner the discal endplate attachment is released. This allows elevation of disc height and attempts deformity correction.

Meticulous care must be taken to avoid endplate violation. Fluoroscopy should be used when spinal instruments such as Curettes, Rasps, and Cobb Elevators are passed into the disc space. Trials are then introduced serially into the disc space, with care taken not to oversize the graft. A long implant that takes advantage of the biomechanical strength of the

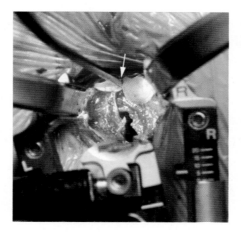

FIG. 10-2   An intraoperative photograph identifying (arrow pointing to Penfield dissector) the anterior longitudinal ligament, taken during a discectomy that was performed during an XLIF procedure. It is very important to assess and reassess the location of this ligamentous structure to avoid entry into the abdomen and potentially avoid vascular injury and/or graft malposition.

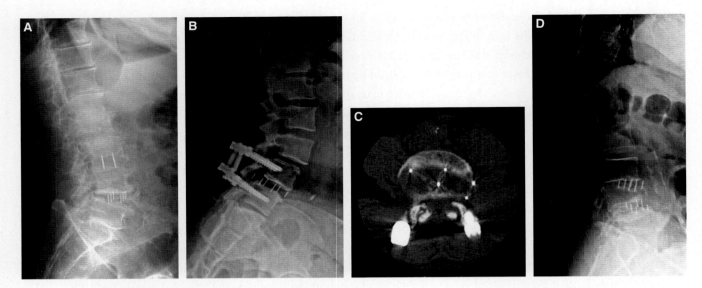

FIG. 10-3   Ideally, grafts should be placed between the anterior and the middle third of vertebral bodies to avoid risk of dislodgement and minimize the risk of neural injury. **A,** Lateral radiograph demonstrating the proper placement of spacers after XLIF. **B,** Lateral radiograph demonstrating a graft that is placed too posteriorly. **C,** Axial computed tomography (CT) image demonstrating the same posteriorly placed graft. **D,** Lateral radiograph showing grafts placed too anteriorly.

dense ring apophysis is recommended. An autologous iliac crest bone graft, or a bone graft replacement such as a bone morphogenetic protein or tricalcium phosphate, may be placed within the spacer before it is implanted into the disc space. The implant should lie at the junction of the middle and anterior thirds of the disc space on lateral fluoroscopy (Fig. 10-3).

CONCLUSION

XLIF is a safe, minimally invasive method of performing interbody fusion above L5. Because it uses the transpsoas approach, it is associated with different complications than is ALIF. Overall, vascular and visceral injuries are less likely to result from XLIF procedures than they are from ALIF procedures. Complications may be minimized by an understanding of the anatomy, vigilant monitoring of the surrounding neurologic structures, a meticulous and thorough discectomy, and appropriate implant placement.

REFERENCES

1. Ozgur BM, Aryan HE, Pimenta L, et al. Extreme Lateral Interbody Fusion (XLIF): A novel surgical technique for anterior lumbar interbody fusion. Spine J 6:435-443, 2006.
2. Enker P, Steffee AD. Interbody fusion and instrumentation. Clin Orthop Relat Res 300:90-101, 1994.

3. Karim A, Mukherjee D, Ankem M, et al. Augmentation of anterior lumbar interbody fusion with anterior pedicle screw fixation: demonstration of novel constructs and evaluation of biomechanical stability in cadaveric specimens. Neurosurgery 58:522-527; discussion 522-527, 2006.

4. Kozak JA, Heilman AE, O'Brien JP. Anterior lumbar fusion options. Technique and graft materials. Clin Orthop Relat Res 300:45-51, 1994.

5. Anand N, Hamilton JF, Perri B, et al. Cantilever TLIF with structural allograft and RhBMP2 for correction and maintenance of segmental sagittal lordosis: long-term clinical, radiographic, and functional outcome. Spine 31:E748-E753, 2006.

6. Christensen FB, Hansen ES, Eiskjaer SP, et al. Circumferential lumbar spinal fusion with Brantigan cage versus posterolateral fusion with titanium Cotrel-Dubousset instrumentation: a prospective, randomized clinical study of 146 patients. Spine 27:2674-2683, 2002.

7. DeBerard MS, Colledge AL, Masters KS, et al. Outcomes of posterolateral versus BAK titanium cage interbody lumbar fusion in injured workers: a retrospective cohort study. J South Orthop Assoc 11:157-166, 2002.

8. Yashiro K, Homma T, Hokari Y, et al. The Steffee variable screw placement system using different methods of bone grafting. Spine 16:1329-1334, 1991.

9. Gumbs AA, Shah RV, Yue JJ, et al. The open anterior paramedian retroperitoneal approach for spine procedures. Arch Surg 140:339-343, 2005.

10. Baker JK, Reardon PR, Reardon MJ, et al. Vascular injury in anterior lumbar surgery. Spine 18:2227-2230, 1993.

11. Rajaraman V, Vingan R, Roth P, et al. Visceral and vascular complications resulting from anterior lumbar interbody fusion. J Neurosurg 91:60-64, 1999.

12. Brau SA. Mini-open approach to the spine for anterior lumbar interbody fusion: description of the procedure, results and complications. Spine J 2:216-223, 2002.

13. Heniford BT, Matthews BD, Lieberman IH. Laparoscopic lumbar interbody spinal fusion. Surg Clin North Am 80:1487-1500, 2000.

14. Inamasu J, Guiot BH. Laparoscopic anterior lumbar interbody fusion: a review of outcome studies. Minim Invasive Neurosurg 48:340-347, 2005.

15. Kaiser MG, Haid RW Jr, Subach BR, et al. Comparison of the mini-open versus laparoscopic approach for anterior lumbar interbody fusion: a retrospective review. Neurosurgery 51:97-103; discussion 103-105, 2002.

16. Thalgott JS, Chin AK, Ameriks JA, et al. Gasless endoscopic anterior lumbar interbody fusion utilizing the B.E.R.G. approach. Surg Endosc 14:546-552, 2000.

17. Sasso RC, Best NM, Mummaneni PV, et al. Analysis of operative complications in a series of 471 anterior lumbar interbody fusion procedures. Spine 30:670-674, 2005.

18. Tiusanen H, Seitsalo S, Osterman K, et al. Anterior interbody lumbar fusion in severe low back pain. Clin Orthop Relat Res 324:153-163, 1996.

19. Farkas JC, Chapuis C, Combe S, et al. A randomised controlled trial of a low-molecular-weight heparin (Enoxaparin) to prevent deep-vein thrombosis in patients undergoing vascular surgery. Eur J Vasc Surg 7:554-560, 1993.

20. Flynn JC, Price CT. Sexual complications of anterior fusion of the lumbar spine. Spine 9:489-492, 1984.

21. Johnson RM, McGuire EJ. Urogenital complications of anterior approaches to the lumbar spine. Clin Orthop Relat Res 154:114-118, 1981.

22. Sasso RC, Burkus JK, LeHuec JC. Retrograde ejaculation after anterior lumbar interbody fusion: transperitoneal versus retroperitoneal exposure. Spine 28:1023-1026, 2003.

23. Tiusanen H, Seitsalo S, Osterman K, et al. Retrograde ejaculation after anterior interbody lumbar fusion. Euro Spine J 4:339-342, 1995.

24. Inoue S, Watanabe T, Hirose A, et al. Anterior discectomy and interbody fusion for lumbar disc herniation. A review of 350 cases. Clin Orthop Relat Res 183:22-31, 1984.

25. Isiklar ZU, Lindsey RW, Coburn M. Ureteral injury after anterior lumbar interbody fusion. A case report. Spine 21:2379-2382, 1996.

26. Scaduto AA, Gamradt SC, Yu WD, et al. Perioperative complications of threaded cylindrical lumbar interbody fusion devices: anterior versus posterior approach. J Spinal Disord Tech 16:502-507, 2003.

27. Elias WJ, Simmons NE, Kaptain GJ, et al. Complications of posterior lumbar interbody fusion when using a titanium threaded cage device. J Neurosurg 93(Suppl 1):S45-S52, 2000.

28. Houten JK, Post NH, Dryer JW, et al. Clinical and radiographically/neuroimaging documented outcome in transforaminal lumbar interbody fusion. Neurosurg Focus 20:E8, 2006.

29. Hackenberg L, Halm H, Bullmann V, et al. Transforaminal lumbar interbody fusion: a safe technique with satisfactory three to five year results. Euro Spine J 14:551-558, 2005.

30. Lowe TG, Tahernia AD, O'Brien MF, et al. Unilateral transforaminal posterior lumbar interbody fusion (TLIF): indications, technique, and 2-year results. J Spinal Disord Tech 15:31-38, 2002.

31. Potter BK, Freedman BA, Verwiebe EG, et al. Transforaminal lumbar interbody fusion: clinical and radiographic results and complications in 100 consecutive patients. J Spinal Disord Tech 18:337-346, 2005.

32. Suwa H, Hanakita J, Ohshita N, et al. Postoperative changes in paraspinal muscle thickness after various lumbar back surgery procedures. Neurol Med Chir (Tokyo) 40:151-154; discussion 154-155, 2000.

33. Gejo R, Matsui H, Kawaguchi Y, et al. Serial changes in trunk muscle performance after posterior lumbar surgery. Spine 24:1023-1028, 1999.

34. Kawaguchi Y, Yabuki S, Styf J, et al. Back muscle injury after posterior lumbar spine surgery. Topographic evaluation of intramuscular pressure and blood flow in the porcine back muscle during surgery. Spine 21:2683-2688, 1996.

35. Kawaguchi Y, Matsui H, Tsuji H. Back muscle injury after posterior lumbar spine surgery. Part 2: histologic and histochemical analyses in humans. Spine 19:2598-2602, 1994.

36. Mayer TG, Vanharanta H, Gatchel RJ, et al. Comparison of CT scan muscle measurements and isokinetic trunk strength in postoperative patients. Spine 14:33-36, 1989.

37. Rantanen J, Hurme M, Falck B, et al. The lumbar multifidus muscle five years after surgery for a lumbar intervertebral disc herniation. Spine 18:568-574, 1993.

38. Sihvonen T, Herno A, Paljärvi L, et al. Local denervation atrophy of paraspinal muscles in postoperative failed back syndrome. Spine 18:575-581, 1993.

39. Villavicencio AT, Burneikiene S, Bulsara KR, et al. Perioperative complications in transforaminal lumbar interbody fusion versus anterior-posterior reconstruction for lumbar disc degeneration and instability. J Spinal Disord Tech 19:92-97, 2006.

40. Hee HT, Castro FP Jr, Majd ME, et al. Anterior/posterior lumbar fusion versus transforaminal lumbar interbody fusion: analysis of complications and predictive factors. J Spinal Disord 14:533-540, 2001.

41. Samudrala S, Khoo LT, Rhim SC, et al. Complications during anterior surgery of the lumbar spine: an anatomically based study and review. Neurosurg Focus 7:e9, 1999.

42. Moro T, Kikuchi S, Konno S, et al. An anatomic study of the lumbar plexus with respect to retroperitoneal endoscopic surgery. Spine 28:423-428; discussion 427-428, 2003.

43. Hollinshead WH, ed. Textbook of Anatomy, 3rd ed. Philadelphia: Harper & Row Publishers, 1974.

44. Bergey DL, Villavicencio AT, Goldstein T, et al. Endoscopic lateral transpsoas approach to the lumbar spine. Spine 29:1681-1688, 2004.

45. Wright N. XLIF—the United States Experience 2003-4. Presented at the Twelfth International Meeting on Advanced Spinal Techniques, Banff, Alberta, Canada, July 2005.

46. Diaz R, Philips F, Pimenta L, et al. XLIF for lumbar degenerative scoliosis: outcomes of minimally invasive surgical treatment out to 3 years post-operatively. Spine J 6:75S, 2006.

11

Clinical Application: Degenerated/Collapsed Disc

Jonathan A. Hyde

Degenerative disc disease is a major source of chronic back pain in the United States, and yet it is one of the most difficult pathologies to manage within the realm of spine surgery. It is a topic that is not only commonly misunderstood, but also misdiagnosed. Many treatments—surgical and nonsurgical alternatives alike—have been described by those attempting to treat this disorder.

Degenerative disc disease is a broad-based term that characterizes most degenerative conditions of the lumbar spine. These conditions include the pathologies most commonly treated—disc prolapse or herniation, spondylolisthesis, degenerative scoliosis, lateral listhesis, and spinal stenosis. When a definitive diagnosis is not readily apparent, a number of descriptive terms such as facet disease, spondylosis, internal disc disruption, black disc disease, vacuum disc disease, and microinstability may be used.

The incidence of low back pain is quite significant, accounting for a large percentage of patient encounters in emergency and primary care settings.[1] In fact, back pain is the most common injury reported within workers' compensation systems. In 1999, the incidence of lower trunk strain or sprain accounted for 10.2% of nonfatal occupational injuries treated in U.S. hospital emergency departments. The annual compensation costs are greater than 5 billion dollars per year, according to data from the 1990s. Worth noting, however, is the fact that more than 90% of patients with acute low back pain have symptoms that resolve within 2 weeks of onset.[2]

As a cause of disability, back pain is the third most common disabling factor, behind heart disease and arthritis. It has been estimated that more than 80% of the U.S. population will experience some form of back pain. The prevalence of active back pain has been estimated to be 18% of the population at any given time.

Back pain is not solely caused by mechanical or neurologic factors. Jarvik et al[3] demonstrated that depression has the highest hazard ratio of any baseline predictor of back pain. Andersson[4] relates that chronic low back pain has become a diagnosis of convenience for many individuals who are disabled for socioeconomic, work-related, or psychological reasons.

Twin studies have been used to ascertain the possible role that genetics plays in the development of low back pain in men.[4,5] The results of exposure-discordant monozygotic and classic twin studies suggest that physical loading specific to occupation and sport has a relatively minor role in disc degeneration.[5] Battie and colleagues,[6] when studying the Finnish Twin Cohort, found a statistically significant genetic correlation for disc height narrowing, duration of the worst pain episode, hospitalizations related to the back, and level of disability within the year previous to the study. The study suggests that disc degeneration is one pathway through which genes influence back pain.

The rates of surgical intervention for lumbar disc disease can vary not only by country, but also by the different regions within each country. Because pain is the primary indication, not functional neurologic deficits, surgery may be substantially driven by factors such as gender, occupation, income, education, and the surgeon's preference.

PATHOPHYSIOLOGY

The development of degenerative disease within the disc has been studied quite extensively, but is still not fully understood. Crock[8] described internal disc disruption as a disabling low back condition caused by alterations within the disc. The changes that occur within the disc parenchyma eventually lead to mechanical and neurologically significant disorders. These changes occur within the nucleus pulposus, as well as the fibrous anular ring.

It is a misconception that disc degeneration is a disease of aging. Degenerative disc disease is instead a spectrum of what apparently is an irreversible, pathologic change to the disc. A cohort study of adolescents with back pain demonstrated a positive correlation between back pain and degenerative disease.[9] Magnetic resonance imaging (MRI) changes were noted to progress in symptomatic adolescents from baseline studies until after the growth spurt.[9]

Yasuma and colleagues[10] demonstrated increased numbers of cartilaginous foci in fissured and ruptured regions of the cartilaginous endplates with age. It is believed that this represents a restorative mechanism.[10] Even with such changes, it was found that degeneration increases with age, with a resultant collapse of the nucleus pulposus and loss of disc height.[10] It has also been believed that the degeneration could be associated with—or could originate from—injury and subsequent repair of the anulus fibrosus. The associated expressions of basic fibroblast growth factor (bFGF), transforming growth factor-beta$_1$ (TGF-β_1), and the associated immunologic response may play a role in this disease process.[11]

According to Adams and Roughley,[12] the process of disc degeneration is an aberrant, cell-mediated response to progressive structural failure. The progression occurs because of the structural failure of the disc—uncoupling of the local mechanical disc cell environment leads to an aberrant disc cell response, which in turn leads to a cascade of cell-mediated responses with further disc disruption.[12] Water is lost from the matrix, and the proteoglycan content changes and diminishes. As cracks and fissures form in the anulus pulposus, the cartilage endplate undergoes thinning, with eventual deformity and sclerosis of the subchondral bone.[13] Disease processes such as herniation with radiculopathy and chronic discogenic pain are associated results from the disc degenerative process.[14]

The natural history of endplate changes was observed over a 3-year period by Kuisma et al.[15] When Modic changes were present, progression to the next level of disease was found in 14% of patients. There was a significant increase in the size of endplate changes in vertebral segments that did not advance by one grade of disease during the follow-up period. These findings suggest that endplate disease may be a progressive—not a stable—radiographic finding.[15]

With resultant degenerative changes of the disc, the biomechanical properties of the spinal motion segment have been shown to be adversely altered. These changes can be correlated with the degree of disease. With grade III and IV degenerative changes, greater segmental motion has been appreciated. As the disease progresses, stabilization eventually occurs, caused by severe disc collapse and the development of osteophytes at the disc margins.[16] When the disc collapses, the neuroforaminal height subsequently is substantially diminished. Morphometric studies performed demonstrated that a disc height loss of only 4 mm was sufficient enough to cause significant foraminal compression, especially with lumbar extension.[17]

The role of supporting ligamentous structure may play a part in the degenerative disc process. In a cadaver study, Aihara and colleagues[18] looked at degeneration above a lumbar transitional vertebra. It was found that the iliolumbar ligament was thinner and weaker than specimens without transitional anatomy. It is believed that instability caused by weak ligamentous support can lead to degenerative changes.[18] This process has been shown to be significantly associated with a higher incidence of herniation and stenosis, especially at the level adjacent to the transitional vertebra.[19,20] These findings could be similar to the development of segmental breakdown above fusions.[21] Conversely, these degenerative changes are also seen in patients who have not had prior spine surgery.[22]

The loss of disc height has also been implicated in the development of instability patterns. Vertical instability has been described in conjunction with conditions such as spondylolisthesis. Disc degeneration produces vertical laxity in both the ligaments and anulus, allowing olisthetic motion in the affected functional spine unit. In turn, the restoration of disc height restores tension to the soft tissues around the disc and results in a spontaneous reduction of the subluxation. Interbody grafting technique was therefore recommended as a treatment for restoring the disc height loss.[23]

Plain radiographic studies may not show significant instability patterns. According to McGregor et al,[24] plain films demonstrated no relationship between spinal motion and the grading of degenerative disease when compared with two different grading systems. MRI studies recently demonstrated the dynamic aspects of disc degenerative processes. The use of the sitting, weight-bearing Fonar MRI has been shown to be superior to recumbent scans to find instability patterns, with the exception of retrolisthesis.[25] Changes in segmental motion without significant changes in lumbar lordosis have been seen on positional MRI between healthy and degenerated discs.[26] Such studies are routinely ordered, occasionally with comparison images, in cases of suspected vertical and sagittal instability.

CLINICAL PRESENTATION

The patient with degenerative disc disease may present with various symptoms, but the most common denominator is a complaint of back pain, often described as a dull ache that tends to act like a band of low back pressure. The symptoms may include radicular complaints that tend to mimic the exiting foraminal nerve of the affected disc space. Occasionally, the patient may complain of hip or groin pain.

Patients may also present with a history of a negative work-up for abdominal or pelvic pain of unknown cause. A vascular work-up may also be indicated, to rule out arterial insufficiency for claudication symptoms. The patient with degenerative disc disease may also present with neurogenic claudication, but with a complaint of back, not radicular, pain.

It is not uncommon for such patients to present with a history of scoliosis or spinal subluxation, with the failure of nonoperative modalities such as chiropractic, physiotherapy, acupuncture, or pain management. They may have undergone procedures such as intradiscal electrothermal therapy or nucleoplasty.[27,28] It is also common for such patients to present with iatrogenic opioid dependence, caused by being told that the ailment causing the chronic pain is inoperable or even without pathology. Behavioral issues such as "learned helplessness" may also be present, which may lead to poor outcomes with or without surgical intervention.[29]

Patients will often relate a specific antecedent event, such as an instance of heavy lifting, or discuss a history of a herniated disc years before. Patients may also complain about pain episodes that originally were infrequent, but now occur on a more regular or continuous basis. The physical examination of such patients is oftentimes relatively normal; a motor function examination rarely shows functional deficits. Femoral and straight-leg raising tests may be indicative of mild muscle tension, without radicular pain production. These patients may show full range of motion, but with crisis pain show severe spasms with limitation. The pain is not reproducible with spinous process or paravertebral point testing. The patients may relate that they feel the symptoms inside the low back, toward the lumbosacral junction, with radiation toward the regions of the bilateral posterior superior iliac spines.

Routine radiograph imaging studies will show space height loss at one or more discs, particularly on lateral plane images. The coronal and sagittal planes may appear normal. Occasionally, all spaces will appear normal, without associated osteophytes or possible instabilities. With more advanced cases, bone-on-bone collapse may be seen. These patients may demonstrate the vacuum disc phenomenon, which may be accentuated by extension imaging.

MRI studies may show various stages of endplate changes, including early-stage disc desiccation. This early desiccation is noted by the loss of T2 signal intensity, a condition known as *the black disc*.[30] The disc may show no significant protrusions or anular tears, but with continued disc collapse one may see a broad-based collapse of the posterior anulus toward the canal or neuroforamina. Herniations, both extrusions and sequestrations, may also occur within the parameters of disc collapse. Large sequestered or extruded herniations may not be addressed, and are not visualized, by use of the extreme lateral transpsoas approach alone.

On both computed tomography (CT) and MRI, visible changes within the endplate regions are consistent with the sclerotic adaptations of advanced disc degeneration. Associated neural canal and lateral recess stenosis may also be verified. In cases of severe facet disease, which causes lateral recess stenosis, the indirect decompression afforded by extreme lateral interbody fusion (XLIF®, NuVasive®, Inc., San Diego, CA) may not fully decompress the anatomic lesion present. In addition, determining the degree of facet disease is especially important for assessing the facet "gapping" that may indicate instability or the possible presence of a synovial cyst.[31] If a symptomatic synovial cyst needs to be excised, a more direct neural canal approach, such as a laminectomy, will also be required.

Fluoroscopic techniques are an extremely important aspect of the work-up for degenerative diseases of the spine.[32] Likewise, transforaminal epidural injections are very useful in the work-up of the pathology. The injection may help therapeutically; more importantly, the technique allows the pathology to be verified diagnostically.[33] In particular, the selective use of these injections for upper lumbar disease has helped diagnose the pain generator for atypical hip and groin symptoms. On occasion, guided facet joint injections are used—mainly for instability syndromes.[34]

Anular tears are associated lesions with degenerative disc changes. Three anular fissure types have been found on cadaveric studies: type 1 with concentric outer tears, type 2 with radial tears, and type 3 with anular insertion tears.[35] MRI may suggest an anular tear, but discography with CT appears to be the best modality for visualization.[36]

The use of discography is a long-disputed radiographic technique used to ascertain an objective source for what is commonly believed to be subjective back pain. The technique is often overused by some as a definitive test to determine the surgical level(s); others use it as a tool to verify pathology.[37] It has been shown that discography is not highly predictive of intradiscal pain-source lesions when compared with unstable spondylolisthesis.[38] My personal use of the technique is to rule out questionable pathologies when determining pain generation on specifically selected patients.[39] I use an unbiased approach to discography by allowing an experienced discographer to perform and interpret the procedure without knowledge of my clinical, working diagnosis. Other surgeons elect to perform the procedures themselves, but clinical and financial biases may potentially affect the results in these circumstances. The eventual interpretation of the data must include pain sensitivity, pain concordance at affected level(s), radiographic interpretation of the discogram (radiograph, and, when available, postdiscogram CT scan), as well as the prediscogram imaging studies and clinical diagnosis.[40,41]

TREATMENT OPTIONS

CONSERVATIVE

The mainstay of nonoperative care for the patient with degenerative disc disease is the use of physiotherapeutic modalities. The majority of patients who present with low back pain secondary to collapsed, degenerative discs respond favorably to an extended course of a back-strengthening program. The modalities usually start with passive techniques, such as massage and myofascial mobilization. Early muscle stretching to hamstring regions may be incorporated at this time, with the exception being patients who have sciatic radicular symptomatology. Active modalities, such as bridging maneuvers and abdominal strengthening, are slowly introduced to build trunk muscle core stabilization. The addition of aerobic training, such as cycling and elliptical machines, allows those patients with previous sedentary lifestyles to build into a long-term home exercise program. I also recommend the use of a walking protocol, starting with a distance of one residential block, then doubling the distance until a daily walking regimen of two miles is accomplished. Chiropractic treatments have been found to be effective for short-term back pain, but no current literature demonstrates efficacy for chronic care.[42,43]

Pharmaceutical agents are used during the treatment period. For the acute onset of pain associated with discogenic disease, I recommend the use of nonsteroidal antiinflammatory drugs (NSAIDs). The use of these medications is associated with risks of bleeding, as well as significant risks of gastritis. Antiulcer medication(s) may be recommended, or formulations combining NSAIDs with such agents may be prescribed. COX-2 formulations, such as celecoxib, are used to minimize gastric symptoms, but may not fully prevent such issues. For more severe cases of acute pain, I recommend a short course of muscle relaxants; such medications often lead to significant drowsiness, so the patients are instructed to avoid activities such as driving or operating heavy equipment while taking the drug. The use of narcotic agents is associated with the risk of dependence issues, but for very severe cases, there may be a role for a short course (1 to 2 weeks) of narcotic medication. The chronic use of opioids is not advised as a treatment for this disorder. Substance use disorders are common in patients taking opioids for back pain, and aberrant medication-taking behaviors occur in up to 24% of cases.[44] Opioids are commonly prescribed by pain management physicians for discogenic disease, but it has been seen that if/when surgery is performed, the patients managed in this fashion tend to require higher peri- and postoperative levels of the narcotic. These patients also tend to have a higher probability of long-term narcotic needs.

For patients who have had poor responses to therapy and oral medications, a trial of epidural steroid injections is recommended. As previously noted, the injections are often given as transforaminal injections, to be more selective to the location of a potential pain generator. When the pain is nonspecific and generally localized to the back, I recommend giving the injection via a translaminar approach. The injections are performed with fluoroscopic guidance, because there is up to a 25.7% rate of inaccurate needle-tip placement with loss of resistance technique.[45]

I do not routinely recommend alternative treatments for discogenic pain, but select studies have shown some beneficial effects in the alternative management of discogenic disease. The role of intradiscal electrothermal therapy (IDET) has been demonstrated to be similar to fusion by Andersson et al,[46] and a statistically significant improvement in pain and function was reported by Saal and Saal.[47] In a prospective nonrandomized study, the role of percutaneous radiofrequency thermocoagulation (nucleoplasty) was shown to be a moderately effective pain-relieving procedure.[48] Conversely, a recent review of the literature has demonstrated that the available evidence does not support the use of radiofrequency thermocoagulation or IDET for discogenic low back pain.[49] The role of vertebral axial decompressive treatments (VAX-D, DRX) has been advertised by the equipment manufacturers and practitioners as effective. Currently, distractive manipulation or traction have not been verified as effective; in fact, there have been reports of progressive lumbar herniation from such treatments.[50-52]

SURGICAL INTERVENTIONS

The use of spine fusion for degenerative disc disease has been found to be a significant help for many patients, with variable results within the literature.[53] The use of posterior in situ fusion with the use of autogenous bone graft was noted to be a procedure that resulted in moderate successes. The surgical approach could be performed through a midline dissection plane with muscle stripping, or through a paramedian approach. The development of posterior pedicle screw instrumentation was noted to increase the fusion rate in the face of lumbar instability.[54] Even with successful posterior fusion, a significant number of patients may continue to suffer from pain generated through micromotion from degenerated collapsed discs.[55]

Interbody graft techniques allow the surgeon to place a structural graft directly within the disc space. The posterior lumbar interbody fusion (PLIF) technique of Cloward allows the surgeon the ability to perform a decompressive laminectomy along with interbody stabilization using a midline approach; this procedure can also be performed using a unilateral transforaminal (TLIF) approach. Interbody space distraction can also be achieved with the use of insert-and-rotate or lordotic-contoured grafts. With the development of tubular and expanding retractor systems, these procedures can be performed using minimally invasive techniques and the pedicle screw hardware can be placed at the same time.[56]

In cases of discogenic disease in which direct decompression is not necessary, it may be decided to use the anterior retroperitoneal approach to place a structural interbody graft. This technique often requires a vascular surgical-approach surgeon, because major blood vessel dissection may be required to safely mobilize these structures. The use of anterior lumbar interbody fusion (ALIF) was found to cause indirect neuroforaminal decompression via the distractive effect of placing the graft.[57] This technique required posterior pedicle-screw or facet-screw instrumentation. The ALIF technique was commonly performed with adjunctive posterior pedicle-screw or facet-screw instrumentation to stabilize the segmental construct. Subsequently, threaded interbody cages, such as BAK, Ray, and LT cages, were used without instrumentation, or stand-alone.[58] The rate of implantation of such devices boomed in the late 1990s, but long-term data suggested that stand-alone ALIF procedures may lead to adverse long-term results.[59,60]

XLIF for Discogenic/Collapsed Lumbar Disease

The use of XLIF has become an important tool in my treatment of discogenic disease at levels above and including L4-5 interspace. At the upper lumbar regions, this approach is accomplished with much less trauma to the vasculature than I have previously seen with anterior approaches close to the renal vessels.

The goals of XLIF in this pathology are the stabilization of the desired level(s), with height restoration and without overdistraction of the disc space (Fig 11-1). I also use this approach to treat patients who have degenerative discs with moderate to severe neuroforaminal stenosis for which disc height correction would significantly increase foraminal volume. If mild to moderate central canal stenosis is noted on preoperative imaging secondary to ligamentum flavum infolding, I use XLIF height restoration to retension the ligament to indirectly decompress the central canal. In my early experience, I would perform a concomitant laminectomy, only to discover that the XLIF relieved the stenosis. Currently, patients are instructed preoperatively about a possible need for laminectomy if residual symptomatic stenosis remains in the postoperative period. In my experience, the use of XLIF with bony lateral recess stenosis will not adequately address that pathology. Also, if severe stenosis is appreciated on preoperative studies, I will routinely perform a concomitant laminectomy after the XLIF is performed.

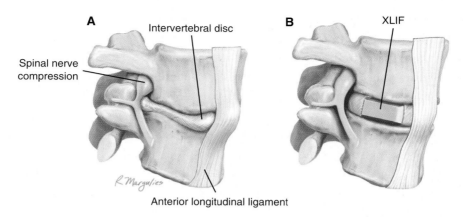

FIG. 11-1 Disc regeneration and restoration. **A,** Preoperative presentation of a degenerated/collapsed disc. **B,** Postoperative correction after the XLIF procedure.

Performing XLIF for discogenic disease has led to a better understanding of the vertical hypermobility that occurs within the collapsed disc. When conducting the preoperative planning on collapsed discs, I will often obtain an extension film to understand if the space demonstrates an opening or vacuum phenomenon. I have found that these preoperative images typically demonstrate less correction than I have seen with operative positioning. The lateral decubitus positioning with lateral flexion—jackknife positioning—tends to place the disc into significant traction. I routinely find that this intraoperative traction verifies my presumptive diagnosis of vertical hypermobility. With experience, one can produce significant height restoration of severely collapsed spaces with just operative positioning.

With the more severe cases, it is common to find the presence of an arthritic bony bar as part of the end-stage aspects of disc collapse. Commonly, the operative position will demonstrate some vertical hypermobility, but without the previously discussed height reduction. Significant releases are required for this condition. On the operative approach side, ipsilateral bone bridging may prevent the passing of the guidewire during the transpsoas passage. I recommend a careful impaction of the blunt initial dissection Dilator with dynamic stimulated and free-run EMG monitoring (NeuroVision®, NuVasive, Inc.) to dock onto the disc space. Dilator steps are then accomplished as per the standard surgical technique (see Chapter 8). Once the MaXcess® Retractor (NuVasive, Inc.) is docked and stabilized, the Dilators are carefully removed. I have found that the impacted Dissector/Dilator Probe acts like a masonry tool, starting a cleavage plane through the osteophyte complex. This is followed by the use of the Cobb Elevators and Kerrison Rongeurs to remove the ossified lateral anulus, providing access for the discectomy.

For significant contralateral osteophyte complexes, I will first attempt a simple release with the long Cobb Elevators, as noted in the standard XLIF technique. This will be followed by use of the insert-and-rotate XLIF disc-space Sizers. I have found these tools to be well-suited to be the initial Distractors when used in the insert (most narrow or flat) position relative to the disc space. Without the rotation maneuvers, I slowly pass the Sizers from 8 mm upward to slowly increase the cleavage plane across the lateral anulus to prevent later body/osteophyte fractures when distraction may be attempted. This technique is also used for those severe disc space conditions in which simple passage of narrow pituitary Rongeurs or Curettes appears to be impossible. Once that contralateral release is performed, I will cautiously use the standard Trial Sizers as final dilation tools.

The XLIF implant selected will depend on intraoperative sizing, as well as on an appreciation of the sagittal balance of the individual patient. The length of the graft will be measured to maximally cover the transverse orientation of the disc space to maximize coverage of the anular ring region. If the space demonstrates a significant preoperative lordosis, or if additional lordosis is required in a multiple-level fusion, I will choose a lordotic implant. If my operative plan involves maximizing the neuroforaminal height, I may opt to avoid lordotic implantation in tight disc spaces to maximize posterior disc space height correction. The biologic implant selected is a surgeon- and patient-specific decision; I have used commercially available bone morphogenic protein in the majority of my patients.

The use of supplemental fixation systems varies from surgeon to surgeon. The initial experience with Pimenta was with stand-alone cage devices. I have used XLIF in many different constructs, such as stand-alone, unilateral and bilateral pedicle screw, facet screw, and anterior screw/rod, as well as two- and four-hole lateral plate constructs. The only significant subsidence I have seen has been in severely osteoporotic bone along with the use of supplemental fixation. I now supplement all osteoporotic interbody fusions, regardless of approach or implant, with some form of vertebral augmentation to prevent subsidence.

The placement of additional fixation is not the focus of this chapter, but I will mention the alternative XLIF approach I have used and shared with colleagues since my first personal cadaveric dissection. This technique allows the simultaneous placement of unilateral percutaneous pedicle screw instrumentation through an alternative retroperitoneal finger-dissection plane. The posterolateral transverse incision plane is routinely located the length of one finger away from the lateral incision site. My variation is making a longitudinal incision in a location similar to that used for a Wiltse incision. This incision allows finger dissection into retroperitoneal space, while also allowing ipsilateral transpedicular percutaneous placement of pedicle screws under fluoroscopic guidance while the patient is in the lateral decubitus position.

The site of this incision is marked before the final preparations and before the operative field is draped. Depending on the location and excursion of the fluoroscopic C-arm, the table may need to be rotated laterally to demonstrate en fosse (oblique) views of the pedicles to be instrumented. The skin location for en fosse percutaneous screw/Jamshidi needle positioning will typically correspond on anteroposterior (AP) visualization to a location just lateral to the tips of the vertebral transverse processes. The finger dissection is easily accomplished in most patients through this incision plane, with the exception being the severely obese patient. In such cases, I will then make the typical transverse finger dissection incision and use the longitudinal incision only for the screws.

PERI- AND POSTOPERATIVE MANAGEMENT

Wound care has not been a significant issue in my XLIF experience. The majority of XLIF wounds are closed with subcuticular Monocryl closures, followed by Steri-Strip closures. The final dressing is clear OpSite, which requires no further wound care until the 2-week postoperative visit. The exceptions are for cases in which the patient's skin quality is extremely poor, as with the elderly. Incisions in such patients are closed with nylon vertical mattress sutures.

I have not had a significant XLIF wound infection in my personal series of cases. All patients are given standard perioperative antibiotics, and mupirocin (Bactroban) nasal ointment is used as an methicillin-resistant *Staphylococcus aureus* (MRSA) prophylaxis. I also use chlorhexidine as my surgical scrub of choice.

Blood loss from the XLIF procedure routinely has been found to be less than 50 cc for a one-level case. Nonetheless, I obtain a hematocrit in the recovery room on postoperative day one for every patient. I have only transfused patients with multiple-level fusions that have required a traditional posterior decompressive approach. The patients with single-level and multiple-level XLIF procedures are mobilized on the hospital floor within 2 to 3 hours after being discharged from the postanesthesia care unit. The majority of patients are discharged on postoperative day one; patients who have had multiple-level or more complex procedures stay in the hospital for an additional 1 or 2 days.

When he or she is discharged, the patient is given a lightweight, adjustable lumbar support. The support is not to be used as a crutch, but as a reminder for the patient to avoid heavy lifting, flexion/extension, and rotation maneuvers. Every patient is instructed to begin a walking protocol, with the expectation that he or she will be walking 1 or 2 miles per day by the 2-week postoperative visit. The patient is instructed to avoid all antiinflammatory medications until directed by the surgeon.

The degree of thigh discomfort varies among patients. All patients are preoperatively instructed in such dysesthesias, which can occur several weeks after the index procedure. I also select the operative side as determined by the location of preoperative pain, as noted by the patient. This operative selection will keep the majority of such postoperative symptoms to the ipsilateral pain location. When such complaints do occur, I use low-dose gabapentin for several weeks. As the symptoms abate, the dosing is slowly weaned.

During the phases of healing, patients may require a short course of physical therapy for lumbar core reconditioning. Radiographic imaging is followed at specific time frames, with a fusion assessment CT scan around the period of the 6-month postoperative visit. For atypical postoperative symptomatology, MRI and/or CT scanning may be used to ascertain any residual or acquired pathologies.

CASE EXAMPLE

A 59-year-old woman with a history of high-blood pressure, noninsulin-dependent diabetes, and thyroid problems presented with chronic back and right-sided leg pain. She had more pain by her right hip, but also started having some left-sided leg discomfort. The majority of the pain was in the back, with a preoperative visual analog scale (VAS) pain score of 10. Preoperatively, she reported weakness, numbness, and tingling in her feet bilaterally, which was worse when sitting and lying down after activities. She found no relief from physical therapy, several spinal blocks, and nonnarcotic and narcotic medications. Her preoper-

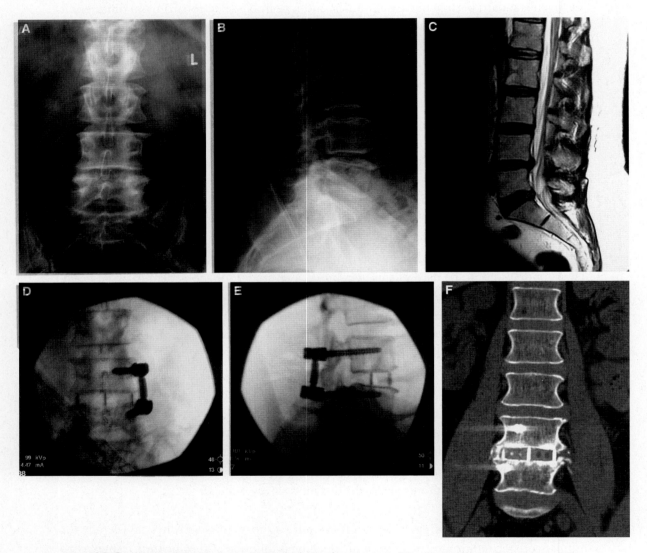

FIG. 11-2 **A** and **B**, Preoperative anteroposterior and lateral radiographs showing diminished disc height at L4-5 with abnormal angular motion. **C**, Preoperative MRI showing a large, broad-based disc herniation with bilateral stenosis. **D** and **E**, Immediate postoperative anteroposterior and lateral radiographs showing significant height restoration of the L4-5 disc space. **F**, A 7-month CT scan demonstrating fusion.

ative MRI scan demonstrates a large, broad-based disc herniation with stenosis that is bilateral in nature. Preoperative anteroposterior, lateral, and flexion/extension radiographs showed diminished disc height at L4-5 with abnormal angular motion. XLIF was chosen as a mechanism for significant height restoration. The procedure was performed with CoRoent® XL (NuVasive, Inc.), bone morphogenic protein, and SpheRx® (NuVasive, Inc.) posterior instrumentation. At 7 months after surgery, the patient had no neurologic deficits, no clinical complaints, and was very satisfied with her surgical result. Her CT scan at this time demonstrated fusion.

CONCLUSION

XLIF has become a significant technique in my practice for treating degenerative lumbar pathologies above L5. The procedure allows a less morbid approach to the anterior aspect of the vertebral segment and has garnered positive responses from my patients. This approach may be used for indirect neuroforaminal correction or in conjunction with traditional open or minimally invasive direct decompressive procedures. XLIF allows the surgeon to place a large surface area interbody fusion device with a short learning curve. Most patients treated with degenerative disc disease are easily mobilized with short hospital stays.

REFERENCES

1. Wiesel SW, Cuckler JM, Deluca F. Acute low back pain: an objective analysis of conservative therapy. Spine 5:324-330, 1980.
2. National Institute for Occupational Safety and Health, June 16, 2007.
   Available at *http://ww2.cdc.gov/risqs/wrinjestimate2.asp.*
3. Jarvik JG, Hollingworth W, Heagerty PJ, et al. Three-year incidence of low back pain in an initially asymptomatic cohort: clinical and imaging risk factors. Spine 31:E1-E3, 2005.
4. Andersson GB. Epidemiological features of chronic low-back pain. Lancet 354:581-585, 1999.
5. Battie MC, Videman T, Parent E. Lumbar disc degeneration: epidemiology and genetic influences. Spine 29:2679-2690, 2004.
6. Battie MC, Videman T, Levalahti E, et al. Heritability of low back pain and the role of disc degeneration. Pain [Epub] Feb 28, 2007.
7. Frymoyer JW. Lumbar disc disease: epidemiology. Instr Course Lect 41:217-223, 1992.
8. Crock HV. A reappraisal of intervertebral disc lesions. Med J Aust 1:983-989, 1970.
9. Erkintalo MO, Saminen JJ, Alanen AM, et al. Development of degenerative changes in the lumbar intervertebral disc: results of a prospective MR imaging study in adolescents with and without low-back pain. Radiology 196:529-533, 1995.
10. Yasuma T, Suzuki F, Koh S, et al. Pathological changes in the cartilaginous plates in relation to intervertebral disc lesions. Acta Pathol Jpn 38:735-750, 1988.
11. Peng B, Hao J, Hou S, et al. Possible pathogenesis of painful intervertebral disc degeneration. Spine 31:560-566, 2006.
12. Adams MA, Roughley PJ. What is intervertebral disc degeneration, and what causes it? Spine 31:2151-2161, 2006.
13. Roberts S, Evans H, Trivedi J, et al. Histology and pathology of the human intervertebral disc. J Bone Joint Surg Am 88:10-14, 2006.

14. Martin ND, Boxell CM, Malone DG. Pathophysiology of lumbar disc degeneration: a review of the literature. Neurosurg Focus 13:E1, 2002.

15. Kuisma M, Karppinen J, Niinimaki J, et al. A three-year follow-up of lumbar spine endplate (Modic) endplate changes. Spine 31:1714-1718, 2006.

16. Tanaka N, An HS, Lim TH, et al. The relationship between disc degeneration and flexibility of the lumbar spine. Spine J 1:47-56, 2001.

17. Mayoux-Benhamou MA, Revel M, Aaron C, et al. A morphometric study of the lumbar foramen. Influence of flexion-extension movements and of isolated disc collapse. Surg Radiol Anat 11:97-102, 1989.

18. Aihara T, Takahashi K, Ogasawara A, et al. Intervertebral disc degeneration associated with lumbosacral transitional vertebrae: a clinical and anatomical study. J Bone Joint Surg Br 87:687-691, 2005.

19. Otani K, Konno S, Kikuchi S. Lumbosacral transitional vertebrae and nerve-root symptoms. J Bone Joint Surg Br 83:1137-1140, 2001.

20. Vergauwen S, Parizel PM, van Breusegem L, et al. Distribution and incidence of degenerative spine changes in patients with a lumbo-sacral transitional vertebra. Eur Spine J 6:168-172, 1997.

21. Park P, Garton HJ, Gala VC, et al. Adjacent segment disease after lumbar or lumbosacral fusion: review of the literature. Spine 29:1938-1944, 2004.

22. Hambly MF, Wiltse LL, Raghavan N, et al. The transition zone above a lumbosacral fusion. Spine 23:1785-1792, 1998.

23. Luk KD, Chow DH, Holmes A. Vertical instability in spondylolisthesis: a traction radiographic assessment technique and the principle of management. Spine 28:819-827, 2003.

24. McGregor AH, Cattermole HR, Hughes SP. Spinal motion in lumbar degenerative disc disease. J Bone Joint Surg Br 80:1009-1013, 1998.

25. Ferreiro Perez A, Garcia Isidro M, Ayerbe E, et al. Evaluation of intervertebral disc herniation and hypermobile intersegmental instability in symptomatic adult patients undergoing recumbent and upright MRI of the cervical or lumbosacral spines. Eur J Radiol 62:444-448, 2007.

26. Karadimas EJ, Siddiqui M, Smith FW, et al. Positional MRI changes in supine versus sitting postures in patients with degenerative lumbar spine. J Spinal Disord Tech 19:495-500, 2006.

27. Gerszten PC, Welch WC, King JT. Quality of life assessment in patients undergoing nucleoplasty-based percutaneous discectomy. J Neurosurg Spine 4:36-42, 2006.

28. Davis TT, Delamarter RB, Sra P, et al. The IDET procedure for chronic discogenic low back pain. Spine 29:752-756, 2004.

29. Chapman SL, Brena SF. Learned helplessness and responses to nerve blocks in chronic low back pain patients. Pain 14:355-364, 1982.

30. Ross JS, Modic MT. Current assessment of spinal degenerative disease with magnetic resonance imaging. Clin Orthop 279:68-81, 1992.

31. Rihn JA, Lee JY, Khan M, et al. Does lumbar facet fluid detected on magnetic resonance imaging correlate with radiographic instability in patients with degenerative lumbar disease? Spine 32:1555-1560, 2007.

32. Abdi S, Datta S, Lucas LF. Role of epidural steroids in the management of chronic spinal pain: a systematic review of effectiveness and complications. Pain Physician 8:127-143, 2005.

33. Manchikanti L. Transforaminal lumbar epidural steroid injections. Pain Physician 3:374-398, 2000.

34. Manchikanti L, Manchikanti KN, Manchukonda R, et al. Evaluation of lumbar facet joint nerve blocks in the management of chronic low back pain: preliminary report of a randomized, double-blind controlled trial: Clinical Trial NCT00355914. Pain Physician 10:425-440, 2007.

35. Yu SW, Haughton VM, Sether LA, et al. Comparison of MR and discography in detecting radial tears of the annulus: a post-mortem study. Am J Neurorad 10:1077-1081, 1989.

36. Bernard TN. Lumbar discography followed by computed tomography. Refining the diagnosis of low-back pain. Spine 15:690-707, 1990.

37. Derby R, Kim BJ, Lee SH, et al. Comparison of discographic findings in asymptomatic subject discs and the negative discs of chronic LBP patients: can discography distinguish asymptomatic discs among morphologically abnormal discs? Spine J 5:389-394, 2005.

38. Caragee EJ, Lincoln T, Parmar VS, et al. A gold standard evaluation of the "discogenic pain" diagnosis as determined by provocative discography. Spine 32:287-288, 2007.

39. Caragee EJ, Paragiodakis SJ, Khurana S. 2000 Volvo Award winner in clinical studies: lumbar high-intensity zone and discography in subjects without low back problems. Spine 25:2987-2992, 2000.

40. Bernard TN. Lumbar discography followed by computed tomography. Refining the diagnosis of low-back pain. Spine 15:690-707, 1990.

41. O'Brien JP. The role of fusion for chronic low back pain. Orthop Clin North Am 14:639-647, 1983.

42. Brunarski DJ. Clinical trials of spinal manipulation: a critical appraisal and review of the literature. J Manipul Physiol Ther 7:243-249, 1984.

43. Haas M, Groupp E, Kraemer DF. Dose-response for chiropractic care of chronic low back pain. Spine J 4:574-583, 2004.

44. Martell BA, O'Connor PG, Kerns RD, et al. Systematic review: opioid treatment for chronic back pain: prevalence, efficacy, and association with addiction. Ann Intern Med 146:116-127, 2007.

45. Bartynski WS, Grahovac SZ, Rothfus WE. Incorrect needle position during lumbar epidural steroid administration: inaccuracy of loss of air pressure resistance and requirement of fluoroscopy and epidurography during needle insertion. AJNR Am J Neuroradiol 26:502-505, 2005.

46. Andersson GB, Mekhail NA, Block JE. Treatment of intractable discogenic low back pain. A systematic review of spinal fusion and intradiscal electrothermal therapy (IDET). Pain Physician 9:237-248, 2006.

47. Saal JA, Saal JS. Intradiscal electrothermal treatment for chronic discogenic low back pain: prospective outcome study with a minimum 2-year follow-up. Spine 27:966-973; discussion 973-974, 2002.

48. Singh V, Piryani C, Liao K. Role of percutaneous disc decompression using coblation in managing chronic discogenic low back pain: a prospective, observational study. Pain Physician 7:419-425, 2004.

49. Urrútia G, Kovacs F, Nishishinya MB, et al. Percutaneous thermocoagulation intradiscal techniques for discogenic low back pain. Spine 32:1146-1154, 2007.

50. Quebec Task Force on Spinal Disorders. A monograph for clinicians. Spine 12:551-559, 1987.

51. Gay RE, Bronfort G, Evans RL. Distraction manipulation of the lumbar spine: a review of the literature. J Manipulative Physiol Ther 28:266-273, 2005.

52. Deen HG, Rizzo TD, Fenton DS. Sudden progression of lumbar disc protrusion during vertebral axial decompression traction therapy. Mayo Clin Proc 78:1554-1556, 2003.

53. Nachemson A, Zdeblick TA, O'Brien JP. Lumbar disc disease with discogenic pain. What surgical treatment is most effective? Spine 21:1835-1838, 1996.

54. Fischgrund JS, Mackay M, Herkowitz HN, et al. 1997 Volvo Award winner in clinical studies. Degenerative lumbar spondylolisthesis with spinal stenosis: a prospective, randomized study comparing decompressive laminectomy and arthrodesis with and without spinal instrumentation. Spine 22:2807-2812, 1997.

55. Weatherley CR, Prickett CF, O'Brien JP. Discogenic pain persisting despite solid posterior fusion. J Bone Joint Surg Br 68:142-143, 1986.

56. Villavicencio AT, Burneikiene S, Bulsara KR, et al. Perioperative complications in transforaminal lumbar interbody fusion versus anterior-posterior reconstruction for lumbar disc degeneration and instability. J Spinal Disord Tech 19:92-97, 2006.

57. Kozak JA, Heilman AE, O'Brien JP. Anterior lumbar fusion options. Technique and graft materials. Clin Orthop Relat Res 300:45-51, 1994.

58. Burkus JK, Schuler TC, Gornet MF, et al. Anterior lumbar interbody fusion for the management of chronic lower back pain: current strategies and concepts. Orthop Clin North Am 35:25-32, 2004.

59. Fenton JJ, Mirza SK, Lahad A, et al. Variation in reported safety of lumbar interbody fusion: influence of industrial sponsorship and other study characteristics. Spine 32:471-480, 2007.

60. Button G, Gupta M, Barrett C, et al. Three- to six-year follow-up of stand-alone BAK cages implanted by a single surgeon. Spine J 5:155-160, 2005.

12

Clinical Application: Junctional Disease of the Lumbar Spine

J. Allan Goodrich ▪ Ildemaro J. Volcan

Junctional lumbar degenerative disease, also known as *adjacent segment disease* or *transitional zone disease,* is the deterioration of a mobile segment directly above or below a previous arthrodesis. Formerly reported infrequently as a consequence of lumbar arthrodesis, the incidence of junctional lumbar disease has increased recently, a result of the accelerating number of fusion cases performed yearly.[1-3] Increases in intradiscal pressure, facet joint loading, and resultant increased mobility are all contributing factors that accelerate degenerative changes.[4-6] Although these changes appear radiographically in almost all fusion cases, clinical symptoms vary remarkably and do not necessarily correlate with imaging studies. Studies with a follow-up of up to 12 years demonstrate that symptoms occur in 5.2% to 18.5% of patients who have had previous fusion surgeries. Higher rates are reported with pedicle screw instrumentation (12.2% to 18.5%), compared with other modes of instrumentation (wires or hooks) or in situ fusion (5.2% to 5.6%).[7] Gillet[8] analyzed the fate of adjacent segments over a 14-year period. Of the patients studied, 75% had a 5-year follow-up. Of this group, 41% developed transitional segment changes; 20% required additional surgery for arthrodesis extension. Although numerous studies document the severity of junctional lumbar degenerative disease, there is no consensus on true risk factors and prevention.

PATHOPHYSIOLOGY

The most common pathologic change caused by a previous fusion is disc space degeneration. On radiographs, this can manifest as disc space narrowing or osteophyte formation. Disc space narrowing and osteophyte formation result in the anterior protrusion of the ligamentum flavum from the posterolateral aspect of the spine into the spinal canal. Other findings include hypertrophy of the facet joints, potential spondylolisthesis, or retrolisthesis, all of which can be severe, as reported by Saxena et al.[9] They also reported that adjacent segment degeneration next to a lumbar fusion may be associated with extreme instability.[9] As disc space narrows in front, the facet joints in the back increase the range of movement, resulting in the enlargement of the ligamentum flavum. In extension, it infolds and encroaches into the spinal canal, contributing to stenosis. Definite risk factors include sagittal malalignment, instrumentation prominence with resulting adjacent facet injury, preexisting degenerative changes, and the patient's age.[10-14] One controversial risk factor is the length of the previous fusion; some authors report this as a definitive risk for transitional disease. However, Ghiselli et al[15] found no correlation between the length of fusion or preoperative arthritic degeneration and the onset of symptomatic transitional disease in their retrospective review of 215 patients. In a retrospective study, Kumar et al[16] reviewed the cases of 83 patients who had been treated for degenerative disc disease with fusions, excluding spondylolisthesis and degenerative scoliosis. Of these patients, 31 (36.1%) developed transitional changes, with a mean follow-up of 5 years. Patients who had normal C7 plumb lines and sacral inclinations had the lowest incidences of transitional disease. There were no differences between men and women, between patients who had only a posterior fusion and those with both posterior lateral and posterior interbody fusions, or between fusions to the sacrum and cases that stopped short of the sacrum. Radiographically, retrolisthesis was the most common manifestation of transitional disease. Sacral inclination was an important factor in adjacent segment deterioration—the more normal the angle, the less likely the patient was to develop the condition.

Cheh et al[17] studied 181 patients who had thoracolumbar and lumbar fusions with pedicle screw fixation; patients were followed for a minimum of 5 years. At follow-up, 133 patients had one- or two-level fusion surgeries, 29 had three- or four-level fusions, and 19 had five- to eight-level fusions. Radiographic evidence of transitional disease was detected in 44% (79) of patients; of these, 56% (44) became clinically symptomatic. The age, length of fusion, type of arthrodesis (circumferential or posterior), and location of proximal, instrumented vertebra were found not to be contributing factors for transitional disease development.

Anterior, posterior midline, and posterolateral fusion shift the center of rotation in individual spinal motion segments, increasing stress on the facet joints and/or discs of adjacent mobile segments. Using in vivo dog models, Dekutoski et al[18] found increased facet joint motion at the proximal free segment. In a progressive study, Axelsson et al[19] learned that uninstrumented, posterolateral fusions increase the mobility of the adjacent segment. Cole et al[20] studied dogs after they developed arthrodesis; they discovered that the condition caused changes in disc metabolism and in the composition of adjacent discs. A control group did not develop such changes.

The presumed risk factors for junctional disease are as follows:
- Older than 60 years of age
- Previous instrumentation
- Length of fusion
- Female
- Loss of coronal/sagittal balance
- Osteopenia
- Preoperative degenerative changes

CLINICAL PRESENTATION

Most patients presenting with junctional disease have had prior surgery from a posterior approach—posterior midline, posterolateral, or transforaminal. Back pain—with or without neurogenic claudication—occurs several months to several years after the initial surgery. The symptoms and physical findings generally correlate with an adjacent level of involvement. An L4-5 fusion, for example, results in radiographic changes at L3-4 that often coincide with symptoms such as back and/or thigh pain or numbness at the L3 or L4 root dermatome. Sensory changes may occur across the anterior/medial knee and leg, with possible depression of the patellar reflex. Most commonly, a typical subjective claudication occurs during ambulation; some relief is experienced with flexion of the spine, such as with leaning forward on a shopping cart while walking in a grocery store. Pain and fatigue ease with rest and time, but it may take 30 minutes or longer, distinguishing it from vascular claudication, which improves quite quickly with rest. As the level of involvement ascends the lumbar spine, more symptoms are experienced in the proximal levels of the spine; these symptoms can be felt in the inguinal region and are sometimes confused with hip pathology.

Plain radiographs often suggest the diagnosis by revealing adjacent disc space collapse, retrolisthesis or spondylolisthesis, osteophyte formation, and facet hypertrophy. Actual canal compromise may be better defined with MRI or CT myelography. In the presence of existing instrumentation, CT with contrast often provides better anatomic detail.

TREATMENT

Conservative measures such as activity modifications and nonsteroidal or analgesic medications may be used initially. Occasionally, injections of steroids and local anesthetics may provide temporary relief; however, surgical intervention is often warranted if symptoms persist.

Traditionally, decompression of adjacent stenosis has been used to alleviate compressive pathology involving the ligamentum flavum and facet joints. However, significant facetectomy is often required to achieve satisfactory nerve root decompression. Therefore adding a fusion to the decompression procedure appears intuitive. Whitecloud et al[21] documented an 80% pseudarthrosis rate when fusion was used to treat transitional disease without instrumentation. However, the study included only 14 patients, and the pseudarthrosis rate decreased to 17% with the use of instrumentation. This finding prompted Whitecloud et al to recommend the use of pedicle screw fixation when revising junctional disease.

Revision using a posterior approach often involves significant dissection of scar tissue at the subadjacent segment, complete with the inherent risks of dural violation. Posterior revisions for junctional disease often result in disappointing clinical outcomes.

A number of nonfusion technologies that treat discogenic-related pathologies have been introduced in the past decade. One potential benefit of these treatments has been the theoretical reduction in transitional segment deterioration. Total-disc arthroplasty, prosthetic nuclear replacements, and posterior stabilization devices are advocated for this purpose. Bertagnoli et al[22] completed a 2-year prospective study that assessed the efficacy of arthroplasty for adjacent segment disease. The patients were between 18 and 67 years old, and the median age was 50. Significant improvements were noted on both the visual analog scale and the Oswestry Disability Index; 86% of the patients reported satisfaction with the outcome at 24 months. Outcome studies with long-term follow-up effects of using dynamic posterior implants for the treatment of transitional disease are not available. Likewise, there is no solid prospective evidence that these devices can either prevent adjacent segment deterioration or manage the condition effectively.[23]

XLIF FOR TRANSITIONAL DISEASES

Minimally invasive techniques that use a posterior approach have been introduced, including transforaminal interbody fusion with either open or percutaneous instrumentation.[24,25] The direct lateral approach provides a virgin surgical avenue where arthrodesis can be performed and avoids the close proximities of the exiting and traversing nerve roots that are encountered using the transforaminal approach. When XLIF cages are used, a much more substantial cross-sectional area is available for grafting purposes. The exteme lateral approach avoids the epidural venous plexus, as well as scar tissue from previous posterior procedures, resulting in less blood loss and decreasing the risk of incidental durotomy. The fusion is compressed biomechanically, and the anterior longitudinal ligament (ALL) is retained; theoretically, this should improve fusion rates (Fig. 12-1).

The XLIF approach is associated with less muscle and bone dissection, which results in less postoperative pain and earlier patient mobilization. This approach may also minimize postoperative pulmonary complications and venous thrombosis.

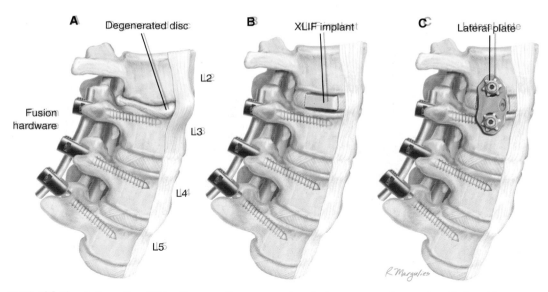

FIG. 12-1 **A,** Junctional disc changes above a previously instrumented posterior fusion. Treatment alternatives include **B,** stand-alone XLIF or **C,** XLIF supplemented with lateral plate fixation.

In our small series, 58 patients (12 of whom had adjacent segment disease) were treated for transitional disease; XLIF involved 20 segments out of a total of 96 arthrodeses performed on the 58 patients (20.8%). Most of the patients had previously undergone instrumented posterolateral fusions associated with decompression procedures for the treatment of lumbar spinal stenosis. Three surgeries treated adjacent segment disease associated with spinal deformity. The patients were an average of 64.5 years old, and the average length of time from the patients' last surgical procedure to XLIF was 69 months. Eleven patients had previous instrumented fusions; only 1 had in situ fusion. However, if the longest two times (10 and 40 years) are eliminated, the average interval between surgeries decreases to 35 months for the remaining 10 patients. Surgical times averaged 2 hours and 10 minutes per case, or 1 hour and 18 minutes per level. The average blood loss was 41 ml per level, or 69 ml per surgery. Hospital stays averaged 2 days if the patient had only an XLIF procedure. The stay increased to an average of 4.7 days if the patient had an additional posterior instrumented fusion. Complications included three levels with endplate fractures, one of which occurred in an obese patient. One patient moved after the incision was made, and the radiographic visualization was lost. The incision was closed and the patient was repositioned; her surgery proceeded as scheduled. Two patients had postoperative proximal thigh dysesthesias; one case resolved within 6 weeks. The other patient had diabetes, and the dysesthesias persisted for 3 months after surgery; the patient also had other comorbidities. All twelve patients were prescribed analgesics preoperatively, and four required narcotic medications postoperatively (three of these patients were prescribed acetaminophen and propoxyphene [Darvocet]); these patients were also being treated for other pain issues (Fig. 12-2). Eleven of the twelve patients reported that they would definitely undergo the XLIF procedure again, based on the pain relief they experienced.

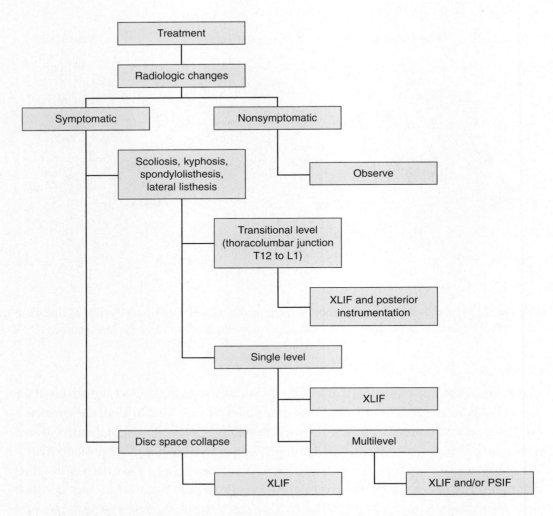

FIG. 12-2   Decision-making algorithm for junctional disease of the lumbar spine.

POSTOPERATIVE MANAGEMENT

Early mobilization is the rule when XLIF is used for a single segment above a previous arthrodesis. A walking program is instituted, and braces are optional. If the junctional disease is associated with a significant coronal or sagittal imbalance, the addition of posterior instrumentation may be necessary, especially as the thoracolumbar junction is treated. General medical interventions such as Venodyne compression devices for deep vein thrombosis prophylaxis can be used, but routine anticoagulation has not been necessary. First-generation cephalosporin or fluoroquinolone may be used within 1 hour of the skin incision being made; these should be continued for 24 hours postoperatively. Patients are released from the hospital when they can tolerate a regular diet, ambulate, and require only oral analgesics—all of which typically occur within 24 hours of surgery. Patients are encouraged to resume their usual activities as their surgical pain resolves, usually 4 to 6 weeks postoperatively. Follow-up includes serial radiographs to assess the fusion, which usually occurs within 3 to 6 months of surgery.

CASE EXAMPLES

CASE 1

A 75-year-old woman presented with a 6-month history of progressive low back pain that radiated to both hips and was worse with weight bearing. Neurologically, there was no focal weakness during the physical examination, but there was a history of neurogenic claudication. A decompressive laminectomy procedure and posterior segmental instrumented fusion at L3-5 were performed during a single surgery in March 2004, a treatment for spinal stenosis and degenerative spondylolisthesis at L4-5 (Fig. 12-3, *A* and *B*). She did well postoperatively until her symptoms recurred. Her comorbidities included obesity, bilateral knee replacement, and right hip replacement. She underwent XLIF of L2-3 for junctional disease 2 years after the primary surgery. During the first surgery, a superior pedicle screw migrated into the L2-3 disc space. During the XLIF procedure, the pedicle screw was accessed, and a cage was inserted over it. She has done relatively well postoperatively and is anticipating a total hip replacement on her left side (Fig. 12-3, *C* and *D*).

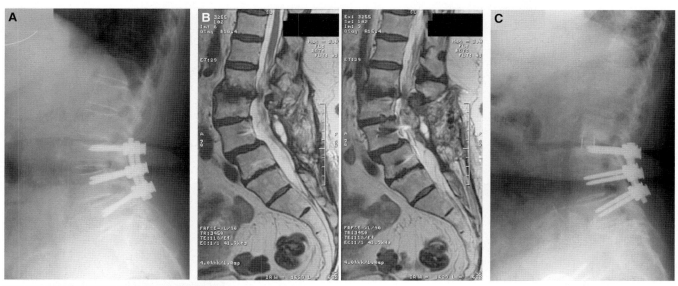

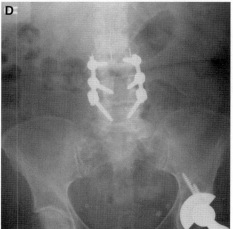

FIG. 12-3 **A,** Preoperative lateral radiograph reveals disc space narrowing with a pedicle screw violating the superior endplate. **B,** Preoperative sagittal MRI reveals disc space narrowing and deterioration at the L2-3 junctional level. **C,** Postoperative lateral radiograph shows the anterior position of the XLIF cage with good disc height restoration. **D,** Postoperative anteroposterior radiograph shows good disc height. The XLIF cage spans from side-to-side, resting on the anular ring.

CASE 2

This 65-year-old woman presented with a long history of low back pain. She had a posterior lateral fusion from L4-sacrum in 1968. She was doing well until 2003, when she developed progressive, unrelenting back pain following a bowel obstruction. She was diagnosed with L1-2 discitis and was treated with antibiotics; her symptoms resolved. She then developed 6 months of worsening lumbar pain, which improved only with recumbency. The tests at this time demonstrated degenerative changes at L2-3 and L3-4 (Fig. 12-4, *A* and *B*). Provocative discography was most positive at L2-3 and, to a lesser extent, at L3-4. The L1-2 level was asymptomatic. Her laboratory results, including white blood cell count and sedimentation rate, were normal. She underwent XLIFs at L2-3 and L3-4 (Fig. 12-4, *C* and *D*). Her postoperative course was unremarkable, and she has recovered nicely.

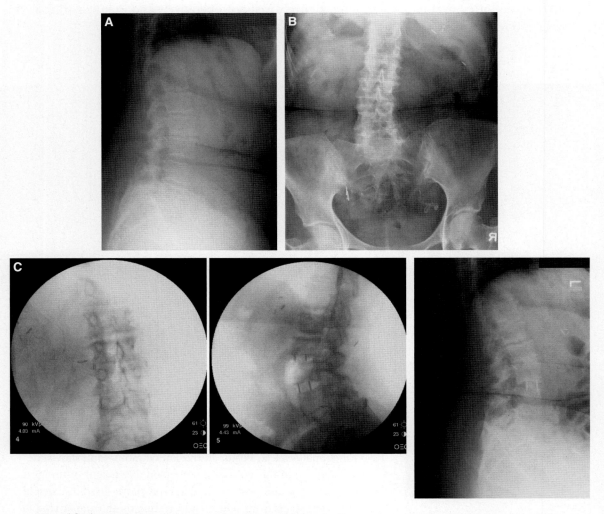

FIG. 12-4   A, Preoperative lateral radiograph reveals disc space narrowing at L1-3 to L3-4. The discogram was positive at L2-3 and L3-4 only. **B,** Preoperative anteroposterior radiograph shows the previous L4-sacrum fusion. **C,** Intraoperative fluoroscopy demonstrates good positioning of the cages with height restoration. **D,** Postoperative radiograph shows the anterior position of the XLIF cages with good disc space height restoration.

CONCLUSION

Transitional disease is common after spinal fusion; radiographically, it is seen in all patients if they are followed long enough. Clinical symptoms, however, develop in only 5.2% to 18.5% of patients who have had fusion surgeries. Symptoms include back pain, with or without neurologic symptoms such as neurogenic claudication. Risk factors for transitional disease are disputed and include sagittal malalignment, length of fusion, use of instrumentation, patient age, and preexisting degenerative disease at the adjacent segment. Decompressive procedures—with or without fusion—have been the standard treatment, with varying degrees of success. Revision surgeries often require extensive dissections through a previous surgical site, resulting in potential risks of incidental durotomy and wound problems. The extreme lateral approach allows access to the adjacent level through a previously untouched route to the spine. Blood loss is minimal, and recovery time appears to be accelerated.

REFERENCES

1. Anderson CE. Spondylolisthesis following spine fusion. J Bone Joint Surg Am 38:1142-1146, 1956.
2. Unander-Scharin L. A case of spondylolisthesis lumbalis aquisita. Acta Orthop Scand 19:536-544, 1950.
3. Weinstein JN, Lurie JD, Olson PR, et al. United States' trends and regional variations in lumbar spine surgery: 1992-2003. Spine 31:2707-2714, 2006.
4. Lee CK, Langeana NA. Lumbosacral spinal fusion: a biomechanical study. Spine 9:574-581, 1984.
5. Ha KY, Schendel MJ, Lewis JL, et al. Effect of immobilization and configuration on lumbar adjacent segment biomechanics. J Spinal Disord 6:99-105, 1993.
6. Weinhoffer SL, Guyer RD, Herbert M, et al. Intradiscal pressure measurements above an instrumented fusion: a cadaveric study. Spine 20:526-531, 1995.
7. Park P, Garton HJ, Gala VC, et al. Adjacent segment disease after lumbar or lumbosacral fusion: review of the literature. Spine 29:1938-1944, 2004.
8. Gillet P. Focus issue: disc arthroplasty. J Spinal Disord Tech 16:338-345, 2003.
9. Saxena A, Baron EM, Anderson DG, et al. Spinal disassociation masquerading as iatrogenic listhesis above a previous fusion. Spine 31:E179-E183, 2006.
10. Rahm MD, Hall BB. Adjacent-segment degeneration after lumbar fusion with instrumentation: a retrospective study. J Spinal Disord 9:932-940, 1996.
11. Wilse LL, Radecki SE, Biel HM, et al. Comparative study of the incidence and severity of degenerative change in the transition zones after instrumented versus noninstrumented fusions of the lumbar spine. J Spinal Disord 12:27-33, 1999.
12. Aota Y, Kumano K, Hirabayashi S. Postfusion instability at the adjacent segments after rigid pedicle screw fixation for degenerative lumbar spinal disorders. J Spinal Disord 8:464-473, 1995.
13. Etebar S, Cahill DW. Risk factors for adjacent-segment failure following lumbar fixation with rigid instrumentation for degenerative instability. J Neurosurg 90:163-169, 1999.
14. Wimmer C, Gluch H, Krismer M, et al. AP-translation in the proximal disc adjacent to lumbar spine fusion: a retrospective comparison of mono- and polysegmental fusion in 120 patients. Acta Orthop Scand 68:269-272, 1997.

15. Ghiselli G, Wang JC, Hsu WK, et al. L5-S1 segment surviorship and clinical outcome analysis after L4-L5 isolated fusion. Spine 28:1275-1280, 2003.
16. Kumar MN, Baklanov A, Chopin D. Correlation between sagittal plane changes and adjacent segment degeneration following lumbar spine fusion. Euro Spine J 10:314-319, 2001.
17. Cheh G, Bridwell K, Lenke L, et al. Risk factors for adjacent segment degeneration following lumbar/thoracolumbar fusion with pedicle screw instrumentation: a minimum 5 year follow up. Presented at the Forty-first Annual Meeting of the Scoliosis Research Society, Monterey, CA, Sept 2006.
18. Dekutoski MB, Schendel MJ, Ogilvie JW, et al. Comparison of in vivo and in vitro adjacent segment motion after lumbar fusion. Spine 19:1745-1751, 1994.
19. Axelsson P, Johnsson R, Strömqvist B. The spondylolytic vertebra and its adjacent segment: mobility measured before and after posterolateral fusion. Spine 22:414-417, 1997.
20. Cole TC, Burkhardt D, Ghosh P, et al. Effects of spinal fusion on the proteoglycans of the canine intervertebral disc. J Orthop Res 3:277-291, 1985.
21. Whitecloud TS III, Davis JM, Olive PM. Operative treatment of the degenerated segment adjacent to a lumbar fusion. Spine 19:531-536, 1994.
22. Bertagnoli R, Yue JJ, Fenk-Mayer A, et al. Treatment of symptomatic adjacent-segment degeneration after lumbar fusion with total disc arthroplasty by using the ProDisc prosthesis: a prospective study with 2-year minimum follow up. J Neurosurg Spine 4:91-97, 2006.
23. Roh JS, Teng AL, Yoo JU, et al. Degenerative disorders of the lumbar and cervical spine. Orthop Clin North Am 36:255-262, 2005.
24. Moskowitz A. Transforaminal lumbar interbody fusion. Orthop Clin North Am 33:359-366, 2002.
25. Lowe TG, Tahernia AD, O'Brien MF, et al. Unilateral transforaminal posterior lumbar interbody fusion (TLIF): indications, technique, and 2-year results. J Spinal Disord Tech 15:31-38, 2002.

13

Clinical Application: XLIF® After Prior Surgery

Eric A. Thomas ▪ J. Allan Goodrich

There is probably no greater challenge in spine surgery than addressing a patient with persisting symptoms after spine surgery. With ever more spine surgeries being performed, especially spine fusions, a variety of postsurgical pathologies may be encountered (Box 13-1).[1-3] These include postlaminectomy instability, pseudarthrosis, recurrent disc herniation, persisting lateral recess stenosis after previous decompression, and junctional stenosis. This chapter reviews these causes, applicable pathophysiology, traditional management (both surgical and nonsurgical), and extreme lateral interbody fusion (XLIF, NuVasive®, Inc., San Diego, CA) applications.

CAUSES

Postlaminectomy instability usually reveals itself by progressive lower back pain with or without a radicular complaint. The symptoms are typically activity related and improve with recumbency. Radiographic evaluation may reveal a wide decompression in anteropos-

---

BOX 13-1   Common Conditions Secondary to Previous Lumbar Spine Surgery (Failed Spine Surgery Syndromes)

Postlaminectomy syndrome

Pseudarthrosis

Junctional syndrome

Recurrent disc herniation

---

terior views and a varying degree of spondylolisthesis in lateral images. Dynamic radiographs are often helpful for revealing increased kyphosis and/or translation at the level or levels involved. Postlaminectomy instability was the second most common cause for reoperation in the National Low Back Pain Study, according to Long.[4] Biomechanical studies have suggested that removal of one third to one half of the facet joints may be undertaken without creating focal instability.[5] Several explanations have been given for progressive postdecompression instability; these include degenerative facet arthropathy, facet resection, and disc and ligamentous changes. Pars interarticularis fracture as a consequence of attenuation or removal during decompression and subsequent stress concentration postoperatively have also been implicated.

A precise definition of instability remains elusive. Certainly translation or increased angulation seen in dynamic radiographs is suggestive, and improvement of symptoms with immobilization may reinforce this suggestion. However, many cases rely on history alone to make a diagnosis. Treatment with arthrodesis and subsequent improvement of symptoms can confirm a diagnosis. However, a reliable study to predict the complete benefits of surgical stabilization still has not been conducted for these situations. Which stabilization technique (that is, in situ fusion, pedicle screw instrumentation, or anterior arthrodesis) is superior for providing predictable pain relief while also minimizing surgical morbidity is subject to debate. Prospective studies are needed to compare the various options—including XLIF—to better identify which method is superior. Diagnosis remains critical because all of these procedures improve stability.

Pseudarthrosis is the most common cause of failure after spine fusion.[5,6] It is often difficult to pinpoint pseudarthrosis as the origin of an individual patient's pain because patients often have evidence of pseudarthrosis on imaging studies without symptoms. Symptoms may include ongoing or worsening low back pain, and imaging studies show no evidence of a fusion mass (posterolateral), radiolucent lines, hardware loosening, or halo formation around the pedicle screws. In general, it takes at least 1 year for a fusion to become mature, and a diagnosis of pseudarthrosis should rarely be entertained until at least 6 months after the operation.

Because pseudarthrosis is one of the most difficult entities to assess in terms of persistent symptoms after fusion surgery, the results of surgically addressing the problem are difficult to predict.[7] Treatment options for posterior lumbar pseudarthrosis include a posterior approach with instrumentation (if it was not performed initially), adjunctive bone grafting (autograft or bone morphogenic proteins), and internal or external electrical stimulation. Repeat posterior surgery may include the addition of an interbody graft using a posterior or transforaminal interbody technique. The limitations of repeat posterior approaches include operating through extensive scar tissue and attempting fusion in a relatively devascularized bed. Additional limitations of the posterior approach include difficulty in improving lumbar lordosis in a flat back without the addition of extensive osteotomies (such as pedicle subtraction or multiple Smith-Peterson osteotomies). However, a posterior approach may be needed because of persistent compressive pathology causing radicular symptoms in addition to mechanical low back pain. Anterior interbody fusion or a combination of techniques (such as 360 degree fusion) involves extensive surgery and accompanying risks of complications.

Junctional syndrome, another category of failed lumbar surgery, involves the progression of the degenerative process into segments adjacent to a previous fusion. Although the condition is nearly 100% detectible in radiographs, clinically relevant symptoms are estimated to occur in only 5.2% to 18.5% of patients.[8] Symptoms may include mechanical low back pain, with or without radicular or neurogenic claudication, depending on the levels involved and the degree of spinal stenosis present. Presumed risk factors for developing junctional syndrome include a patient being older than 60 years, length of fusion (increasing number of functional spine units), loss of coronal/sagittal balance, osteopenia, and preoperative degenerative changes.

Traditional approaches for treating junctional syndrome include reexploration through the previous operative bed, with the intention of decompression, and arthrodesis with instrumentation. Additional anterior interbody fusions might be performed in some compromised patients, such as smokers, those with inflammatory conditions such as rheumatoid arthritis, or those who take steroids or medications that interfere with bone graft healing (Box 13-2).

Recurrent disc herniation rates vary in the literature from 6% to 16%.[9,10] Patients with persistent normal disc height may experience recurrent herniation, but this is unusual. Subsequent degenerative changes may evolve slowly over time. If there is internal disc disruption, reexploration and further disc excision predictably leads to aggravation of the symptoms, and fusion surgery is required.[7] Isolated disc resorption may occur after disc excision, resulting in marked loss of disc height. These cases may respond to interbody fusion techniques.

BOX 13-2   Risk Factors for Pseudarthrosis

Patient Factors	*Surgical Factors*
Poor nutrition	Inadequate preparation of fusion bed
Smoking	Inadequate bone grafting
Diabetes	Poor-quality bone graft
Connective tissue disease	Inadequate instrumentation
Metabolic bone disease	Kyphotic deformity
Medications	
Steroids	
Anticonvulsants (for example, phenytoin [Dilantin])	
NSAIDs	

From Moshirfar A, Rand FF, Jenis LG, et al. Complications of lumbosacral and spinopelvic fusion. In Howard A, Lewis G, eds. Complications of Spinal Surgery: Treatment and Prevention. Philadelphia: Lippincott Williams & Wilkins, 2006, pp 135-141.

NONOPERATIVE TREATMENT OPTIONS

Many patients who have persistent symptoms after lumbar surgery should be managed initially with a trial of medications or activity modification. In some compromised patients, conservative measures may fail to alleviate pain; for these individuals, both diagnostic and therapeutic spinal injections may be used. A team approach, including treatments by an experienced pain management physician, can often avoid further surgical interventions. If a specific origin of a patient's ongoing complaints cannot be found, another surgical procedure is unlikely to be effective. In certain situations, a spinal cord stimulator for chronic pain therapy may be more beneficial. Medical issues associated with increased blood loss and operative time include cardiopulmonary complications.

XLIF AFTER PREVIOUS SURGERY

XLIF after a failed surgery offers several major advantages (Fig. 13-1). If there is instability following posterior decompressive surgery or pseudarthrosis after previous posterior fusions above L5-S1, a new approach through previously undissected tissue may be used to place a stabilizing interbody graft. Circumventing previous hardware insertion may decrease blood loss, operative time, and medical issues associated with them. The removal of the previous total disc replacement (as described by Pimenta et al[11]) avoids the scarring and large-vessel adherence that are commonly encountered with repeat anterior approaches.

Junctional syndrome is also amenable to the XLIF approach. The distraction of the collapsed interspace and relief of redundant anular and ligamentous intrusion into the canal may provide indirect decompression from the adjacent stenosis. Extension of the previous posterior instrumentation may be avoided, thus reducing surgical exposure and its resulting morbidity.

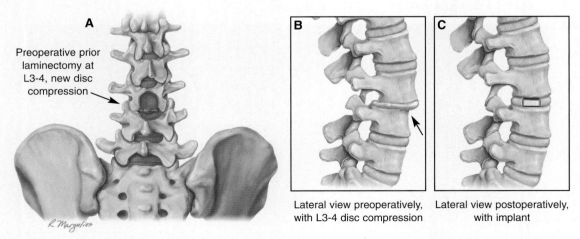

A Preoperative prior laminectomy at L3-4, new disc compression

R. Margulies

B Lateral view preoperatively, with L3-4 disc compression

C Lateral view postoperatively, with implant

FIG. 13-1   A and **B,** Preoperative disc collapse and lateral listhesis with laminectomy. **C,** Postoperative correction with restored disc height.

CASE EXAMPLES

POSTLAMINECTOMY INSTABILITY

A 64-year-old man underwent lumbar laminectomy for stenosis 4 years previously (Fig. 13-2, *A*). He developed increasing, debilitating mechanical back pain that was unresponsive to conservative care. Preoperative radiographs showed significant disc collapse, loss of lordosis, and instability (Fig. 13-2, *B* and *C*). A single-level XLIF was performed at L3-4, improving segmental height and angulation by placing the graft in the anterior half of the disc space (Fig. 13-2, *D* and *E*). The patient recovered well from the surgery and had significant back pain relief; the site appeared to be fused at his 9-month follow-up visit.

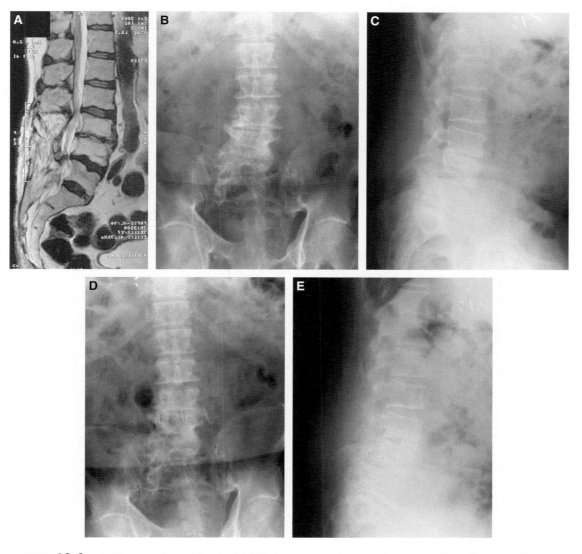

FIG. 13-2 **A,** Preoperative midsagittal MRI showing previous laminectomy, disc collapse, and persistent posterior bulging into the canal at L3-4. **B** and **C,** Preoperative anteroposterior (AP) and lateral radiographs reveal collapse and instability at L3-4. **D** and **E,** AP and lateral radiographs 9 months after surgery show restoration of disc height and segmental lordosis.

PSEUDARTHROSIS

A 70-year-old woman presented with a 10-year history of back and right leg pain after a posterolateral fusion performed in 1993. She had a bone growth stimulator placed in 1995 after apparent pseudarthrosis, and her implants were removed in 1997. Flexion/extension radiographs from her examination showed gross motion (Fig. 13-3, *A* and *B*). The surgical treatment included XLIF at L4-5 to stabilize the segment and avoid the posterior scar tissue from her multiple previous surgeries (Fig. 13-3, *C* and *D*). The procedure was uneventful, and the patient was discharged from the hospital, pain free, 18 hours after surgery.

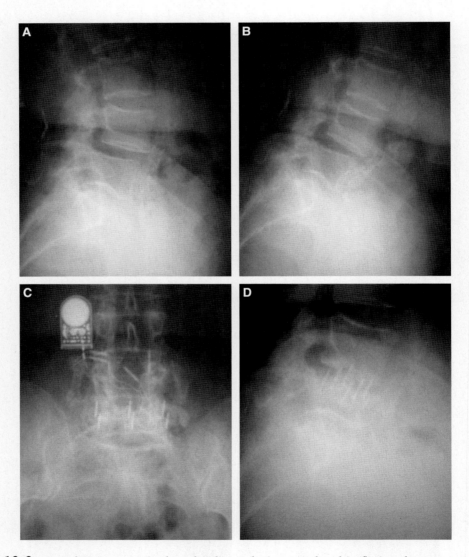

FIG. 13-3   A and **B**, Preoperative lateral radiographs in neutral and in flexion show gross motion indicative of pseudarthrosis of previous posterolateral fusion at L4-5. **C** and **D**, AP and lateral radiographs reveal XLIF graft placement at L4-5 to stabilize the nonunion.

JUNCTIONAL SYNDROME

A 63-year-old man with a previous laminectomy and posterior interbody fusion at L4-5 presented with debilitating back and leg pain. Preoperative imaging showed disc space collapse and degenerative scoliosis above the previous fusion site from L1-2 to L3-4 (Fig. 13-4, *A* and *B*) with significant multilevel central stenosis, as shown on the myelogram (Fig. 13-4, *C*). XLIF was performed from L1 to L4, with revision of posterior pedicle screw fixation and augmentation from T11 to L5. Disc heights were restored, and sagittal and coronal alignments improved significantly, all of which was maintained at the 9-month follow-up (Fig. 13-4, *D* and *E*).

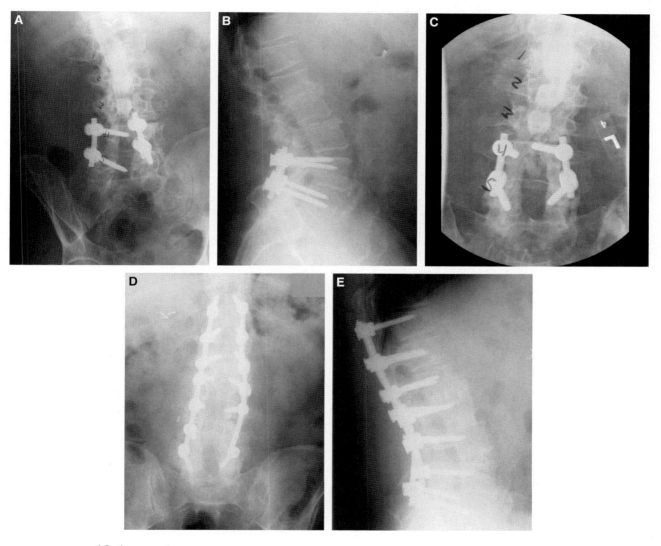

FIG. 13-4 **A** and **B,** Preoperative AP and lateral radiographs highlight the previous decompressive posterior lumbar interbody fusion (PLIF) procedure at the L4-5 level with new collapse at multiple levels above. **C,** A myelogram reveals occlusion of the canal at multiple levels above the previous L4-5 fusion. **D** and **E,** AP and lateral radiographs 9 months after surgery show continued restoration of disc space and alignment.

RECURRENT DISC HERNIATION

A 58-year-old man presented with combined low back and groin pain radiating into the upper thigh. He had undergone several previous back surgeries, and preoperative imaging showed degenerative disc disease with a recurrent herniated disc and stenosis at L2-3 on the right side (Fig. 13-5, *A* and *B*). XLIF at L2-3 was uneventful, taking about an hour to perform, and the patient was walking the same day and was discharged from the hospital the next day. His leg and back pain had improved significantly at the 6-month follow-up (Fig. 13-5, *C* and *D*).

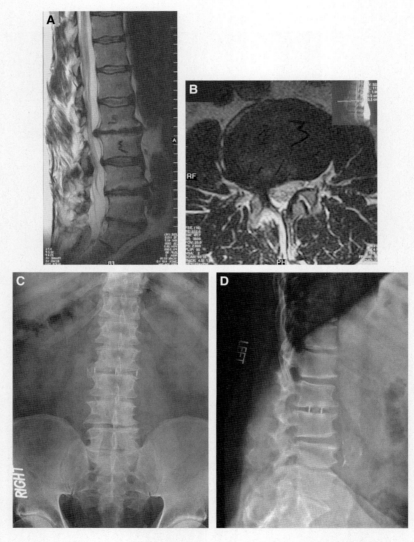

FIG. 13-5   A and **B,** Preoperative sagittal and axial MRI reveals right-sided reherniation and stenosis at L2-3 in a patient who had a previous decompressive surgery at the same level. **C** and **D,** AP and lateral radiographs 6 months after surgery show maintenance of disc height.

CONCLUSION

Failed back syndrome, including postlaminectomy instability, pseudarthrosis, junctional syndrome, and recurrent disc herniation with disc space collapse, may all be adequately addressed using the XLIF approach. However, a second-stage posterior procedure may be necessary if there are extruded disc fragments and pseudarthrosis in high-risk cases. Usually the pathology can be handled adequately from the extreme lateral approach only.

REFERENCES

1. Burton CV, Kirkaldy-Willis WH, Yong-Hing K, et al. Causes of failure of surgery on the lumbar spine. Clin Orthop Relat Res 157:191-199, 1981.
2. Slipman CW, Shin CH, Patel RK, et al. Etiologies of failed back surgery syndrome. Pain Med 3:200-214, 2002.
3. Waguespack A, Schofferrman J, Slosar P, et al. Etiology of long-term failures of lumbar spine surgery. Pain Med 3:18-22, 2002.
4. Long DM. Failed back syndrome. In Kostuik JP, ed. Failed Spinal Surgery (State of the Art Reviews: Spine), vol 11. Philadelphia: Hanley & Belfus, 1997, pp 439-452.
5. DePalma AF, Rothman RH. The nature of pseudarthrosis. Clin Orthop Relat Res 59:113-118, 1968.
6. Frymoyer JW, Hanley EN Jr, Howe J, et al. A comparison of radiographic findings in fusion and nonfusion patients ten or more years following lumbar disc surgery. Spine 4:435-440, 1979.
7. Kostuik JP. Failures after spinal fusion. In Kostuik JP, ed. Failed Spinal Surgery (State of the Art Reviews: Spine), vol 11. Philadelphia: Hanley & Belfus, 1997, pp 589-645.
8. Park P, Garton HJ, Gala VC, et al. Adjacent segment disease after lumbar or lumbosacral fusion: review of the literature. Spine 29:1938-1944, 2004.
9. Cauchoix J, Ficat C, Girard B. Repeat surgery after disc excision. Spine 3:256-259, 1978.
10. O'Sullivan MG, Connolly AE, Buckley TF. Recurrent lumbar disc protrusion. Br J Neurosurg 4:319-325, 1990.
11. Pimenta L, Diaz RC, Guerrero L. Charité lumbar artificial disc retrieval: use of a lateral minimally invasive technique: technical note. J Neurosurg Spine 5:556-561, 2006.

14

Clinical Application:
Degenerative Spondylolisthesis

Paul Fuchs · Chad M. Kessler

The intact neural arch of spondylolisthesis was first described in 1950 by MacNab[1] when he correlated the pathoanatomy with the clinical description of degenerative spondylolisthesis. Spondylolisthesis was later broken down into a five-part classification system, which was initially described by Newman[2] and later revised by Wiltse et al.[3]

The term *spondylolisthesis* derives from the Greek terms *spondulos,* referring to the vertebral body, and *olisthesis,* meaning 'slippage or sliding down.' The condition typically results from long-standing intersegmental instability, and is also believed to result from a failure of the apophyseal joints—most commonly those at the L4-5 level—to resist shear forces; this allows the vertebral body to displace anteriorly with relation to its subjacent vertebra. Numerous studies have explored the epidemiology of degenerative spondylolisthesis. MacNab's research in 1950 revealed that degenerative spondylolisthesis most commonly occurs in the sixth decade.[1] In the mid-1970s, Rosenberg[4] described predisposing factors for degenerative spondylolisthesis. The cadaveric portion of this study revealed that degenerative spondylolisthesis was almost six times more prevalent in females than in males, and three times more common in black females than in white females. He also noted that the L4-5 level was by far the most common level in which spondylolisthesis occurred. This was followed by the L5-S1 and L3-4 levels, respectively. The average amount of slippage was only 14%, with no slippage exceeding 30%. Rosenberg postulated that the more stable L5-S1 segment led to an increased concentration of stress on the L4-5 level, acting as a predisposing factor to slippage. This hypothesis is further supported by the increased incidence of the condition in patients with prior fusion at L5-S1.[5] This chapter focuses on the pathophysiology and clinical presentation of degenerative spondylolisthesis; various treatment options are also discussed.

PATHOPHYSIOLOGY

Degenerative spondylolisthesis is usually the result of long-standing instability that results from a combination of disc degeneration and facet-joint degeneration. An increase in the incidence of spondylolisthesis has been noted in women who have previously undergone oophorectomy.[6] It was theorized by Imada et al[6] that all oophorectomies lead to decreasing serum estrogen levels, thus decreasing the elasticity of fibrous connective tissue. Pregnancy and obesity, with their losses of abdominal muscle tone, are also related causes.[7]

Changes in facet joint anatomy have been studied with relation to degenerative spondylolisthesis, and it has been noted that an increase in the facet angle relative to the coronal plane leads to a higher incidence of spondylolisthesis. Boden at al[8] used magnetic resonance imaging (MRI) to map out the mean orientation of the lumbar facet joints in patients with degenerative spondylolisthesis compared with asymptomatic controls. This study confirmed that an increasing sagittal orientation of the facets at all levels of the lumbar spine led to an increased incidence of degenerative spondylolisthesis, especially at the fourth and fifth lumbar vertebrae. This study concluded that facet angles exceeding 45 degrees at the L4-5 level were associated with as much as a 25-fold increase in the incidence of spondylolisthesis. The relative stability of the L5-S1 segment, with its coronally oriented facets, leads to increased shear forces at the L4-5 level. Iatrogenic fusion, disc space collapse and degeneration, and sacralization of the L5 segment have all been associated with a higher rate of degenerative spondylolisthesis at the L4-5 segments.[9]

As degenerative changes progress in the apophyseal joints, shear forces are not adequately restrained, and microfractures may occur with remodeling. As the disc continues to degenerate, forward displacement of the vertebral body may be noted, along with loss of disc integrity and ligamentous stretching. However, there have been no findings to suggest that overall joint laxity plays a significant role.[10] With vertebral body displacement, the spinal canal and intervertebral foramen can become compromised. If the central canal has preexisting congenital tightness, then significant stenosis may occur as the intact neural arch steadily impinges on the dural sac. The continued degenerative and osteophytic changes of the apophyseal joints further compromise the lateral recesses, leading to radicular symptoms and/or neurogenic claudication in some patients. Disc degeneration and loss of disc height—along with the buckling of ligamentum flavum and subsequent ligamentous laxity—allow the hypermobility to progress. It has been noted that degenerative spondylolisthesis rarely exceeds 30%. Synovial cysts may also develop at the degenerative segment, further compromising the area available for the nerve roots.

The natural history of degenerative spondylolisthesis has not been extensively studied. Matsunaga et al[11,12] noted no specific correlation between the amount of radiographic slippage and the development of clinical symptoms over a 5-year period. It has been noted that a severe loss of disc height seems to lessen the chance of significant progression of the slippage.

Further clinical studies also found that patients without neurologic deficits at initial evaluation remained free of neurologic deficits throughout a 10-year follow-up period.[12] Of patients with lower extremity symptoms on initial evaluation, 86% experienced some improvement with time. However, more than a third of these patients experienced recurrent symptoms. Neurogenic claudication noted at the time of the initial evaluation led to progression of symptoms over time in patients who were not treated surgically.

CLINICAL PRESENTATION

Intermittent episodes of moderate-to-severe low-back pain seem to be the most common presenting complaint in degenerative spondylolisthesis. The back pain may or may not be accompanied by radicular symptoms or neurogenic claudication. Patients often have difficulty standing or walking for extended periods of time. Discomfort is typically present in the low lumbar region, extending into the buttock area, and can be characterized by aching, weakness with heaviness, and numbness or burning sensations.[13] These lower extremity complaints are often the reason for the patient's initial evaluation with a spine specialist.

Frequently, patients report an improvement in symptoms when in a flexed or sitting position; symptoms are often aggravated when the spine is extended—when the patient stands. In addition, patients often have lower extremity symptoms and/or back pain at night, which can disturb sleep patterns. These lower extremity symptoms often lead to an eventual need for surgical intervention.

The physical examination findings in patients with degenerative spondylolisthesis are often subtle and inconsistent. The range of motion in the lumbar spine may be normal, and a palpable step-off at the unstable segment is rarely noted, except in very thin patients. The L5 nerve root is commonly affected, and this may be demonstrated by some weakness in the extensor hallucis longus (EHL). Reflexes are often blunted, and stretch signs are rarely present. Bladder dysfunction related to the stenosis or degenerative spondylolisthesis is very rare.

The differential diagnosis in degenerative spondylolisthesis includes vascular claudication caused by peripheral vascular disease. A good vascular examination should be undertaken, and arterial flow studies should be performed if necessary. Peripheral neuropathy may also be confused with the neurologic complaints associated with degenerative spondylolisthesis. A history of diabetes, hypersensitivity, and sensory changes in a stocking/glove-type distribution can help differentiate peripheral neuropathy from the neurologic complaints that are associated with spinal stenosis. Degenerative hip or knee disease and metastatic disease should also be ruled out during the work-up for degenerative spondylolisthesis.

Plain radiographs taken with the patient in a standing position can often aid a surgeon in making the diagnosis of degenerative spondylolisthesis. Dynamic flexion extension radiographs have been shown to assist in making the diagnosis in some circumstances, and several authors have suggested recumbent flexion and extension views for those patients who are unable to stand for radiographs.[14]

In patients with primarily back pain, plain radiographs should suffice. However, in patients with neurologic symptoms, further evaluation is warranted. Advanced imaging, like magnetic resonance imaging (MRI), is still indicated for patients who have back pain—if only to exclude other diagnoses that may contribute to back pain without neurologic symptoms or findings. MRI currently provides the greatest detail with regard to the status of the spinal canal and clearly reveals most degenerative spondylolisthesis. Both sagittal and axial images assist the surgeon in evaluating the degree of central lateral recess and foraminal stenosis. Computed tomography (CT) myelogram may also be used when MRI is contraindicated (for example, in patients with pacemakers). A bone scan is rarely part of the initial evaluation of degenerative spondylolisthesis.

TREATMENT

One should exhaust nonoperative treatments before considering surgical intervention. Conservative treatment regimens include physical therapy, aerobic conditioning, antiinflammatories, pain medications, muscle relaxants, and/or weight reduction.[15-17] Using aggressive pain management and/or physiatry can be beneficial when exhausting all conservative measures. In addition, a patient may benefit from receiving recommendations about such things as appropriate lifting techniques and preventing long-term standing and/or sitting. A large percentage of these patients can be significantly deconditioned and may have difficulty walking short distances because they are aerobically out of shape. Encouraging a patient to exercise can have a positive affect, regardless of whether that patient is being treated conservatively or is a candidate for potential surgery.

NONSURGICAL
Aerobic Conditioning

Physical therapy is a first-line treatment for symptoms associated with degenerative spondylolisthesis. Core strengthening with isometric exercises can restore muscle function. Traction can offer relief of both low-back and radicular-type symptoms; however, long-term relief associated with traction is difficult to predict. Other modalities used in conjunction with physical therapy are deep-tissue massage, stretching (particularly the hamstrings), and transcutaneous electrical nerve stimulation (TENS). Low-impact exercises such as walking are ideal because they do not require significant exertion and can be performed by most patients with degenerative spondylolisthesis. In those patients who are truly limited in their walking, bicycling, swimming, or other low-impact aerobic conditioning may be suggested. Patients who are truly limited in their walking because of neurogenic claudication may find cycling to be easier than walking, because the flexed position of bicycling relieves the pressure on the nerves. Exercise is beneficial for overall health, and patients who are in good aerobic condition have a tendency to recover more quickly from back injuries and have a lower chance of developing chronic, debilitating back conditions.

Medication

Antiinflammatories should be used as a first-line treatment for symptoms associated with degenerative spondylolisthesis. Current COX-2 inhibitors cause less gastric upset and can improve overall function of patients.[18] If side effects occur, such as stomach upset or a bleeding ulcer, or if it is not approved by the patient's primary care physician, use of the medication should be curtailed.

Narcotic-based analgesics should be prescribed only on a short-term basis during severe episodes of pain. If it is recognized that a patient is becoming dependent on analgesics, or if the pain associated with degenerative spondylolisthesis cannot be treated with occasional analgesics, then other treatment options need to be discussed with the patient.

Low doses of antidepressants have been shown to improve the neuropathic pain and chronic nerve pain that can be associated with degenerative spondylolisthesis. Once again, however, overuse and dependence on antidepressant medicines for neuropathic pain should be discouraged.

Weight Reduction

Weight reduction can positively affect a patient's overall health and can help improve symptoms associated with degenerative spondylolisthesis. Although weight reduction can potentially have a larger impact on reducing low-back pain, it might not have as much of an impact on reducing the neurologic symptoms associated with degenerative spondylolisthesis.

Epidural Injections

The use of epidural injections remains somewhat controversial. Some studies note that epidural injections do not have any significant, positive, long-term affect on degenerative spondylolisthesis. However, epidural injections are, at the very least, a temporizing option for patients. Patients who are frail or debilitated, or those who have health issues that would contraindicate potential surgical intervention, may benefit from epidural steroid injections.[19,20]

Other Considerations

Patients who present with degenerative spondylolisthesis can also have myriad other medical conditions. Patients in this age population commonly have comorbidities such as hypertension, diabetes, obesity, cardiac arrhythmias, and cardiomyopathies. In addition, because of their loss of independence, psychological and emotional issues could also be present. It is helpful to use a multidisciplinary approach with a spine surgeon, physical therapist, physiatrist, and primary care physician to help a patient gain both acceptable function and relief from symptoms.[21] A concerted effort should be made by the entire multidisciplinary team to exhaust all conservative measures. However, if symptoms persist and the patient's overall function is compromised, surgical intervention should be considered to help restore function and prevent a prolonged debilitated state.

SURGICAL
Lumbar Spine Decompression-Laminectomy

The standard lumbar laminectomy consists of a midline incision and exposure of the vertebral segment that is to be decompressed. The lumbar lamina is removed out to the margin of the pedicle laterally, from the most proximal segment to the most distal segment. A significant portion of patients have enlarged facets that often need to be either partially resected or undercut to adequately decompress the lateral recesses. Although the lumbar decompression can adequately decompress the neural elements, it is also possible for the slippage to progress and for the symptoms to recur.

A metaanalysis study was performed by Mardjetko et al[22] that included a multitude of papers published between 1970 and 1993. The study revealed that patients who underwent a concomitant arthrodesis had results superior to those patients who did not. Ongoing pain or recurrence of pain is a concern in patients who undergo isolated decompression without fusion. Some surgeons report that this is potentially caused by the radical wide decompression with facetectomies. Patients with unilateral pain that is more radicular and those with minimal back pain can potentially undergo unilateral laminotomies with decompression of the lateral recess. Maintaining the posterior elements and posterior interspinous ligaments can possibly prevent further slippage, allowing adequate treatment of the presenting symptom.

Lumbar Decompression With Noninstrumented Posterolateral Fusion

A landmark study by Herkowitz and Kurz[23] compared decompression alone with decompression and noninstrumented posterolateral fusion in the treatment of patients with degenerative spondylolisthesis with stenosis. The study reported superior results when a concomitant posterolateral fusion was performed with a decompression. In the fused group, 96% of patients had a satisfactory outcome; only 44% in the unfused group had similar results. Herkowitz and Kurz concluded that in situ arthrodesis—when associated with decompression—was far superior to decompression alone; they then recommended the combination of arthrodesis and decompression. This study also concluded that even if a patient develops a pseudarthrosis without solid fusion, the results would be far superior to decompression alone.

The decompression technique is carried out using the standard midline approach. The laminectomy with partial facetectomy is carried out to free the emerging nerve roots that may be compressed by the superior and/or inferior facet.[24] The amount of facetectomy really depends on the severity of the stenosis. In the presence of severe stenosis, both the superior and inferior facets should be aggressively resected. However, if the stenosis is more moderate in the lateral recesses, then a less extensive facetectomy should be performed. A total facetectomy should be avoided because it is usually unnecessary and can potentially promote further slippage even when a fusion is performed. Posterolateral fusion requires meticulous exposure of the transverse processes and lateral wall of the pars.

The surgeon must decide which graft material to use. Graft options include autogenous bone graft from the iliac crest—which can be associated with wound-healing complications in the elderly population—or local autogenous bone graft from the laminectomy site. Other options include using bone graft extenders such as calcium phosphate crystals, demineralized bone matrix, and allograft bone chips (see Chapter 7).

Lumbar Decompression and Posterolateral Fusion With Pedicle Screw Instrumentation

Some surgeons use pedicle screws when performing a decompression and posterolateral fusion. They propose that the pedicle screws lower the chances of the patient needing to wear a brace, shorten the hospital stay, and reduce postoperative pain. In addition, internal fixation has been shown by several authors to increase the fusion rate and decrease the amount of stress that is placed on the fusion segment.[25] Pedicle screws can also help prevent further slippage of the spondylolisthetic segment.

Fischgrund et al[10] conducted a prospective randomized study analyzing the effectiveness of decompressive laminectomy and posterolateral fusion, both with and without instrumentation, in patients with degenerative spondylolisthesis. In those patients who underwent a noninstrumented fusion, 85% experienced good or excellent results, and in those who underwent an instrumented fusion, 76% experienced either good or excellent results. Although a larger percentage of patients in the noninstrumented group experienced excellent or good results, a successful arthrodesis was definitely seen more often in those patients who had undergone instrumented fusion. It was also noted that an excellent or good result was still seen even when there was a pseudarthrosis after a noninstrumented fusion. In a meta-analysis study by Mardjetko et al,[22] the patients who had laminectomies with instrumented and/or noninstrumented fusion had a higher satisfactory rate than those with laminectomy alone. As with the study by Fischgrund et al,[10] the fusion rate was higher in those with an instrumented fusion.

In the end, the decision to use pedicle screws is the surgeon's choice. The surgeon must seriously evaluate the patient's concomitant comorbidities when considering instrumentation possibilities. Placing instrumentation can require longer operative times and more blood loss. Some authors have reported the complication rate to be higher with instrumentation. Most studies in the literature support the belief that the clinical outcome for patients with degenerative spondylolisthesis is more predictable and improves if concomitant posterolateral fusion is performed. Although using pedicle screws improves the fusion rate, there are no strong data showing that the clinical outcome is better with instrumentation.

Posterior Lumbar Interbody Fusion

Interbody devices can be used in conjunction with or without posterolateral fusion and pedicle screw instrumentation. Placing an interbody device improves fusion rate and provides anterior column support. Increasing the intervertebral height and providing anterior column support can reverse vertebral slipping and progression. The restoration of foraminal height can decrease the nerve root compression secondary to foraminal stenosis. Some surgeons believe, anecdotally or otherwise, that placing interbody devices—thereby improving lumbar lordosis—can prevent future adjacent-level breakdowns. Additionally, interbody fusion can prevent the need for a wide dissection and exposure of the transverse processes associated with a posterolateral fusion. This can possibly decrease operative time and blood loss. At this time, the prospective studies investigating whether this type of procedure can yield improved surgical and clinical outcomes are limited.

Anterior Lumbar Interbody Fusion

Proponents of anterior lumbar interbody fusion for the treatment of degenerative spondylolisthesis report satisfactory results.[26,27] A significant amount of support for anterior lumbar interbody fusion for the treatment of degenerative spondylolisthesis is seen in the Japanese literature. Tanaka et al[26] reported that those patients who have a single-level lesion and experience leg pain with walking and standing—but not in the resting position—are good candidates for anterior lumbar interbody fusion. Takahashi et al[27] reported that patients who get a good result from a molded-body orthosis and improve in a flexed position are also good candidates for anterior lumbar interbody fusion. Anterior lumbar interbody fusion can provide an indirect decompression, restore intervertebral height, and reduce slippage of the diseased segment, thereby improving the patient's symptoms. Proponents of this technique also report improved foraminal area, lordosis, and fusion rates because of the large surface area and anterior compression on the graft. When patients have severe end-stage lumbar central and lateral recess stenosis with marked overgrowth of the lumbar facets, a posterior decompression is often needed.[28]

Satomi et al[28] used CT scanning after myelography to establish a staging system for degenerative spondylolisthesis. The early stages of degenerative spondylolisthesis, in which there is no major involvement of the facet joints, are more amenable to anterior lumbar interbody fusion than the later stages. They noted that anterior lumbar interbody fusion was not as effective in cases in which the superior articular process of the lower vertebrae was contributing to neural compression and involved in the clinical symptoms.

XLIF® FOR DEGENERATIVE SPONDYLOLISTHESIS

Extreme lateral interbody fusion (XLIF, NuVasive®, Inc., San Diego, CA) is a novel option for the treatment of degenerative spondylolisthesis.[29] As with other fusion techniques, a multitude of structural improvements in the diseased segments can be accomplished. The interbody device, which has a large surface area, extends across the ring apophysis bilaterally, providing excellent structural support. Major improvements in the intervertebral height, foraminal volume, and lumbar lordosis can be accomplished after placing either a parallel or lordotic graft (Fig. 14-1). Additionally, because both the anterior and posterior longitudinal ligaments remain intact, the listhesis can be reduced through ligamentotaxis and restoration of intervertebral height. The technique described can be performed through a minimally invasive approach using a lateral portal. This technique offers less bleeding than traditionally seen with an open posterior approach, and it also minimizes muscle stripping and denervation of the posterior lumbar musculature, thereby decreasing postoperative pain. Because of the minimally invasive nature of the technique, the lengths of the hospital stay and recovery time are decreased. In addition, because of the excellent exposure of the lateral intervertebral space with the lateral portal, a much larger interbody device can be placed than those used with the standard posterior lumbar interbody technique or transforaminal interbody technique. The operative dissection (2 to 3 cm) and surgical time are far less than those associated with the standard anterior retroperitoneal approach. Technically, placing the cage as far posterior as feasible provides the best reduction of the listhesis.

To treat degenerative spondylolisthesis, XLIF can be performed in a stand-alone mode, with a lateral plate and screws, and/or with posterior pedicle screw instrumentation. The degree of central and/or lateral recess stenosis can help the XLIF surgeon decide whether posterior decompression is necessary; this can be performed adjunctively as either an open procedure

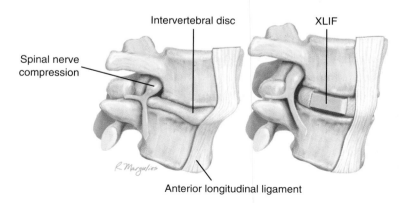

FIG. 14-1 Degenerative spondylolisthesis is corrected with an XLIF procedure, which provides restoration of disc height and ligamentotaxis. Note improvements in the intervertebral height, the forminal area, and in the correction of the listhesis.

or a microprocedure. As mentioned in the previous section, an interbody device spans a very large surface area across the ring apophysis. This allows excellent anterior column support and resultant indirect decompression of the stenotic segment; there is also a strong likelihood of reduction of the listhesis. If the surgeon determines that the patient needs additional support and fixation—as seen in patients with osteoporosis—a lateral plate can be placed through the portal. The lateral plate offers additional stability and can prevent subsidence. Posterior pedicle screw placement can also be considered if added fixation is necessary. With this application, pedicle screw placement via either the percutaneous or minimally invasive approach is ideal. If severe central and lateral recess stenosis is present, posterior decompression with laminectomy could be completed during a single surgery or in a staged fashion.

POSTOPERATIVE MANAGEMENT

The patient is mobilized on the day of surgery with the assistance of a physical therapist. Traditionally the patient is discharged home when he or she is able to void, ambulate under his or her own power, and when the pain is controlled. A normal diet usually can be followed without concern, because there has been no manipulation of the intestines during surgery. If a patient has undergone a one-level XLIF and he or she has no major comorbidities, it is not unusual for that patient to be discharged the day of surgery or the next day. Once discharged, the patient is started on an aggressive walking program. The walks are increased each week by 5-minute increments, until the goal of walking between 45 minutes and 1 hour each day is met. Lifting more than 20 pounds and extreme bending are prohibited until radiographic signs of fusion are seen. If a stand-alone procedure has been performed, a rigid lumbosacral orthosis (LSO) is used for the first 3 months, and if pedicle screws have been placed, the surgeon's preferred orthosis is used.

CASE EXAMPLE

A 50-year-old woman presented with neurogenic claudication and L4-5 degenerative spondylolisthesis (Fig. 14-2). MRI confirmed lumbar stenosis and L4-5 facet disease, which correlates with the patient's symptoms. She had an L4-5 XLIF with percutaneous pedicle screw instrumentation to stabilize and indirectly decompress the segment. She is shown postoperatively. She has returned to clerical work and has experienced a significant improvement in her symptoms.

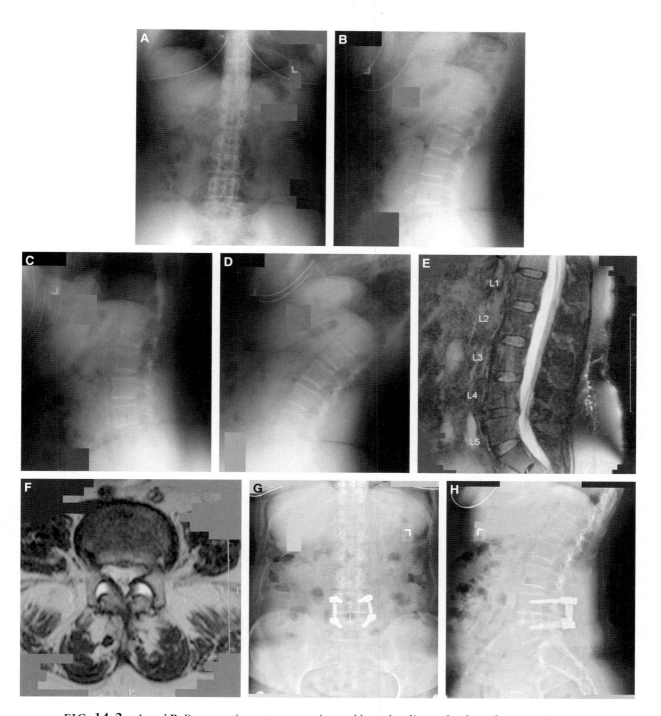

FIG. 14-2 **A** and **B,** Preoperative anteroposterior and lateral radiographs show degenerative spondylolisthesis. **C** and **D,** Anterolisthesis of L4 on L5 is evident on the preoperative flexion and extension radiographs. **E,** The preoperative sagittal T2 MRI demonstrates L4 reduced on L5. **F,** The preoperative axial T2 MRI shows L4-5 subarticular stenosis and abundant fluid in the facet joints. **G** and **H,** Postoperative anteroposterior and lateral radiographs show correction of the alignment.

CONCLUSION

Degenerative spondylolisthesis is common in patients in the sixth decade and older. It is very likely that the development of degenerative spondylolisthesis is caused by anatomic factors such as ligament laxity, degenerative changes of the intervertebral disc, and facet joint orientation. The first line of treatment should be conservative. Surgical intervention should only be considered when conservative measures have been extensively exhausted. Patients with degenerative spondylolisthesis traditionally present with remote episodes of back pain, have developed leg pain, and have resultant neurogenic claudication. It is ideal to distinguish neurogenic claudication from vascular claudication. In degenerative spondylolisthesis, the main presenting symptoms are pain and difficulty with ambulation; both lower extremities are normally involved. Patients commonly report that forward flexion and the "walking with a cart" position will often relieve their symptoms. Sitting also relieves the symptoms associated with claudication. Traditionally the patient's neurologic examination is normal.

It is generally accepted in today's literature that a decompression in conjunction with posterolateral fusion provides the best clinical results. Many physicians prefer to use pedicle screw instrumentation to increase the fusion rate, decrease the need for bracing, and decrease postoperative pain. The literature supports that the use of pedicle screw instrumentation does indeed increase the fusion rate, but there is no definitive proof that the clinical outcome is more successful with pedicle screw instrumentation than without.

The XLIF technique is a novel approach that offers yet another option in the treatment of degenerative spondylolisthesis. XLIF (with or without lateral plate and screws) offers a one-stage procedure to indirectly decompress and reconstruct the diseased segment with moderate stenosis. With moderate stenosis *and* a dynamic component to the spondylolisthesis, extreme lateral interbody fusion with lateral plate or with percutaneous pedicle screws provides a minimally invasive treatment for the diseased segment and can improve the patient's symptoms. In patients who have a more end-stage degenerative spondylolisthesis with severe lumbar stenosis and marked facet arthropathy, the addition of a direct posterior decompression is determined based on the surgeon's experience and preference.

REFERENCES

1. MacNab I. Spondylolisthesis with an intact neural arch: the so-called pseudo-spondylolisthesis. J Bone Joint Surg Br 32:325-333, 1950.
2. Newman P. Stenosis of the lumbar spine and spondylolisthesis. Clin Orthop Relat Res 115:116-121, 1976.
3. Wiltse LL, Newman PH, Macnab I. Classification of spondylolisis and spondylolisthesis. Clin Orthop Relat Res 117:23-29, 1976.

4. Rosenberg NJ. Degenerative spondylolisthesis. Predisposing factors. J Bone Joint Surg Am 57:467-474, 1975.

5. Brown MD, Lockwood JM. Degenerative spondylolisthesis. Instr Course Lect 32:162-169, 1983.

6. Imada K, Matsui H, Tsuji H. Oophorectomy predisposes to degenerative spondylolisthesis. J Bone Joint Surg Br 77:126-130, 1995.

7. Sanderson PL, Frasier RD. The influence of pregnancy on the development of degenerative spondylolisthesis. J Bone Joint Surg Br 78:951-954, 1996.

8. Boden SD, Riew KD, Yamaguchi K, et al. Orientation of the lumbar facet joints: association with degenerative disc disease. J Bone Joint Surg Am 78:403-411, 1996.

9. Lin K, Jenis LG. Degenerative lumbar spondylolisthesis. Semin Spine Surg 15:150-159, 2003.

10. Fischgrund JS, Mackay M, Herkowitz HN, et al. 1997 Volvo Award Winner in Clinical Studies. Degenerative lumbar spondylolisthesis with spinal stenosis: a prospective, randomized study comparing decompressive laminectomy and arthrodesis with and without spinal instrumentation. Spine 22:2807-2812, 1997.

11. Matsunaga S, Sakou T, Morizono Y, et al. Natural history of degenerative spondylolisthesis: pathogenesis and natural course of the slippage. Spine 15:1204-1210, 1990.

12. Matsunaga S, Ijiri K, Hayashi K. Nonsurgically managed patients with degenerative spondylolisthesis: a 10- to 18-year follow-up study. J Neurosurg 93(Suppl 2):S194-S198, 2000.

13. Cauchoix J, Benoist M, Chassaing V. Degenerative spondylolisthesis. Clin Orthop Relat Res 115:122-129, 1976.

14. Whiffen JR, Neuwirth MG. Degenerative spondylolisthesis. In Bridwell KH, Dewald RL, eds. The Textbook of Spinal Surgery, vol 2. Philadelphia: JB Lippincott, 1991, pp 657-674.

15. Koes BW, Scholten RJ, Mens JM, et al. Efficacy of non-steroidal anti-inflammatory drugs for low back pain: a systematic review of randomised clinical trials. Ann Rheum Dis 56:214-223, 1997.

16. Magora A. Conservative treatment in spondylolisthesis. Clin Orthop Relat Res 117:74-79, 1978.

17. Shekelle PG, Adams AH, Chassin M, et al. The Appropriateness of Spinal Manipulation for Low-Back Pain: Indications and Ratings by a Multidisciplinary Expert Panel. Santa Monica, CA: RAND Corp, 1991.

18. Taylor R. Nonoperative management of spinal stenosis. In Herkowitz HN, Garfin SR, Eismont FJ, et al, eds. Rothman-Simeone The Spine, vol 2, 5th ed. Philadelphia: Saunders Elsevier, 2006, pp 1010-1014.

19. Boachie-Adjei O. Conservative management of spondylolisthesis. Semin Spine Surg 1:106-115, 1989.

20. Rosen CD, Kakanovitz N, Bernstein R, et al. A retrospective analysis of the efficacy of epidural steroid injections. Clin Orthop Relat Res 288:270-272, 1988.

21. Capner N. Spondylolisthesis. Br J Surg 19:347-386, 1932.

22. Mardjetko SM, Connolly PJ, Shott S. Degenerative lumbar spondylolisthesis. A meta-analysis of literature 1970-1993. Spine 19(Suppl 20):S2256-S2265, 1994.

23. Herkowitz HN, Kurz LT. Degenerative lumbar spondylolisthesis with spinal stenosis. A prospective study comparing decompression with decompression and intertransverse process arthrodesis. J Bone Joint Surg Am 73:802-808, 1991.

24. Postacchini F, Cinotti G, Perugia D, et al. The surgical treatment of central lumbar stenosis. Multiple laminotomy compared with total laminectomy. J Bone Joint Surg Br 75:386-392, 1993.

25. Zdeblick TA. A prospective, randomized study of lumbar fusion. Preliminary results. Spine 18:1983-1991, 1993.

26. Tanaka M, Nakahara S, Koura H, et al. Minimally invasive anterior lumbar interbody fusion for degenerative spondylolisthesis. Seikeigeka 50:1384-1388, 1995.

27. Takahashi K, Kitahara H, Yamagata M, et al. Long-term results of anterior interbody fusion for treatment of degenerative spondylolisthesis. Spine 15:1211-1215, 1990.

28. Satomi K, Hirabayashi K, Toyama Y, et al. A clinical study of degenerative spondylolisthesis. Radiographic analysis and choice of treatment. Spine 17:1329-1336, 1992.

29. Ozgur BM, Aryan HE, Pimenta L, et al. Extreme lateral interbody fusion (XLIF): a novel surgical technique for anterior lumbar interbody fusion. Spine J 6:435-443, 2006.

15

Clinical Application: Degenerative Scoliosis

Frank M. Phillips ▪ Michael J. Lee ▪ Daniel K. Park

Adult scoliosis is more than 10 degrees of spine curvature in a skeletally mature individual. De novo lumbar scoliosis is thought to develop primarily as a consequence of spinal degeneration and occurs in adulthood without a previous history of scoliosis. The deformity develops as a result of asymmetric disc collapse, vertebral body wedging, and facet arthropathy with loss of facet joint competence. These changes may result in spinal instability and a scoliotic deformity that is often accompanied by the loss of lumbar lordosis. Anterolisthesis may accompany degenerative scoliosis, and rotatory listhesis occurs in up to one third of patients, typically at the L3-4 level. These pathologic features may narrow the spinal canal, causing spinal stenosis that typically manifests with neurogenic claudication symptoms.

EPIDEMIOLOGY

The prevalence of symptomatic degenerative scoliosis has been estimated to be between 2.5% and 7.5% of the population, depending on the age group.[1-3] Recent studies suggest that in an asymptomatic population older than 60 years the prevalence may be as high as 68%.[4] Kobayashi and colleagues[5] prospectively followed 60 patients between the ages of 50 and 84 who had no evidence of scoliosis. During a 12-year follow-up period, 22 of the patients developed de novo scoliosis. Marty-Poumarat et al[6] reported that, in patients with de novo scoliosis, the progression of the curve occurs at a linear rate of 1.64 degrees per year, which is greater than the progression seen in idiopathic scoliosis (0.82 degrees per year).

CLINICAL PRESENTATION

Low back pain is a common presenting symptom of patients with degenerative scoliosis.[1,7] Patients with scoliotic lumbar curves are more likely to have back pain than patients with scoliotic thoracic curves.[8] Generalized back pain may be related to muscle fatigue secondary to imbalance related to the spinal deformity. Pain within the concavity of the curve may be caused by facet arthropathy, disc degeneration, and/or spinal instability. In addition to back pain, patients may also present with symptoms of neurogenic claudication secondary to central, lateral recess, or foraminal stenosis. Liu et al[9] confirmed that the L3 and L4 roots are more strongly compressed by foraminal or extraforaminal stenosis at the concave side of the curve, whereas the L5 and S1 roots are affected by lateral recess stenosis on the convex side of the compensatory curve. Rotatory listhesis is believed to predict back pain as well as radicular symptoms.

A spinal examination of patients with degenerative scoliosis should include a thorough neurologic examination. If there has been a change in bowel or bladder behavior, the examiner should also assess perianal sensation, rectal tone, and the bulbocavernosus reflex. If a patient's history is suggestive of myelopathy, long-tract signs and gait should be assessed to rule out other neurologic conditions. In patients with a history suggestive of claudication, vascular status in the lower extremities should be examined to rule out other potential causes.

The examiner should also assess the overall balance and flexibility of the spine in the coronal and sagittal planes. Pelvic obliquity, waist and shoulder asymmetry, and leg length discrepancy should be evaluated. All patients should also be examined for coexisting hip and knee arthritis and associated contractures.

RADIOGRAPHIC EVALUATION

Standard full-spine standing radiographs should be obtained for any patient with scoliosis. This allows assessment of the patient's global balance in both the coronal and sagittal planes. If the decision has been made to proceed with surgical management, side-to-side bending radiographs may be considered to determine curve flexibility. Bending radiographs in the sagittal plane may also be considered if there is a kyphotic deformity.

Magnetic resonance imagining (MRI) is the gold standard for assessing the extent and location of spinal stenosis in patients with neurogenic claudication. Sagittal MRI images may be useful to assess for foraminal stenosis. In cases for which an MRI is contraindicated, a computed tomography (CT) myelogram can assess for neural compression.

TREATMENT OPTIONS

NONOPERATIVE MANAGEMENT

Nonoperative management of degenerative scoliosis consists primarily of antiinflammatory and analgesic medication, modification of activities, and physical therapy, which usually consists of core-strengthening exercises and cardiovascular conditioning. In general, narcotics should be avoided except for acute pain episodes. When neurocompressive symptoms are present, epidural or nerve root steroid injections can provide diagnostic information as well as symptomatic relief. Recently, Riew et al[10] suggested that most patients with lumbar spinal stenosis who have successful injection treatment for radiculopathy tend to avoid surgery for at least 5 years. Although epidural steroid injections for lumbar stenosis can provide short-term relief, the long-term efficacy of such injections is not well defined. Delport et al[11] retrospectively analyzed 140 patients with lumbar stenosis. After steroid injection treatment, only one third of this group had pain relief lasting more than 2 months. Conversely, Botwin et al[12] reported more than a 50% improvement in pain and a 64% functional improvement after 12 months in a similar population.

OPERATIVE MANAGEMENT

In older patients with degenerative scoliosis, surgery has been primarily offered when nonoperative measures have failed to relieve severe claudication symptoms. Progressive or profound neurologic deficits, which are extremely uncommon, may necessitate surgical intervention. Surgical treatment should be tailored to the patient, based on the severity of his or her symptoms, the deformity, and the patient's overall health, activity level, and expectations of surgery. A surgeon should evaluate numerous factors before considering surgical treatment for degenerative scoliosis. The primary complaints and presumed symptom generators should be carefully identified. In addition, the patient's medical status must be carefully evaluated—medical comorbidities are common in older patient populations, and patients must be medically optimized before surgical intervention. A patient's ability to tolerate surgical procedures also affects the extent of possible surgery. Finally, there are spinal anatomic factors that impact the type of surgical procedure, such as:

- Degree of scoliosis
- Global spinal balance
- Degree and location of spinal stenosis
- Presence of anterolisthesis or rotatory listhesis
- Health of the intervertebral discs
- Bone quality

A patient with radiculopathy or neurogenic claudication, a relatively minor degree of scoliosis (less than 20 degrees), and no anterolisthesis or rotatory listhesis may be treated with a limited decompressive procedure without concomitant fusion. Epstein et al[13] and Nachemson[14] reported acceptable results after performing decompression alone in adult patients with degenerative scoliosis; however, these studies were not well controlled. Frazier et al[15] reported a series of 19 patients with curves greater than 15 degrees; 15 underwent decompression without fusion. Although a direct comparison of patients with and without fusion was not performed, the study suggested that curve magnitude was associated with poorer outcomes.

In patients with more significant scoliosis and/or coexistent anterolisthesis or lateral listhesis, fusion should be considered to prevent progression of the deformity after the destabilizing effects of a laminectomy. In addition, when the spine is destabilized by the extent of bony resection required for effective decompression, fusion should be performed. Preoperative predictors of a more aggressive scoliosis with a higher likelihood of progression include curves of greater magnitudes (>20 degrees), rotatory listhesis (typically L3-4), abnormal motion in bending films, sagittal plane instabilities, and lumbar flat back. These findings are more likely to lead to fusion being performed at the time of decompression. Ideally, the fusion should span the apex of any scoliosis, which often requires fusion from L2 to L5. If the curve extends more proximally, or if there is advanced degeneration with kyphotic deformity in the upper lumbar spine, the fusion may need to be extended to the thoracic spine. With significant spinal decompensation or L5 vertebral tilt, fusion may need to be extended to the sacrum. Supplemental spinal instrumentation in the form of pedicle screw constructs has been shown to increase fusion rates. But these increased fusion rates must be balanced against the risks of hardware failure with osteoporosis, which is frequently present in this patient population. Surgeries of this magnitude in this population are also quite morbid, with a significant risk of complications.

Traditionally, fusion procedures for treating degenerative scoliosis consist of posterior instrumentation, with or without interbody fusion. There are, however, few quality studies documenting outcomes of surgical treatment for this condition. Reports of degenerative scoliosis surgical treatment are retrospective case series. In 1992, Marchesi and Aebi[16] reported a series of 27 patients treated with posterior pedicle instrumentation. They reported better than 50% average correction, few complications, and a 4% pseudarthrosis rate. In 1994, Grubb et al[17] reported on 25 adults with degenerative scoliosis who were treated surgically with posterior procedures. At 2 years of follow-up, 70% of patients reported pain reduction. In 1999, Zurbriggen et al[18] reported on 30 patients with degenerative scoliosis of the lumbar spine who were treated with posterior instrumented fusion. Good to excellent results were reported by 29 patients (96.3%) at a mean follow-up of 59 months. Some authors have reported superior outcomes for combined posterior and interbody fusion over posterior fusion alone. McPhee and Swanson[19] evaluated 21 patients, 11 of whom were treated with interbody and posterior fusion. They found that combined interbody and posterior procedures yielded a higher fusion rate, greater deformity correction, and superior functional results. Grubb et al[17] reported a 40% pseudarthrosis rate in patients with degenerative scoliosis who were treated with posterior-only instrumented fusion, whereas all patients with anteroposterior fusions healed.

These procedures for degenerative scoliosis are associated with long operative times, high blood loss, and extended hospitalization. As the surgical magnitude increases—especially when anterior approaches are combined with posterior surgery—morbidity, complications, and recovery times increase substantially. Zheng et al[20] reported an average hospitalization of 6.2 days, estimated blood loss of 1073 ml, and operative time of 280 minutes in patients undergoing multisegment lumbar decompression fusions. In this study, degenerative scoliosis was found to be associated with longer operative times and higher intraoperative blood loss. In addition, the number of levels fused was significantly associated with length of hospital stay, operative time, blood loss, and volume of blood transfusion. A recent study examined complications in lumbar spine surgery in 161 elderly patients.[21] It found only five major complications in the population, including pulmonary embolism, myocardial infarction, urosepsis, epidural hematoma, and retroperitoneal hematoma. No deaths were reported. In addition to these five major complications, 23 minor complications occurred, including ileus, confusion, urinary retention, urinary tract infection, and deep vein thrombosis. The purpose of this study was to determine whether there was a different complication rate in elderly patients undergoing lumbar fusion with or without instrumentation. The authors did not find a difference, but they did observe that more than four levels of surgery was significantly associated with the occurrence of major complications.

XLIF® FOR DEGENERATIVE SCOLIOSIS

The extreme lateral interbody fusion (XLIF) procedure (NuVasive®, Inc., San Diego, CA) employs a minimally invasive retroperitoneal approach to the interbody space through the psoas muscle. In general, the nerve roots tend to reside in the posterior third of the psoas, so a transpsoas approach should ideally be within the anterior half of the psoas.[22,23] When traversing the psoas muscle, electromyography (EMG) monitoring (NeuroVision® JJB System [NuVasive, Inc.]) is performed to assess the proximity of extraforaminal nerve roots and/or lumbar plexus traveling within the psoas muscle. If monitoring indicates proximity, the Dilator should be redirected. Once the Dilator has safely crossed the psoas muscle to the level of the interspace, sequential Dilators are passed over the initial Dilator, and the final Retractor is placed. EMG monitoring should be used throughout this approach to avoid nerve root injury. After placement of the Retractor, the disc space is prepared, and the interbody device is placed. If interbody fixation is tenuous, then posterior fixation with percutaneous pedicle screws should be performed to augment the segment rigidity.

The XLIF approach for treating degenerative scoliosis may offer various clinical advantages over more traditional techniques. The less invasive nature of this surgery offers the patient more substantial advantages than large instrumented fusion techniques. The minimal dissection and stripping of the XLIF procedure result in less surgical time, less bleeding, and potentially less postoperative pain. This approach also obviates the need for an access surgeon for retroperitoneal interbody access. For correcting scoliotic deformities, the XLIF procedure straightens and derotates the spine through bilateral anular release, placement of a large implant across the disc space spanning the ring apophysis, and the effects of ligamentotaxis. Segmental interbody implant placement realigns the endplates to a horizontal position, restores disc and foraminal heights, and indirectly decompresses the neural elements (Fig. 15-1). Sagittal balance is also corrected and maintained by placement of an implant, either lordotic or nonlordotic, in the anterior half of the disc space. In addition, the interbody space provides a superior environment for fusion compared with the posterolateral gutter used for posterior approaches.

The principle of providing indirect neural decompression by restoring disc height and foraminal volume using an interbody fusion is well established. Indeed, this approach is routinely employed in the cervical spine for treating foraminal stenosis from osteophytes or disc material. However, this treatment has been less extensively studied in the lumbar spine. Vamvanij et al[24] performed a cadaveric study to examine increases in the canal and foraminal cross-sectional areas after interbody device placement in the lumbar spine. A 33.14% increase in the cross-sectional canal area and a 41.03% increase in the foraminal area were observed when a distraction plug was placed from a lateral approach. Further research is required to determine the degree of spinal stenosis that can be treated with indirect decompression using the XLIF technique.

The XLIF technique was first presented by Luiz Pimenta in 2001[25] as a minimally invasive procedure for interbody fusions above L5. A series of the first 145 cases performed in the

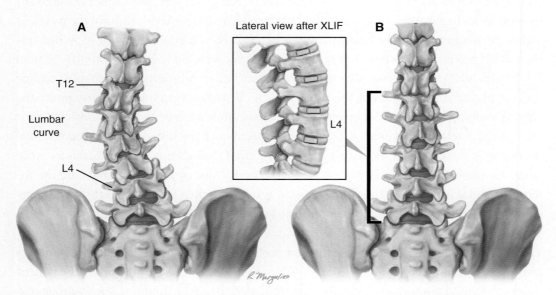

FIG. 15-1   Degenerative scoliosis and restoration. **A,** Preoperative presentation of degenerative scoliosis. **B,** Postoperative presentation after XLIF correction.

United States, by 20 surgeons across the country, was presented by Neill Wright in 2005.[26] Indications for XLIF surgery in this series included degenerative disc disease, recurrent disc herniation, low-grade degenerative spondylolisthesis, pseudarthrosis, and adjacent level degeneration, among others. The study demonstrated the safety and reproducibility of the procedure as well as the minimally invasive benefits: the average operative time was 74 minutes, the average blood loss was less than 100 ml, the average hospital stay was 1 to 2 days, and no major or lasting complications were reported.

As interest and experience with the technique have grown, so too have the indications and potential for applications from the lateral approach. Adult scoliosis, in particular, has been of growing interest, because the XLIF approach offers a less invasive and therefore more tolerable surgical option for patients who often present with significant comorbidities that can complicate the large, invasive reconstructive surgeries that have traditionally been performed for this condition.

POSTOPERATIVE RESULTS

In 2004, Pimenta[27] presented a prospective evaluation on the application of XLIF to treat degenerative scoliosis in his first 12 patients. Patients recovered quickly with no serious complications, and the scoliosis corrections ranged from 18 degrees to 3 degrees, with an average improvement in lumbar lordosis of 14 degrees. Others have since reported similar results,[28,29] and Pimenta continues to present updated follow-up data on the degenerative scoliosis population with his prospective case series. At the most recent presentation, the results included 51 patients reaching 3 years postoperative follow-up with maintenance of deformity correction and symptom resolution.[30] Hsu et al[31] recently presented their results using XLIF for adult deformity correction. In their series, 43 patients encompassing 79 levels were treated with XLIF for a variety of spinal disorders over a 4-year period; of these, 28 patients (59 levels) were diagnosed with a coronal plane deformity including adolescent idiopathic scoliosis and degenerative scoliosis or sagittal plane deformity including focal kyphosis or spondylolisthesis. Fourteen patients received the XLIF procedure for degenerative disc disease without deformity. No major complications occurred, and the authors specifically noted no permanent neurologic deficits, major vessel injuries, bowel injuries, or venous thromboemboli (VTE). Blood loss and hospital stays were reduced compared with open surgical techniques, and VAS improved by an average of 65%. Two cases of prolonged anterior thigh pain on the operative side occurred in the degenerative disc cohort, but the pain resolved by 3 months. One patient required reoperation for a prominent graft and subsequently for subsidence of an L4-5 cage in a long construct to L5. The authors concluded that XLIF is a safe and effective method for anterior release and interbody fusion with spinal deformity.

COMPLICATIONS

Complications related specifically to the XLIF approach have been observed, such as anterior thigh pain, which is usually transient. This may relate to the dissection of the psoas muscle or may reflect neurapraxia related to retraction of the intrapsoas nerves. Isolated cases of neurologic deficit have been reported after XLIF, with most of these being transient sensory changes. Access to the L4-5 disc using the XLIF technique may be compromised by the iliac crest obstructing direct lateral access to the disc. Thoughtful positioning of the patient with lateral bending of the torso may help facilitate the XLIF technique in most situations. When treating patients with degenerative scoliosis, the deformity may dictate the optimal side from which to access the spine. The L4-5 level is typically more easily accessed from within the concavity of the curve.

Because the XLIF technique for treating degenerative scoliosis is a relatively recent development, a number of questions remain to be answered. The amount of stenosis that is amenable to indirect decompression through disc space distraction is unknown. It is likely that, in addition to the XLIF procedure, some patients with more severe spinal stenosis may require direct decompression of the neural elements, which may be accomplished with a minimally invasive posterior decompression. The necessity for supplemental posterior instrumentation to enhance construct rigidity after XLIF is uncertain. Concerns for stand-alone XLIF include the risk of subsidence (particularly for patients with osteoporosis) and pseudarthrosis. These risks need to be balanced against the added morbidity and risks of posterior pedicle screw instrumentation in older patients. If there is concern for the stability of the XLIF construct, it is advisable to add supplemental posterior instrumentation. The role for a novel lateral plate applied using the XLIF approach requires further study.

CASE EXAMPLES

CASE 1: STAND-ALONE

A 64-year-old woman with a history of high blood pressure presented with back pain on a self-reported scale of 7 out of 10, accompanied by leg pain (2 out of 10), and a slight quadriceps deficit (strength 4 out of 5). Preoperative imaging showed degenerative scoliosis of 28 degrees, encompassing mainly the L2-3, L3-4, and L4-5 levels, with lateral listhesis of the L3 vertebral body (Fig. 15-2, *A*), loss of lumbar lordosis (kyphotic by 3 degrees [Fig. 15-2, *B*]), and stenosis at the L2-3 and L3-4 levels (Fig. 15-2, *C*). The operative plan included correction of lateral listhesis at L3, restoration of disc height at L4-5, and improvement in coronal and sagittal balance through a left-sided XLIF from L2-3 to L4-5. It was discussed with and agreed to by the patient that direct posterior decompression would be performed in a second surgery only if symptoms persisted, and that posterior instrumentation would be performed in a second surgery only if loss of correction or pseudarthrosis occurred. The surgery was performed uneventfully, and the patient was ambulating within 5 hours of surgery and discharged home on postoperative day 2. She complained of significant left thigh pain that lasted for 1 week, after which it completely resolved. She had no complaints at the 6-week visit, at which point she had returned to work. Postoperative images showed correction of the scoliosis from 28 degrees to 14 degrees (Fig. 15-2, *D*), and improvement of sagittal alignment from 3 degrees kyphosis to 11 degrees lordosis (Fig. 15-2, *E*). A 6-month CT scan revealed good progression of fusion. The patient was last seen at 9 months postoperatively, with continued complete resolution of symptoms. She was working and extremely happy with the results.

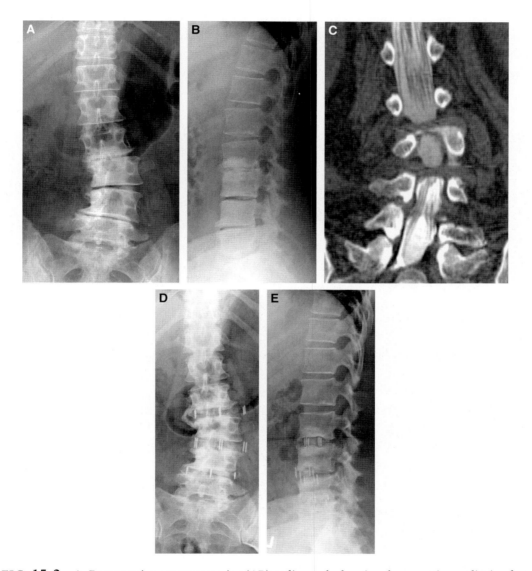

FIG. 15-2 **A,** Preoperative anteroposterior (AP) radiograph showing degenerative scoliosis of 28 degrees at L2-3, L3-4, and L4-5 with lateral listhesis of the L3 vertebral body. **B,** Preoperative lateral radiograph showing loss of lumbar lordosis. **C,** A preoperative CT scan showing stenosis at the L2-3 and L3-4 levels. **D,** Postoperative AP radiograph showing correction of the scoliosis from 28 degrees to 14 degrees. **E,** A postoperative lateral radiograph showing improvement in the sagittal alignment from 3 degrees kyphosis to 11 degrees lordosis.

CASE 2: INSTRUMENTED, WITH DIRECT DECOMPRESSION

This 76-year-old woman with coronary artery disease and hypertension presented with chronic low back pain and neurogenic claudication. She had a two-block walking tolerance and 4 out of 5 strength in her left and right tibialis anterior and left extensor hallucis longus. Preoperative imaging showed 34 degrees of scoliosis with significant axial rotation from L1 to L5, lateral listhesis at L3-4 (Fig. 15-3, *A*), and significant herniation at L2-3 (Fig. 15-2, *B* and *C*). The surgical plan included XLIF from L2 through L5 to decrease the morbidity of the anterior exposure and blood loss. A posterior laminectomy of L2 through L5 and instrumentation of T11 through L5 were added for stabilization and maintenance of deformity correction (Fig. 15-3, *D* and *E*). The patient was ambulatory on postoperative day 2 and was discharged home from the hospital on postoperative day 7.

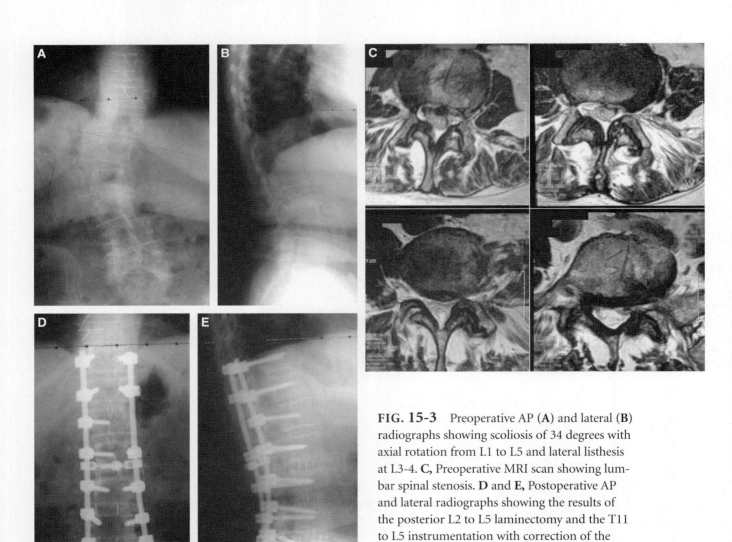

FIG. 15-3   Preoperative AP (**A**) and lateral (**B**) radiographs showing scoliosis of 34 degrees with axial rotation from L1 to L5 and lateral listhesis at L3-4. **C,** Preoperative MRI scan showing lumbar spinal stenosis. **D** and **E,** Postoperative AP and lateral radiographs showing the results of the posterior L2 to L5 laminectomy and the T11 to L5 instrumentation with correction of the scoliosis.

CONCLUSION

There are few data regarding the surgical management of lumbar degenerative scoliosis. The XLIF procedure is a relatively new technique, and long-term follow-up is needed to assess the efficacy of XLIF in treating degenerative scoliosis. Although there are no direct comparative studies, multilevel XLIF appears to have advantages over traditional posterior fusion, with or without interbody fusion, with regard to operative time, hospitalization, blood loss, and postoperative pain.

REFERENCES

1. Kostuik JP, Bentivoglio J. The incidence of low-back pain in adult scoliosis. Spine 3:268-273, 1981.
2. Perennou D, Marcelli C, Herisson C, et al. Adult lumbar scoliosis. Spine 19:123-128, 1994.
3. Vanderpool DW, James JI, Wynne-Davies R. Scoliosis in the elderly. J Bone Joint Surg Am 51:446-455, 1969.
4. Schwab FJ, Ashok D, Lorenzo G, et al. Adult scoliosis: prevalence, SF-36, and nutritional parameters in an elderly volunteer population. Spine 30:1082-1085, 2005.
5. Kobayashi T, Atsuta Y, Takemitsu M, et al. A prospective study of de novo scoliosis in a community based cohort. Spine 31:178-182, 2006.
6. Marty-Poumarat C, Scattin L, Marpeau M. Natural history of progressive adult scoliosis. Spine 32:1227-1234, 2007.
7. Jackson RP, Simmons EH, Stripinis D. Incidence and severity of back pain in adult idiopathic scoliosis. Spine 8:749-756, 1983.
8. Jackson RP, Simmons EH, Stripinis D. Coronal and sagittal plane spinal deformities correlating with back pain and pulmonary function in adult idiopathic scoliosis. Spine 14:1391-1397, 1989.
9. Liu H, Ishihara H, Kanamori M, et al. Characteristics of nerve root compression caused by degenerative lumbar spinal stenosis with scoliosis. Spine J 3:524-529, 2003.
10. Riew KD, Park JB, Cho YS, et al. Nerve root blocks in the treatment of lumbar radicular pain. A minimum five-year follow-up. J Bone Joint Surg Am 88:1722-1725, 2006.
11. Delport EG, Cucuzzella AR, Marley JK, et al. Treatment of lumbar spinal stenosis with epidural steroid injections: a retrospective outcome study. Arch Phys Med Rehabil 85:479-484, 2004.
12. Botwin KP, Gruber RD, Bouchlas CG, et al. Fluoroscopically guided lumbar transforaminal epidural steroid injections in degenerative lumbar stenosis: an outcome study. Am J Phys Med Rehabil 81:898-905, 2002.
13. Epstein JA, Epstein BS, Jones MD. Symptomatic lumbar scoliosis with degenerative changes in the elderly. Spine 4:542–547, 1979.
14. Nachemson A. Adult scoliosis and back pain. Spine 4:513–517, 1979.
15. Frazier DD, Lipson SJ, Fossel AH, et al. Associations between spinal deformity and outcomes after decompression for spinal stenosis. Spine 22:2025–2029, 1997.
16. Marchesi DG, Aebi M. Pedicle fixation devices in the treatment of adult lumbar scoliosis. Spine 17(Suppl 8):S304-S309, 1992.
17. Grubb SA, Lipscomb HJ, Suh PB. Results of surgical treatment of painful adult scoliosis. Spine 19:1619-1627, 1994.
18. Zurbriggen C, Markwalder TM, Wyss S. Long-term results in patients treated with posterior instrumentation and fusion for degenerative scoliosis of the lumbar spine. Acta Neurochir (Wien) 141:21-26, 1999.

19. McPhee IB, Swanson CE. The surgical management of degenerative lumbar scoliosis. Posterior instrumentation alone versus two stage surgery. Bull Hosp Jt Dis 57:16-22, 1998.

20. Zheng F, Cammisa FP Jr, Sandhu HS, et al. Factors predicting hospital stay, operative time, blood loss, and transfusion in patients undergoing revision posterior lumbar spine decompression, fusion, and segmental instrumentation. Spine 27:818-824, 2002.

21. Cassinelli EH, Eubanks J, Vogt M, et al. Risk factors for the development of perioperative complications in elderly patients undergoing lumbar decompression and arthrodesis for spinal stenosis: an analysis of 166 patients. Spine 32:230-235, 2007.

22. Ebraheim NA, Xu R, Huntoon M, et al. Location of extraforaminal lumbar nerve roots: an anatomic study. Clin Orthop 340:230-235, 1997.

23. Gu Y, Ebraheim NA, Xu R, et al. Anatomic considerations of the posterolateral lumbar disk region. Orthopedics 24:56-58, 2001.

24. Vamvanij V, Ferrara LA, Hai Y, et al. Quantitative changes in spinal canal dimensions using interbody distraction for spondylolisthesis. Spine 26:13-18, 2001.

25. Pimenta L. Lateral endoscopic transpsoas retroperitoneal approach for lumbar spine surgery. Presented at the Eighth Brazilian Spine Society Meeting, Belo Horizonte, Brazil, May 2001.

26. Wright N. XLIF: the United States experience 2003-2004. Presented at the International Meeting on Advanced Spinal Techniques, Banff, Canada, July 2005.

27. Pimenta L. A new minimally invasive surgical technique for adult degenerative scoliosis. Poster presented at the International Meeting on Advanced Spinal Techniques, Bermuda, July 2004.

28. Ozgur B, Aryan H, Taylor W. Adult degenerative scoliosis repair via an extreme lateral interbody fusion technique (XLIF). Poster presented at the International Meeting on Advanced Spinal Techniques, Banff, Canada, July 2005.

29. Ozgur B, Aryan H, Taylor W. Five-level combined thoracoscopic and extreme lateral interbody fusion (XLIF) for adult degenerative scoliosis repair: case report. Poster presented at the International Meeting on Advanced Spinal Techniques, Banff, Canada, July 2005.

30. Diaz R, Phillips F, Pimenta L. XLIF for lumbar degenerative scoliosis: outcomes of minimally-invasive surgical treatment out to 3 years post-op. Presented at the North American Spine Society Annual Meeting, Seattle, WA, Sept, 2006.

31. Hsu V, Akbarnia B, Van Dam B, et al. eXtreme lateral interbody fusion for adult deformity: the safety, early benefits, and results of a novel approach to the spine. Presented at the International Meeting on Advanced Spinal Techniques, Paradise Island, Bahamas, July 2007.

16

Clinical Application: Complex Deformity

R. Shay Bess ▪ Behrooz A. Akbarnia
Darrel S. Brodke ▪ Ramin Bagheri

Complex adult spinal deformity is a general term that includes coronal and sagittal plane deformities of variable causes, such as residual childhood idiopathic, congenital, and neuromuscular spinal deformities presenting in the adult; degenerative scoliosis secondary to disc and facet degeneration; posttraumatic deformities; and iatrogenic deformity secondary to wide laminectomy or spinal arthrodesis with lumbar hypolordosis (iatrogenic flat back). Adult spinal deformity is a growing medical challenge. It has been estimated that approximately 6% of adults over 50 years of age have scoliosis and that approximately 500,000 adults in the United States have scoliotic curves greater than 30 degrees.[1,2] The treatments for adult spinal deformities are markedly different from the treatments for childhood spinal deformities. Children with spinal deformities often present with minimal symptoms, minimal disability, and few or no medical comorbidities. Consequently, management focuses on preventing curve progression and the future sequelae that result from the deformity. Affected adults, however, have been shown to demonstrate greater function limitations, greater daily analgesic use, and less satisfaction with their appearance compared with unaffected individuals.[3-8] Therefore the goals of management of adult spinal deformity include the restoration of coronal and sagittal balance, providing pain relief, and improving the quality of life.

A discussion of the variety of nonoperative and operative options for treating adult spinal deformities is unfortunately beyond the scope of this chapter. However, this discussion provides a brief overview of the clinical and radiographic assessment of adult patients with spinal deformities and focuses on indications and options for anterior column support, emphasizing the benefits of lateral access to the anterior column in this population. Supporting biomechanical data for lateral interbody fusion are also presented.

INITIAL ASSESSMENT

A thorough history and physical examination should be obtained to assess the cause and duration of the patient's deformity, previous treatment, recent deformity progression, any recent increase in pain and/or disability, and the distribution of back and leg pain. Symptoms of radiculopathy and neurogenic claudication should be elucidated. The patient's comorbidities, nicotine use, and functional status are also obtained. Increased comorbidities and associated debilitation may cause patients to have an apparent physiologic age that exceeds their chronologic age, which may result in poor toleration of the demands of an extensive reconstructive surgery.[1,9-12] Treating physicians may want to consider nonoperative or appropriate limited operative treatment in this frail patient population. Conversely, if the patient's physiologic age appears to be equal to or less than the chronologic age, a discussion of more extensive reconstructive procedures should take place. If a nonoperative treatment is chosen, patients with thoracic curves that exceed 50 degrees or lumbar curves that exceed 30 degrees should be counseled that they are at risk for curve progression.[13,14]

RADIOGRAPHIC EVALUATION

Optimal radiographic evaluation of adult spinal deformities includes standing 36-inch cassette anteroposterior and lateral radiographs of, at minimum, C7 to the pelvis and femoral heads. This film allows assessment of the patient's coronal and sagittal balance, measurement of spinopelvic parameters, and simultaneous visualization of the primary and secondary scoliotic curves in the functional standing position. Supine and side-bending films are also recommended to assess the flexibility of the patient's deformity and to help differentiate structural from compensatory curves. A lateral bolster hyperextension radiograph delineates the flexibility of sagittal deformities and helps the treating physician to decide whether postural reduction of the deformity provides correction or if more extensive interbody reconstruction or osteotomy procedures are needed.

As with other spinal disorders, advanced diagnostic imaging, including magnetic resonance imaging (MRI) and computed tomography (CT) myelography, should be used to evaluate for neural element compression in patients with radicular or claudication symptoms. Although MRI is currently the standard diagnostic modality used to assess neural compression, scoliotic vertebral rotation may confound MRI findings. In this setting, CT myelography may better delineate foraminal, apical, and lateral recess stenosis, although the benefits of myelography should be weighed against the invasive nature of this examination. MRI also allows assessment of intervertebral disc degeneration. Information gained from CT and MRI, in combination with radiographic evidence of disc degeneration, helps in the decision to include or exclude cephalad and caudad vertebral levels in the spinal arthrodesis.[15]

OPERATIVE TREATMENT AND CONSIDERATIONS FOR ANTERIOR COLUMN SUPPORT

Segmental spinal instrumentation has revolutionized the treatment of spinal deformities. Pedicle screw (PS) constructs, in particular, have demonstrated improved coronal and sagittal correction compared with traditional hook-and-wire constructs.[16-25] Despite technical advances in PS instrumentation, structural anterior column support combined with posterior spine fusion (PSF) has many benefits when treating a spinal deformity. These benefits include the creation of a load-sharing environment for segmental implants that increases the endurance limit of the construct; reduction of lateral olisthesis; restoration of segmental lordosis; improved sagittal balance; and improved fusion rates in clinical scenarios that are challenging for successful arthrodesis (for example, revision spine surgery, deficient posterior elements after a wide laminectomy, and chronic nicotine use).[26-28] The absolute indications for combined anterior-posterior spine fusion (APSF) versus those for stand-alone anterior spine fusion (ASF) or PSF are unclear. Historically, anterior release and structural interbody fusion, as the anterior portion of the APSF procedure, have demonstrated greater fusion rates, greater coronal correction, and greater maintenance of physiologic lumbar lordosis than stand-alone PSF. Traditionally, patients who are candidates for the combined approach include those with thoracolumbar and lumbar (TL/L) coronal deformities greater than 45 degrees, deformities with an apical translation greater than 3 cm from the center sacral vertebral line (CSVL), lateral olisthesis (greater than 5 mm) of the apical vertebrae, and rigid sagittal deformities with less than 20 degrees of lordosis (Table 16-1).[28-30] APSF has also been recommended for patients with constructs that cross the lumbosacral junction, because pseudarthrosis rates as high as 15% to 20% have been reported when performing stand-alone posterior arthrodesis across the lumbosacral junction.[31]

The following approaches are available to access the interbody space and achieve structural anterior column support: anterior lumbar interbody fusion (ALIF), posterior lumbar interbody fusion (PLIF), transforminal lumbar interbody fusion (TLIF), and, more recently, the

TABLE 16-1   Historical Indications for Combined APSF in Thoracolumbar and Lumbar Deformity.[27-30]

Condition	Radiographic Value
Coronal deformity	Cobb angle greater than 45 degrees
Apical translation	More than 3 cm from the CSVL
Lateral olisthesis	Greater than 5 mm
Sagittal deformity	Less than 20 degrees of lordosis in the Cobb angle measured from T12 to S1

CSVL, Center sacral vertical line.

lateral approach to the interspace (extreme lateral interbody fusion [XLIF®], NuVasive®, Inc., San Diego, CA). In this chapter, we review reports on the traditional methods used to approach the lumbar interspace and describe the early experiences of XLIF, used to achieve anterior column support in adult patients with TL/L deformities.

APPROACHES TO THE ANTERIOR COLUMN IN TL/L DEFORMITY

Traditionally, the anterior procedure for large TL/L deformities has included a thoracoabdominal approach, multilevel lumbar discectomy, and structural interbody grafting. Structural interbody grafting has demonstrated lower pseudarthrosis rates and improved maintenance of lordosis compared with morselized autograft or iliac crest autografting in the anterior column.[32] However, the value of multilevel ASF has recently been questioned. A number of studies have demonstrated increased morbidity associated with an extensive anterior or anteriolateral approach and have questioned the need for multilevel anterior dissection when using PS constructs.[33-36] Using the Scoliosis Research Society (SRS) Morbidity and Mortality database over a 3-year period, Coe et al[37] reported on the complications associated with performing spine fusions on patients with adolescent idiopathic scoliosis (AIS). The overall complication rate for all procedures was 5.7% (363 complications per 6334 spine fusions). Of the 4369 patients who underwent PSF, 221 (5.1%) had complications, whereas 82 of the 801 (10.1%) patients who underwent combined APSF had complications ($p < 0.0001$). To our knowledge, there are no studies that compare the radiographic and clinical outcomes of APSF with PSF for adult spinal deformities. However, if the surgical morbidities reported for patients with AIS are extrapolated to adult scoliosis, the complications for a large, multilevel APSF procedure will undoubtedly be greater in the adult population, because the overall surgical complication rate reported for adults treated for spinal deformity is approximately 25% to 30%.[11] Complications may be even greater if the spine is exposed more than once.[38]

The link between nutrition and wound healing is a critical issue that must be considered for adult patients with spinal deformities who undergo surgical treatment. Lenke et al[39] prospectively analyzed the length of time required for patients to return to their preoperative nutritional baselines after they have undergone spinal reconstructions. The authors found that normalization to baseline nutritional status occurs, on average, within 6 weeks. Patients who underwent fusion of more than 10 spine levels and those undergoing APSF were at an increased risk for prolonged normalization (more than 12 weeks) to baseline.

Kim et al[40] reported on the morbidity of adult scoliosis patients who received a thoracolumbar (TL) approach as part of an APSF. Of these patients, 25% rated the pain over the TL scar as moderate to severe, 50% reported bulging of the TL scar, and 25% reported limitations in their activities of daily living because of the anterior incision. Consequently, many surgeons have begun to reconsider extensive multilevel ASF combined with PSF procedures for TL/L deformities and are pursuing alternative, less invasive procedures for anterior column support. These alternatives include a paramedian approach for low lumbar (L4-5 and L4-S1) ASF, a multilevel PLIF or TLIF at the base of the construct, and, more recently, a multilevel lateral approach and interbody fusion (XLIF).

Good results have been reported using a retroperitoneal paramedian approach to provide access to the low lumbar spine (L4-5 and L5-S1). This approach provides structural anterior column support to the foundation of a long thoracolumbar construct and increases fusion rates across the lumbosacral junction. The approach also preserves the abdominal viscera within the peritoneal envelope and minimizes operative intestinal trauma, which in turn may reduce the formation of visceral adhesions, shorten the duration of postoperative ileus, and reduce intravenous fluid requirements (as compared with a transperitoneal approach).[41] The paramedian retroperitoneal approach may be used to achieve exposure from the sacrum to L2 and is associated with less postoperative muscle pain than a standard flank approach. Dissection proximal to L2 is prevented by the renal vessels.[42,43] PLIF and TLIF may also be used to approach the lower lumbar interbody space and provide a foundation for long constructs. The advantage of using PLIF or TLIF for interbody fusion in patients with large TL/L deformities is that a 360-degree fusion can be achieved in a single-stage, all-posterior approach.[44] This eliminates the need to choose between a same-day or staged procedure and between an initial anterior and posterior procedure. The all-posterior approach is also useful for patients in whom an anterior approach is challenging, including patients who have undergone abdominal procedures and obese patients. The need for nasogastric suction is also eliminated, and the amount of postoperative ileus is reduced. Additionally, the risk of retrograde ejaculation in men caused by damage to the hypogastric plexus at L5-S1 is eliminated. When comparing combined anterior and posterior approaches for APSF with TLIF and PSF, combined approaches have been associated with increased costs, increased operating room time, greater blood loss, longer hospital and intensive care unit stays, and a greater incidence of perioperative complications.[45,46]

Lateral interbody fusion is emerging as a viable alternative for achieving anterior column support in patients with thoracolumbar deformity. The interspaces from T12-L1 to L4-5 can be approached retroperitoneally via a transpsoas lateral approach to the interspace. The benefits of a lateral approach include less tissue dissection and a smaller incision than with a conventional thoracolumbar approach and greater access to cephalad lumbar disc spaces than with a paramedian approach. Consequently, the complications and morbidity of an anterior approach are reduced. The lateral approach also requires that less tissue be dissected, improving the postoperative nutritional status and resulting in faster wound healing. Because the lateral approach maintains the anterior longitudinal ligament (ALL), and because of the stability generated by the CoRoent® interbody cage (NuVasive, Inc.), patients who initially undergo multilevel XLIF as part of a staged spinal reconstruction are able to mobilize between the lateral and posterior stages. Bess et al[47] reported that stand-alone XLIF increased flexion/extension stiffness by 457%, increased lateral bending stiffness by 375%, and increased axial rotation stiffness by 179%, compared with the intact spine. Consequently, physicians can more confidently mobilize patients between stages after a stand-alone interbody fusion, reducing the risk for pneumonia, deep vein thrombosis, and decubitus ulcers. This is not possible with multilevel, stand-alone ALIF, because of the risk of implant dislodgement. Stand-alone ALIF can be supplemented with anterior or lateral instrumentation; however, the additional implants necessitate further dissection and impede any deformity correction that is generated during the posterior part of the procedure. Lateral interbody fusion also minimizes the risk of device displacement during the posterior procedure; stand-alone ALIF devices can become displaced when the patient is being placed in a prone position or during the posterior procedure. Additionally, if the patient becomes unstable or if complications occur during the XLIF procedure, the surgeon can confidently convert a planned same-day procedure to a staged procedure without the worry of unstable interbody implants.

Many of the complications of ALIF can be avoided by performing PLIF or TLIF for interbody fusions. However, posterior-based procedures are unable to provide the primary benefits of ALIF for deformity correction—an extensive discectomy and release, a large graft for better sagittal and lateral olisthesis correction, and increased space for interbody fusion. Additionally, multilevel (three levels or more) PLIF or TLIF is time consuming and may be associated with excessive blood loss and neural retraction. PLIF and TLIF are also challenging if the patient has had previous lumbar decompression; the surgeon often must dissect through an extensive dural scar, even when performing TLIF. Consequently, XLIF is able to provide the benefits of both ALIF and PLIF/TLIF and minimize the negative aspects of these procedures. However, the techniques for and outcomes of patients undergoing multilevel XLIF for TL/L deformities require additional study. Diaz et al[48] and Ozgur et al[49] have reported good preliminary results using XLIF for degenerative lumbar scoliosis; however, these studies had a limited number of patients, small curve magnitudes (less than 20 degrees), and short-term follow-ups (1 year).[50]

Multilevel XLIF for Adult Thoracolumbar Deformity

The techniques for approaching the lateral spine and applying XLIF to TL/L deformities are the same as for a spine with minimal deformity; however, the margin for error is smaller, and the fundamentals for XLIF must be followed closely (Fig. 16-1).

SAME-DAY VERSUS STAGED PROCEDURES

The decision to perform a staged or same-day procedure depends on the extent of the planned procedure and the physiologic age of the patient. We prefer to perform the XLIF procedure first, because we believe that the coronal and sagittal correction provided by the

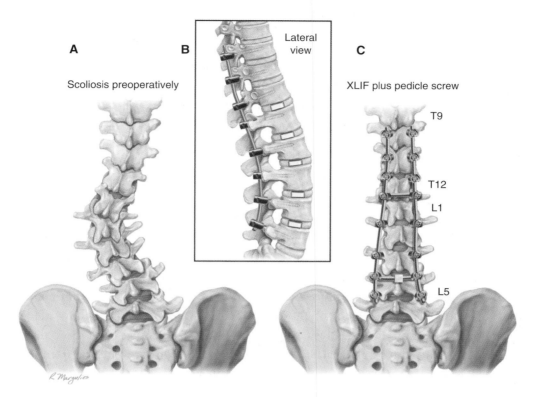

FIG. 16-1 **A,** Thoracolumbar scoliosis before surgery. **B** and **C,** After correction with multilevel XLIF.

XLIF procedure is maximized by placing the XLIF interbody grafts before securing the spine with posterior segmental implants. Although XLIF has been used as a stand-alone procedure, we always combine XLIF with segmental posterior spinal arthrodesis if an adult patient has a complex TL/L scoliosis curve greater than 30 degrees.

Reduced morbidity and reduced postoperative complications have been described when combined reconstructions are performed as same-day rather than as staged procedures.[51-54] Studies have suggested that when performing complex reconstructions in a staged fashion, patients are malnourished from the first stage and are at increased risk for complications from the second surgical procedure. However, large, multilevel, complex spinal reconstructions often require prolonged operative times, resulting in excessive blood loss and prolonged anesthesia. These may be more practical as staged procedures, because surgeon- and patient-related complication rates have been shown to increase in procedures extending beyond 12 hours. Lapp et al[55] evaluated patients undergoing same-day or staged spinal reconstruction surgery (with more than 10 levels) who were randomized to receive or not receive total parenteral nutrition (TPN). Patients who underwent staged APSF reconstructions with TPN administration showed statistically less nutritional depletion and fewer major complications than those who underwent same-day reconstructions with or without TPN. The authors recommended considering staging surgeries and administering TPN after each stage if the procedure time is anticipated to be 10 hours or more and blood loss more than 2000 ml.

CONCAVITY OR CONVEXITY APPROACH

The decision to approach the lumbar curve from the concavity or convexity is best determined by the flexibility of the lumbar curve and the alignment of the L4-5 interspace. The benefits of approaching the deformity from the convexity include the proximity of the vertebral interspace to the skin surface, because the disc spaces are closer to the skin surface than in the concavity. The disc spaces are also wedged open in the convexity compared with the concavity. Additionally, bridging osteophytes are often present in the concavity, and may obscure the disc space, creating an obstacle when approaching the intervertebral disc space. A primary benefit of approaching the interspace from the curve's concavity is the favorable angle of the disc spaces. The cephalad and caudad interspaces are tilted into the concavity. This is especially beneficial at L4-5, because the orientation of the disc space tilts the L4-5 interspace away from the pelvis on the concavity and into the pelvis on the convexity. Therefore the orientation of the L4-5 disc space may preclude an approach from the convexity, because the pelvis and iliac crest may obscure the interspace. The L4-5 orientation, however, may be flexible, so that if, on the preoperative lateral bending films (and when positioning the patient on the operative table), the L4-5 disc space comes to lie above the iliac crest, the deformity can be approached from the convexity. This prevents the need to flip the patient and perform the XLIF procedure from both sides.

Preoperative lateral bending films may demonstrate that the deformity is flexible in the coronal plane and corrects appreciably compared with the standing films. In this scenario, the curve can easily be approached from the concavity, because, as mentioned in the previous paragraph, an approach from the concavity facilitates access to the L4-5 interspace. If the curve is rigid, however, it will likely be easier to access the interspaces across the convexity, and, if necessary, perform the L4-5 XLIF from the contralateral (concave) side.

PATIENT POSITIONING

Patient positioning is crucial. Care and time must be taken to ensure that the spine is approached from a direct lateral position. Because the scoliotic spine is rotated, the surgeon must take into account the respective axial deformity and align the patient in a true lateral position. If the approach to the interspace is not directly lateral in each level, the instruments used to perform the discectomy and the interbody device will be directed ventrally, through the ALL into the abdomen, or dorsally, into the spinal canal. The pedicles, as viewed in the AP plane, are the best landmark for a true lateral position. Patients with spinal deformities may have had prior lumbar procedures and may have deficient or absent posterior elements. Consequently, the spinous processes may not be available for reference as a landmark to determine vertebral rotation. The pedicles are a consistent landmark, and their presence allows the surgeon to safely approach the interspace in the setting of a prior lumbar decompression. Instead of rotating the fluoroscope, we recommend rotating the patient and operative table when aligning the interspace to ensure that the disc space is perpendicular to the floor. In this manner, the fluoroscope and surgeon work directly perpendicular to the disc space, which is aligned perpendicular to the floor. This positioning reduces the amount of instrument misdirection, because the surgeon is always working perpendicular to the floor. As each successive interspace is approached, the table must be rotated accordingly to account for axial vertebral rotation, ensuring that each level is perpendicular to the floor. The surgeon must also account for lateral tilt and olisthesis of the scoliotic spine to ensure that the disc space is approached from a true lateral position in the coronal plane, as well as the axial plane. Adjusting the tilt of the table at each disc space corrects the deformity visible on the lateral fluoroscopic view and allows the surgeon to safely approach the disc space without compromising the vertebral endplates.

NUMBER OF INTERSPACES TO XLIF

No hard rule is available regarding the number of interspaces to fuse. When performing a multilevel XLIF to correct adult deformities, we recommend that the apex of the curve and the base of the construct be fused. The maximal amount of coronal and sagittal correction occurs when releasing the disc space and performing XLIF across the apex of the curve. Additionally, the base of the construct requires an interbody fusion to prevent pseudarthrosis. Sequential correction often occurs with multilevel XLIF; therefore it may not be necessary to perform XLIF from end vertebra to end vertebra across the curve. As the case progresses, the amount of correction obtained should be assessed and, if possible, the cephalad levels limited. It is important to note, however, that the TL junction has the highest rate of pseudarthrosis after surgery for adult spinal deformities; these levels will likely benefit from interbody fusion and an associated higher fusion rate.[56]

POSTERIOR FUSION

We routinely perform a posterior segmental instrumented spinal arthrodesis in conjunction with multilevel XLIF. Inclusion of the cephalad and caudad stable vertebrae within the arthrodesis limits the risk of postoperative curve decompensation. However, as indicated previously, the benefit of performing multilevel XLIF before the posterior arthrodesis is that the number of fusion levels may be reduced secondary to coronal and sagittal correction resulting from the initial XLIF procedure. Including the L5-S1 space within the arthrodesis is debatable. Guidelines for including L5-S1 have been described previously.[15,28,31]

POSTOPERATIVE MANAGEMENT

Patients are mobilized on postoperative day 1. Early mobilization reduces the risk for perioperative pulmonary and skin complications and encourages the return of bowel and bladder function. If the XLIF and posterior arthrodesis procedures are not performed on the same day, we continue to mobilize patients and encourage ambulation after stand-alone XLIF interbody procedures until the posterior procedure is performed. We believe that the initial stability provided by the XLIF interbody grafts and retention of the ALL during the technique allow safe interval mobilization with minimal risk for graft dislodgement. This is an additional benefit of multilevel XLIF over standard multilevel ALIF, because patient ambulation in the setting of a stand-alone initial multilevel ALIF would undoubtedly lead to graft dislodgement.

Postoperative bracing is debatable. No study definitively supports or refutes the use or duration of a postoperative brace.[57-59] The theoretical benefit of rigid external support must be weighed against the biomechanical disadvantages of the brace's distance from the spine, brace discomfort, and the risk of skin breakdown.

Patients are followed on a routine postoperative basis—usually at 2 to 4 weeks to check the wound; at 1, 3, 6, and 12 months postoperatively; and yearly thereafter. Radiographs are obtained at each visit. Patients are evaluated clinically and radiographically for signs and symptoms of perioperative complications, including infection, implant dislodgement, adjacent-segment degeneration, proximal- and distal-junction kyphosis, and pseudarthrosis. Studies have indicated that patients need to be followed clinically and radiographically for at least 5 years or more to confirm solid arthrodesis.[56]

CASE EXAMPLE

This 59-year-old woman presented with adult idiopathic scoliosis (Fig. 16-2). Her T12-L4 left lumbar curve measured 53 degrees and bent to 41 degrees. The preoperative MRI showed degeneration of the L4-5 disc. Surgery included a five-level XLIF at T12-L1, L1-2, L2-3, L3-4, and L4-5, and posterior spine fusion with instrumentation from T10-L5. She is shown 1 year postoperatively.

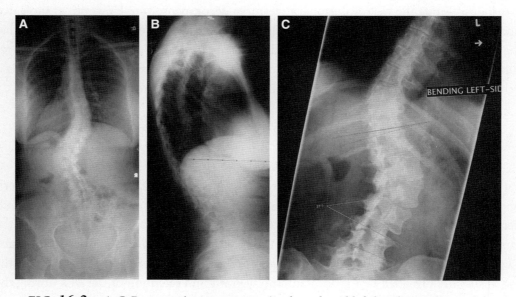

FIG. 16-2   **A-C,** Preoperative anteroposterior, lateral, and left-bending radiographs.

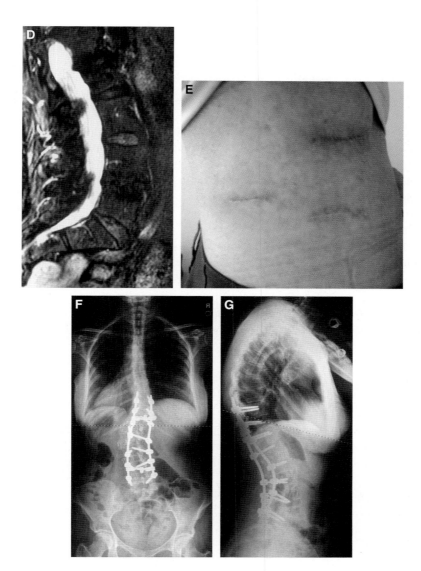

FIG. 16-2, cont'd   **D,** Preoperative MRI. **E,** The patient is shown 6 months postoperatively. **F** and **G,** Anteroposterior and lateral radiographs obtained 1 year postoperatively.

CONCLUSION

Multilevel XLIF combined with instrumented PSF provides excellent coronal and sagittal correction in adult patients with TL/L spinal deformities. The technique allows a multilevel, structural interbody fusion to be performed with minimal soft tissue dissection, avoiding many of the morbidities of a multilevel open ALIF and allowing a more extensive release and placement of a larger interbody graft than posterior interbody procedures. Multilevel XLIF is a more viable alternative to interbody fusion than conventional techniques and is our preferred method for soft tissue release and interbody fusion for most adult TL/L deformities.

REFERENCES

1. Bradford DS, Tay BK, Hu SS. Adult scoliosis: surgical indications, operative management, complications, and outcomes. Spine 24:2617-2629, 1999.

2. Vanderpool DW, James JI, Wynne-Davies R. Scoliosis in the elderly. J Bone Joint Surg Am 51:446-455, 1969.

3. Berven S, Deviren V, Demir-Deviren S, et al. Studies in the modified Scoliosis Research Society Outcomes Instrument in adults: validation, reliability, and discriminatory capacity. Spine 28:2164-2169; discussion 2169, 2003.

4. Ascani E, Bartolozzi P, Logroscino CA, et al. Natural history of untreated idiopathic scoliosis after skeletal maturity. Spine 11:784-789, 1986.

5. Nilsonne U, Lundgren KD. Long-term prognosis in idiopathic scoliosis. Acta Orthop Scand 39:456-465, 1968.

6. Deviren V, Berven S, Kleinstueck F, et al. Predictors of flexibility and pain patterns in thoracolumbar and lumbar idiopathic scoliosis. Spine 27:2346-2349, 2002.

7. Weinstein SL. Bristol-Myers Squibb/Zimmer award for distinguished achievement in orthopaedic research. Long-term follow-up of pediatric orthopaedic conditions. Natural history and outcomes of treatment. J Bone Joint Surg Am 82:980-990, 2000.

8. Glassman SD, Bridwell K, Dimar JR, et al. The impact of positive sagittal balance in adult spinal deformity. Spine 30:2024-2029, 2005.

9. Daubs MD, Lenke LG, Cheh G, et al. Adult spinal deformity surgery: complications and outcomes in patients over age 60. Spine 32:2238-2244, 2007.

10. Grubb SA, Lipscomb HJ, Suh PB. Results of surgical treatment of painful adult scoliosis. Spine 19:1619-1627, 1994.

11. Linville DA, Bridwell KH, Lenke LG, et al. Complications in the adult spinal deformity patient having combined surgery. Does revision increase the risk? Spine 24:355-363, 1999.

12. Hu SS, Berven SH. Preparing the adult deformity patient for spinal surgery. Spine 31:S126-S131, 2006.

13. Korovessis P, Piperos G, Sidiropoulos P, et al. Adult idiopathic lumbar scoliosis. A formula for prediction of progression and review of the literature. Spine 19:1926-1932, 1994.

14. Weinstein SL, Ponseti IV. Curve progression in idiopathic scoliosis. J Bone Joint Surg Am 65:447-455, 1983.

15. Kuhns CA, Bridwell KH, Lenke LG, et al. Thoracolumbar deformity arthrodesis stopping at L5: fate of the L5-S1 disc, minimum 5-year follow-up. Spine 32:2771-2776, 2007.

16. Luhmann SJ, Lenke LG, Kim YJ, et al. Thoracic adolescent idiopathic scoliosis curves between 70 degrees and 100 degrees: is anterior release necessary? Spine 30:2061-2067, 2005.

17. Kim YJ, Lenke LG, Cho SK, et al. Comparative analysis of pedicle screw versus hook instrumentation in posterior spinal fusion of adolescent idiopathic scoliosis. Spine 29:2040-2048, 2004.

18. Suk SI, Lee CK, Kim WJ, et al. Segmental pedicle screw fixation in the treatment of thoracic idiopathic scoliosis. Spine 20:1399-1405, 1995.

19. Brown CA, Lenke LG, Bridwell KH, et al. Complications of pediatric thoracolumbar and lumbar pedicle screws. Spine 23:1566-1571, 1998.

20. Liljenqvist U, Lepsien U, Hackenberg L, et al. Comparative analysis of pedicle screw and hook instrumentation in posterior correction and fusion of idiopathic thoracic scoliosis. Eur Spine J 11:336-343, 2002.

21. Lenke LG. Debate: resolved, a 55 degrees right thoracic adolescent idiopathic scoliotic curve should be treated by posterior spinal fusion and segmental instrumentation using thoracic pedicle screws: pro: thoracic pedicle screws should be used to treat a 55 degrees right thoracic adolescent idiopathic scoliosis. J Pediatr Orthop 24:329-334; discussion 338-341, 2004.

22. Suk SI, Lee CK, Min HJ, et al. Comparison of Cotrel-Dubousset pedicle screws and hooks in the treatment of idiopathic scoliosis. Int Orthop 18:341-346, 1994.

23. Suk SI, Kim WJ, Lee SM, et al. Thoracic pedicle screw fixation in spinal deformities: are they really safe? Spine 26:2049-2057, 2001.

24. Bess RS, Lenke LG, Bridwell KH, et al. Comparison of thoracic pedicle screw to hook instrumentation for the treatment of adult spinal deformity. Spine 32:555-561, 2007.

25. Dobbs MB, Lenke LG, Kim YJ, et al. Anterior/posterior spinal instrumentation versus posterior instrumentation alone for the treatment of adolescent idiopathic scoliotic curves more than 90 degrees. Spine 31:2386-2391, 2006.

26. Lowe TG. Anterior column support: mesh versus graft. In Lenke LG, ed. Modern Anterior Scoliosis Surgery. St Louis: Quality Medical Publishing, 2004, pp 37-50.

27. Bridwell KH. Indications and techniques for anterior-only and combined anterior and posterior approaches for thoracic and lumbar spine deformities. Instr Course Lect 54:559-565, 2005.

28. Bridwell KH. Load sharing principles: the role and use of anterior structural support in adult deformity. Instr Course Lect 45:109-115, 1996.

29. Bridwell KH. Degenerative scoliosis. In Bridwell KH, DeWald RL, Kim WH, et al, eds. The Textbook of Spinal Surgery, 2nd ed. Philadelphia: Lippincott Williams & Wilkins, 1997, pp 777-798.

30. Kostuik JP. Adult scoliosis. In Bridwell KH, DeWald RL, Kim WH, et al, eds. The Textbook of Spinal Surgery, 2nd ed. Philadelphia: Lippincott Williams & Wilkins, 1997, pp 733-776.

31. Bridwell KH. Lumbosacral junction and sacrum stabilization. In Kim DH, ed. Spinal Instrumentation: Surgical Techniques. New York: Thieme, 2005.

32. Ouellet JA, Johnston CE II. Effect of grafting technique on the maintenance of coronal and sagittal correction in anterior treatment of scoliosis. Spine 27:2129-2135; discussion 2135-2136, 2002.

33. Kim YJ, Lenke LG, Bridwell KH, et al. Pulmonary function in adolescent idiopathic scoliosis relative to the surgical procedure. J Bone Joint Surg Am 87:1534-1541, 2005.

34. Vedantam R, Lenke LG, Bridwell KH, et al. A prospective evaluation of pulmonary function in patients with adolescent idiopathic scoliosis relative to the surgical approach used for spinal arthrodesis. Spine 25:82-90, 2000.

35. Wong CA, Cole AA, Watson L, et al. Pulmonary function before and after anterior spinal surgery in adult idiopathic scoliosis. Thorax 51:534-536, 1996.

36. Graham EJ, Lenke LG, Lowe TG, et al. Prospective pulmonary function evaluation following open thoracotomy for anterior spinal fusion in adolescent idiopathic scoliosis. Spine 25:2319-2325, 2000.

37. Coe JD, Arlet V, Donaldson W, et al. Complications in spinal fusion for adolescent idiopathic scoliosis in the new millennium. A report of the Scoliosis Research Society Morbidity and Mortality Committee. Spine 31:345-349, 2006.

38. Nguyen HV, Akbarnia BA, Van Dam BE, et al. Anterior exposure of the spine for removal of lumbar interbody devices and implants. Spine 31:21, 2006.

39. Lenke LG, Bridwell KH, Blanke K, et al. Prospective analysis of nutritional status normalization after spinal reconstructive surgery. Spine 20:1359-1367, 1995.

40. Kim YB, Lenke LG, Kim YJ, et al. The morbidity of an anterior thoracolumbar approach in adult patients with greater than five-year follow-up. Presented at the Forty-First Annual Meeting of the Scoliosis Research Society. Monterey, CA, Sept 2006.

41. Westfall SH, Akbarnia BA, Merenda JT, et al. Exposure of the anterior spine, technique, complications, and results in 85 patients. Am J Surg 154:700-704, 1987.

42. Sicard GA, Reilly JM, Rubin BG, et al. Transabdominal versus retroperitoneal incision for abdominal aortic surgery: report of a prospective randomized trial. J Vasc Surg 21:174-181; discussion 181-183, 1995.

43. Dewald CJ, Millikan KW, Hammerberg KW, et al. An open, minimally invasive approach to the lumbar spine. Am Surg 65:61-68, 1999.

44. Harms J, Rolinger H. [A one-stager procedure in operative treatment of spondylolistheses: dorsal traction-reposition and anterior fusion (author's transl)] Z Orthop Ihre Grenzgeb 120:343-347, 1982.

45. Whitecloud TS III, Roesch WW, Ricciardi JE. Transforaminal interbody fusion versus anterior-posterior interbody fusion of the lumbar spine: a financial analysis. J Spinal Disord 14:100-103, 2001.

46. Hacker RJ. Comparison of interbody fusion approaches for disabling low back pain. Spine 22:660-665; discussion 665-666, 1997.

47. Bess RS, Bacchus K, Vance R, et al. Lumbar Biomechanics with Extreme Lateral Interbody Fusion (XLIF®) Cage Construct. Presented at the Fourteenth International Meeting on Advanced Spine Techniques, Paradise Island, Bahamas, July 2007.

48. Diaz R, Phillips FM, Pimenta L. Minimally-invasive fusion (XLIF) in the treatment of symptomatic degenerative lumbar scoliosis. Presented at the Twenty-First Annual Meeting of the North American Spine Society. Philadelphia, Sept 2005.

49. Ozgur BM, Aryan HE, Yoo K, et al. Adult degenerative scoliosis repair via an extreme lateral interbody fusion technique (XLIF). Presented at the Seventy-Third Annual Meeting of the American Association of Neurological Surgeons. New Orleans, April 2005.

50. Hsu V, Akbarnia BA, Van Dam B, et al. Extreme lateral interbody fusion (XLIF): evaluation of safety and short-term results. Presented at the Fourteenth International Meeting on Advanced Spine Techniques, Paradise Island, Bahamas, July 2007.

51. Mandelbaum BR, Tolo VT, McAfee PC, et al. Nutritional deficiencies after staged anterior and posterior spinal reconstructive surgery. Clin Orthop Relat Res 234:5-11, 1988.

52. Shufflebarger HL, Grimm JO, Bui V, et al. Anterior and posterior spinal fusion. Staged versus same-day surgery. Spine 16:930-933, 1991.

53. Viviani GR, Raducan V, Bednar DA, et al. Anterior and posterior spinal fusion: comparison of one-stage and two-stage procedures. Can J Surg 36:468-473, 1993.

54. Ogilvie JW. Anterior and posterior spinal surgery: same-day, staged, anterior first, posterior first, or simultaneous? Instr Course Lect 45:99-100, 1996.

55. Lapp MA, Bridwell KH, Lenke LG, et al. Prospective randomization of parenteral hyperalimentation for long fusions with spinal deformity: its effect on complications and recovery from postoperative malnutrition. Spine 26:809-817; discussion 817, 2001.

56. Kim YJ, Bridwell KH, Lenke LG, et al. Pseudarthrosis in adult spinal deformity following multisegmental instrumentation and arthrodesis. J Bone Joint Surg Am 88:721-728, 2006.

57. Resnick DK, Choudhri TF, Dailey AT, et al. Guidelines for the performance of fusion procedures for degenerative disease of the lumbar spine. IX. Brace therapy as an adjunct to or substitute for lumbar fusion. J Neurosurg Spine 2:716-724, 2005.

58. Connolly PJ, Grob D. Bracing of patients after fusion for degenerative problems of the lumbar spine—yes or no? Spine 23:1426-1428, 1998.

59. Fidler MW, Plasmans CM. The effect of four types of support on the segmental mobility of the lumbosacral spine. J Bone Joint Surg Am 65:943-947, 1983.

17

Clinical Application: Revision Surgery

Andrew Cappuccino ▪ Luiz Pimenta

In 1991, Obenchain[1] was the first to describe minimally invasive laparoscopic lumbar discectomy. The field of minimally invasive spine surgery is rapidly evolving as surgeons strive to eliminate transperitoneal exposure and its potential risks. The motivation for these efforts has been the hope of minimizing the well-described complications associated with direct anterior surgery.[2-6] Since its introduction in the literature,[7] extreme lateral interbody fusion (XLIF®, NuVasive®, Inc., San Diego, CA) has grown in acceptance and popularity as a minimally invasive direct lateral retroperitoneal approach to the anterior lumbar spine that may be used for all applications of anterior spine surgery.

Ozgur et al[7] elegantly describe the treatment of simple and complex pathologic conditions of the lumbar spine above the L4-5 level using a minimally open approach with maximal access transpsoas technology. The success of such surgery depends heavily on continuous neural monitoring to avoid injury to nerves of the lumbosacral plexus lateral to the spine. Once surgeons have mastered this exposure, they can easily perform direct approaches to the anterior column to correct both degenerative and deformity-related pathologic conditions of the lumbar spine.

The lateral transpsoas approach avoids the major potential pitfalls of revision anterior retroperitoneal or transperitoneal surgery. Anterior revisions can be technically challenging

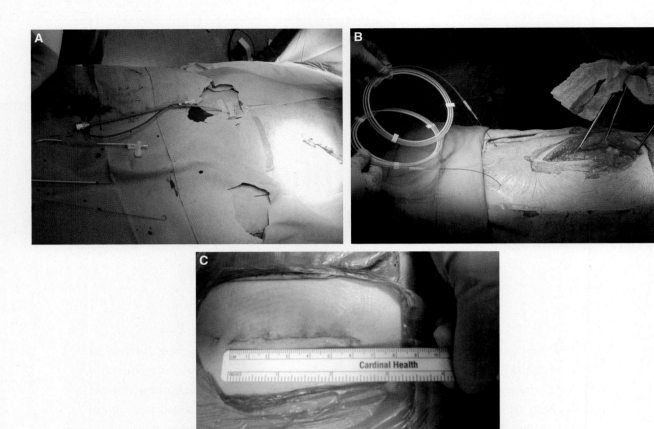

FIG. 17-1   A and **B,** Inferior vena cava (IVC) filter and catheterization of both femoral veins may be necessary in anterior revision approaches as a precautionary step. **C,** A 5 cm incision used for lateral revision surgery, without catheters or bleeding. This is favorable when compared with the open anterior revision approach. Even without complications, anterior revision approaches cause significant morbidity.

and require significant preparation and skill to avoid complications (Fig. 17-1, *A* and *B*). In addition, these revisions often result in morbidity (Fig. 17-1, *C*). Bergey et al[8] describe the significant complication rates (11%) of the endoscopic approach, while Nguyen et al[9] report a general surgical complication rate of 40% and a vascular complication rate as high as 57% in their series of anterior reexposure of the lumbar spine for removal of spine implants. For these reasons, the minimally invasive retroperitoneal transpsoas approach makes good sense and can spare significant morbidity when used properly.

With XLIF, two small incisions are used to enter the retroperitoneal space. The surgeon then obtains access to the lateral aspect of the iliopsoas muscle through blunt digital dissection. Real-time dynamic neurologic surveillance is maintained with the NeuroVision® JJB Nerve Monitoring System (NuVasive, Inc.) (Fig. 17-2).

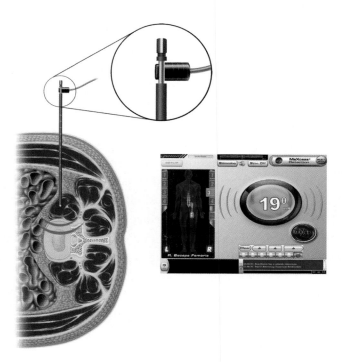

FIG. 17-2 The use of NeuroVision monitoring to traverse the psoas muscle is important to the safety of the approach. Dynamic EMG stimulation is provided through the access Dilators; this provides discrete threshold identification and the identification of nerve proximity and direction, thereby affording guidance around the nerves of the lumbosacral plexus during the approach.

INDICATIONS AND CONTRAINDICATIONS

Indications for the XLIF procedure as a revision strategy have included removal of failed total disc replacement (TDR) prostheses[10] as well as removal of failed interbody grafts (impacted or threaded cages and allografts). Partial corpectomies have been performed as well as anterior column stabilization after osteotomies using the XLIF approach. Anterior instrumentation in the form of plate/bolt or screw/rod stabilization has been successfully completed with this technique.

Contraindications to this approach include pathology at L5-S1, lumbar spondylolisthesis of grade III or higher, or any condition that would preclude a patient's undergoing general anesthesia. Relative contraindications include previous bilateral retroperitoneal surgery, pregnancy, bilateral retroperitoneal scarring, or bony pathology that precludes fusion surgery, such as osteopenia, osteoporosis, chronic autoimmune disease, and steroid dependence.

SURGICAL TECHNIQUE

The approach steps of the surgical technique are the same in revision procedures as for primary procedures and include attention to patient positioning and safe transpsoas exposure.

PATIENT PREPARATION

An antibiotic is administered for prophylaxis, and deep vein thrombosis (DVT) precautions are instituted. Markings are done, as described in Chapter 8. General anesthesia is induced, electromyographic (EMG) monitoring leads are placed, and (optionally) a Foley catheter is inserted. The patient is placed in the lateral decubitus position (either left or right) on a bendable radiolucent operative table that can be adjusted to the jackknife position. All bony prominences should be well-padded. Fluoroscopic true anteroposterior and lateral radiographs are obtained before the patient is prepared and draped. The patient is then secured to the table with 3-inch tape; the table should be jackknifed to maximally expose the lateral access between the base of the twelfth rib and the iliac crest. The table should not be moved until surgery has been completed on the target level (except to maintain true anteroposterior and lateral positioning) or until the next level is to be prepared, if necessary.

EXPOSURE

Once the surgical site is identified fluoroscopically, finger dissection is used just posterolateral to the direct lateral incision site to access the retroperitoneal space. The muscle fibers are carefully spread and the surgeon's finger is advanced until a loss of muscular resistance indicates that the retroperitoneal space has been reached. At this point—especially in revision surgeries—great care should be taken to avoid abrupt advancement so no injury occurs to the peritoneum or adjacent viscera. With caution, even scarred retroperitoneal fat can be swept free from the iliopsoas muscle, which may have a smoother than normal surface when palpated in revision surgery. Using standard landmarks (including the transverse processes, retropsoas recess, and lateral iliopsoas), the surgeon can easily access the targeted disc space, sweeping the index finger up to the inside abdominal wall under the direct lateral skin mark to ensure that a safe pathway exists between the abdominal wall and the psoas muscle.

An incision is made at this location and the initial NeuroVision® Dilator (NuVasive, Inc.) can be safely introduced. The index finger that is inside the retroperitoneal space is used to guide the dilating probes down to the lateral wall of the psoas muscle. Under fluoroscopic guidance, the probe is placed on the lateral aspect of the psoas and a Twitch Test is performed with the NeuroVision system to ensure that the muscle paralytic agent from anesthesia induction has completely worn off. It is imperative in revision surgery to have very precise neural monitoring and an understanding of how to sound out, directly dissect, retract, and protect the nerve roots within the psoas and lumbosacral plexus.

With sequential dilating cannulas, the surgeon exposes the lateral aspect of the targeted disc. Even in revision surgery the lateral anulus usually remains intact, and a sharp guidewire can be used to pierce this anulus. Once the guidewire and Dilators are in place, the MaXcess® Retractor (NuVasive, Inc.) can be positioned, which can be verified with the handheld direct current EMG probe. For revision procedures, the MaXcess Retractor should be anchored as far posterior as safely possible using the Standard Shim in the posterior Blade, and the Retractor is then carefully deployed in the cephalocaudal direction until a desired working portal is achieved. With the use of standard discectomy instruments and specific revision instrumentation designed by NuVasive, Inc., various procedures are possible, such as revision of a failed total disc replacement (TDR) (both keel and nonkeel based), revision of a failed fusion, a deformity, and anterior column stabilization after an osteotomy. For any of these procedures, strict attention to the fluoroscopic images is necessary to avoid injuries to vascular or visceral structures adjacent to the spine. Therefore the operative table is continually readjusted to maintain the initial position and perspective once the baseline position is established, because the patient may have a tendency to shift position during revision surgery as forces are applied to effect the procedure. A final free-run EMG should be tested before closure; if available, motor evoked potentials should also be tested.

Revision of Failed TDR (Both Keel and Nonkeel Based)

Once wide exposure is achieved, the complete lateral anular remnant should be removed as well as any osteophytes (Fig. 17-3, *A* through *D*). The TDR prosthesis should be exposed

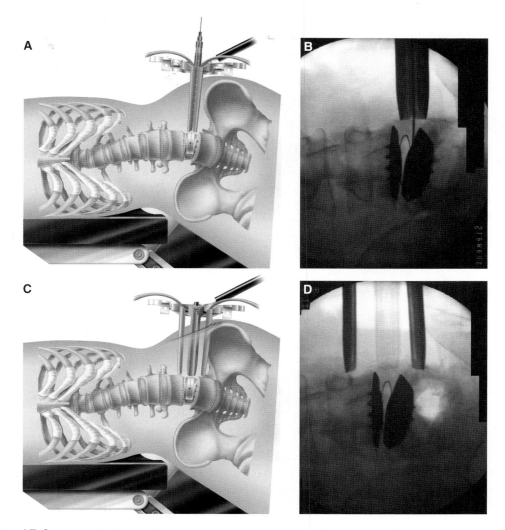

FIG. 17-3 **A** and **B,** The MaXcess system is used with NeuroVision-enabled blunt Dilators to gently split the fibers of the psoas muscle without nerve injury until the disc space is reached. **C** and **D,** The MaXcess Retractor is advanced over the Dilators, rigidly locked to the surgical table, and expanded over the disc space.

Continued

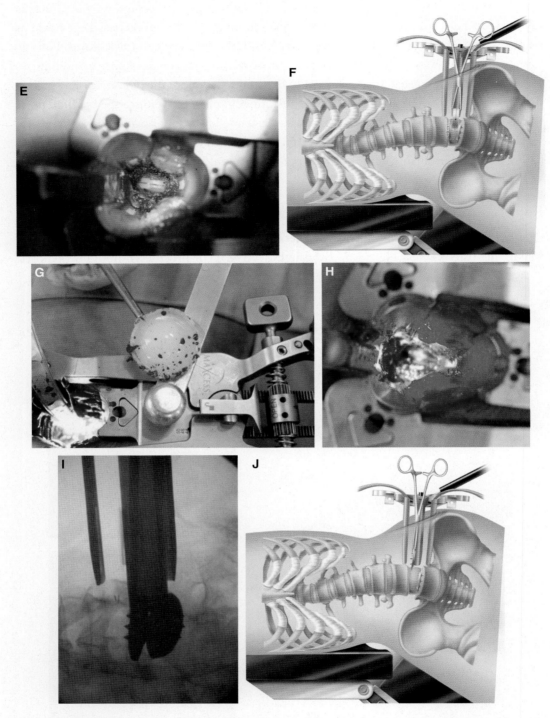

FIG. 17-3, cont'd   **E,** The polyethylene core is visualized. **F** and **G,** The polyethylene core is easily grasped and removed using a Kocher clamp. **H,** The device endplates are visualized after removal of the core. **I** and **J,** The metal endplates are pried loose from their bony attachment without much force using an osteotome and can be grasped and removed from the disc space with a Kocher clamp.

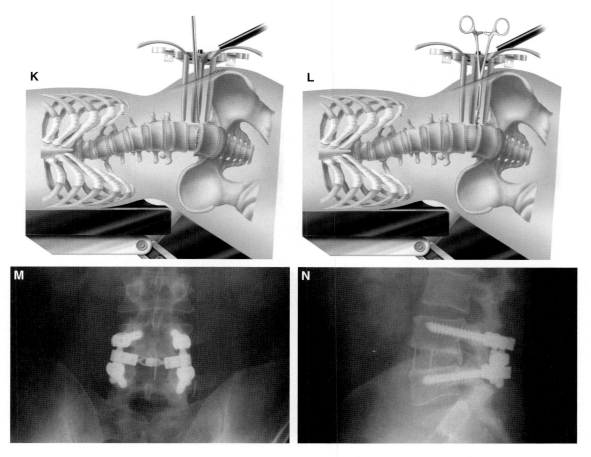

FIG. 17-3, cont'd K and L, Endplate loosening and removal is repeated for the second surface using an osteotome and Kocher clamp. **M,** One year postoperative anteroposterior (AP) and **N,** lateral radiographs of a patient after TDR explantation and 360-degree fusion.

and the lateral rim of the endplates inspected. All soft tissue should be removed from between the endplates and the core of the prosthesis exposed (Fig. 17-3, *E*). In a nonkeeled prosthesis, the endplate Distractor from the revision instrument system should be placed on the metallic endplates and a careful distraction performed. This will unlock the polyethylene core, which can then be removed using a Kocher clamp or extracting forceps from the revision instrument systems (Fig. 17-3, *F* through *H*). After the polyethylene core is removed, the metal endplates are pried loose from their bony attachment with an osteotome. Next, a Kocher clamp is used to grasp and remove the endplates from the disc space (Fig. 17-3, *I* through *L*). After the implant is removed, the area is fused, as in this patient (Fig. 17-3, *M* and *N*). Two-level cases can be revised in the same manner (Fig. 17-4, *A* through *D*).

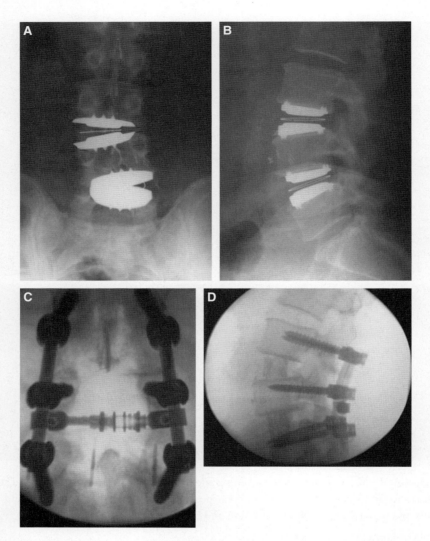

FIG. 17-4   A 42-year-old male underwent an L3-4, L4-5 disc replacement for discogenic back pain. The two-level arthroplasty decompensated over 6 months and led to severe low back pain and right leg radiculopathy. Eight months after surgery, he underwent explantation of the Charité prostheses, at L3-4 and L4-5, as seen in the preoperative radiographs (**A** and **B**). The right-sided revision surgery lasted approximately 1 hour and 45 minutes; the artificial discs were removed, and 16 mm high-lordotic PEEK CoRoent® (NuVasive, Inc.) cages were installed. During the same surgery, he underwent posterior L3-5 decompression and fusion with SpheRx® (NuVasive, Inc.) variable-angled screw instrumentation. The total operative time was 3 hours and 15 minutes. **C** and **D,** Radiographs taken 6 months postoperatively; the patient was doing extremely well, with no back pain.

In a keeled prosthesis, Pimenta[11] described a hemicorpectomy to remove the keel from the superior endplate of the disc space. Then the inferior endplate can be lifted with simple osteotomes from the inferior vertebral body (Fig. 17-5). The disc space, now completely evacuated, can be fused with an interbody graft, and the partial lateral corpectomy is transfixed with screw/rod or screw/plate instrumentation (Fig. 17-6, *A* through *D*). It is recommended that after a revision disc replacement, instrumentation be used subsequent to a complete resection of the anterior longitudinal ligament.

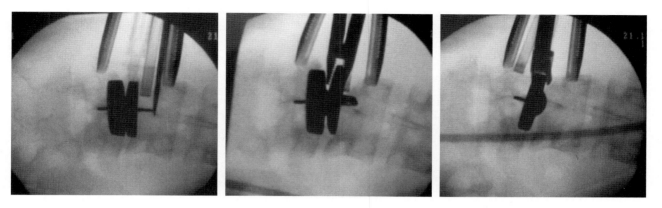

FIG. 17-5　A keeled total disc replacement device can be removed by partial selective corpectomy and removal of the endplates through the defect.

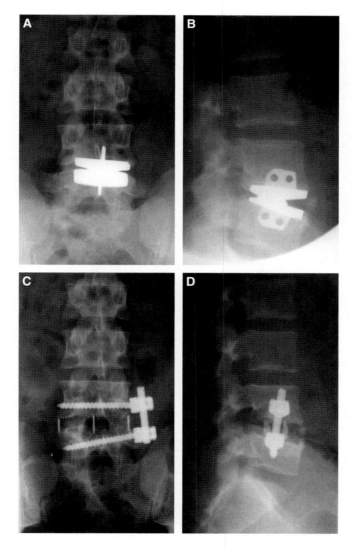

FIG. 17-6　**A** and **B,** Prerevision anteroposterior and lateral radiographs of a patient with a keeled TDR device. **C** and **D,** Same patient after removal of the device and revision to fusion using lateral instrumentation to repair the partial corpectomy defect in the superior vertebra.

Revision of Failed Fusion

The same exposure and approach should be used to revise a failed anterior fusion. Once this exposure has been achieved, lateral osteophytes and bone should be removed using standard discectomy instruments until the impacted or threaded fusion cage is encountered (Fig. 17-7, *A* through *D*). For impacted cages, a simple circumscription with osteotomes, mallets, and pituitary rongeurs is performed. The cages can be removed en bloc or fractured for easier removal. Under fluoroscopic guidance, complete excavation of the disc space should be performed and the contralateral anular remnant released (Fig. 17-7, *E* and *F*). The remaining space is contoured with broad, flat osteotomes and ring curettes to ensure a flat surface for structural interbody grafting (Fig. 17-7, *G* and *H*). Anterior instrumentation is applied when possible, using screw/rod instrumentation or bolt/plate instrumentation, and supplemental posterior segmental instrumentation should be used to augment stability (Fig. 17-7, *I* and *J*).

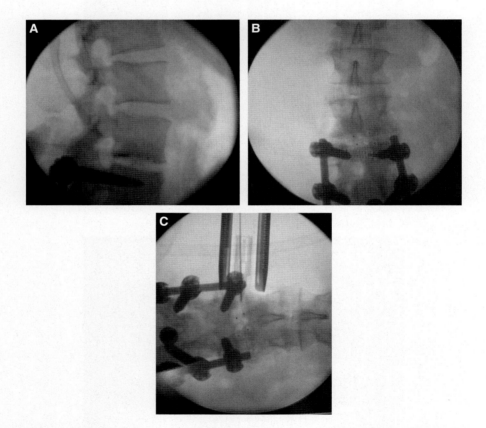

FIG. 17-7   A and **B,** A 37-year-old male with multiple anterior and posterior low back surgeries who underwent a stand-alone PLIF at L3-4 above a solid instrumented L4-S1 fusion. This led to pseudoarthrosis at L3-4 and severe mechanical back pain. At the time of revision, a transpsoas approach was used to remove the failed carbon fiber cages at L3-4 and implant a large PEEK impacted cage with lateral bolt-plate fixation. **C,** Localizing radiograph with the MaXcess Retractor anchored in the disc space, in preparation for the removal of the pseudarthrosis.

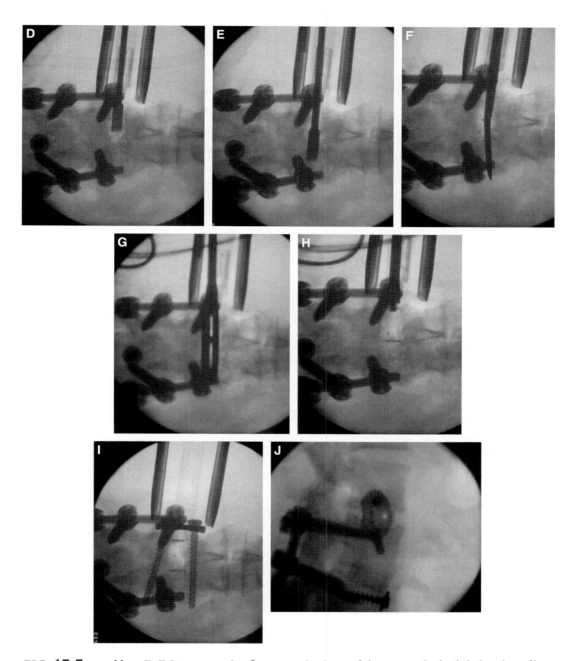

FIG. 17-7, cont'd   **D-F,** Intraoperative fluoroscopic views of the removal of a failed carbon fiber cage in the disc space of L3-4 using osteotomes, elevators, and pituitary rongeurs. **G,** Intraoperative trialing of a large impacted PEEK cage to check for stability of the L3-4 segment. **H,** AP fluoroscopic view of the final impacted PEEK cage in position at the L3-4 disc space. **I** and **J,** The final AP and lateral fluoroscopic views of lateral plate instrumentation transfixing the revised fusion at L3-4, all of which was completed through a 3 cm lateral incision. The total operative time was 1 hour and 30 minutes, with a 150 cc blood loss. Radiographs shown are three months postoperative. The patient had a good result with significant relief of back pain.

If previous pedicle screw instrumentation is in place, disc space revision can be performed and the pedicle screw instrumentation replaced in an exchange procedure, thus enabling a two-stage instead of a three-stage procedure. In the case of threaded cages, previously existing pedicle screws must be removed before the anterior column is addressed. This will allow better interbody distraction and potentially less vertebral body resection during the revision procedure. To revise threaded cages, the Spreader/Distractor from the NuVasive revision system can be used to spread the vertebral bodies. Subsequent partial superior and inferior corpectomy may be necessary to remove embedded cages. In this case, a large implant, often larger than 16 mm, may be necessary, and it is advisable to have an expandable cage available at the time of any revision surgery.

Deformity

In the treatment of failed deformity surgery, where multiple pseudarthroses exist and the deformity is progressive, especially with instability (such as lateral listhesis), the XLIF technology can be used to reduce the listhesis and stabilize the failed posterior fusions. This is usually done at multiple levels and may be done as an additive to existing instrumentation for failed fusion, or with revision or adjunctive instrumentation in cases with significant instability.

Anterior Column Stabilization After Osteotomy

Correcting a spinal deformity with the use of osteotomy has gained great popularity among spine surgeons. Most often, the anterior column is not addressed. Stabilizing the anterior column after the osteotomy is simple and beneficial for maintaining the correction of the deformity and to speed the healing at the osteotomized level. This is true for pedicle subtraction osteotomies, closing wedge osteotomies, and Smith-Peterson osteotomies. In performing transpsoas techniques for these applications, the operating surgeon should become comfortable with the management of spine segmental vessels and direct nerve root dissection within the substance of the psoas.

CLOSURE

After successfully completing the procedure and irrigating the surgical field, a decision can be made as to whether closed drainage is necessary. Final fluoroscopy should be done to evaluate the results of the procedure before closure. Once images are procured, the table should be returned to the neutral lateral position to facilitate closure. Closure should be in multiple layers including the lateral abdominal wall, the subcutaneous tissue, and skin. A standard dressing can be applied. The patient can then be returned to the supine position, awakened when medically ready, and transported to the recovery room, or positioned for a secondary approach as necessary.

POSTOPERATIVE MANAGEMENT

All patients should be placed in a rigid brace after revision surgery. Few require intensive care management, and then usually because of preexisting medical conditions. The diet can be advanced as tolerated, and patients should be mobilized on the morning of postoperative day one in physical therapy. The hospital stay is determined by the patient's ability to perform activities of daily living, ambulate independently with or without an assistive device, tolerate a regular diet, and use only oral analgesics for pain management (which is usually minimal postoperatively).

COMPLICATIONS

In our personal series of 40 revision lumbar surgeries using lateral retroperitoneal transpsoas techniques, the most common complication was anterior thigh pain and/or numbness, which occurred approximately 25% of the time. This resolved spontaneously, from 5 days to 3 months and 18 days after revision surgery. It is believed that this pain occurs from mobilization of the iliopsoas muscle. Presently we attempt to minimize the pain by administering pregabalin (Lyrica) 75 mg twice daily for 5 days preoperatively and 5 days postoperatively. There was one femoral nerve palsy, believed to be an L3 nerve root stretch, that was undetected intraoperatively, was confirmed by EMG postoperatively, and did not resolve leading to a 2.5% neurologic complication rate. We have noted no paralyses or bladder, bowel, ureteral, or visceral injuries. There were no cases of retrograde ejaculation (0% compared with 14% reported in the literature for revision anterior surgery). There was one major vascular injury that required conversion to a laparotomy and vascular surgical intervention, leading to a 2.5% major vascular complication rate, compared with 57% seen in a series by Nguyen et al.[9] There were no mortalities (compared with 7.1% in Nguyen's series[9]). Blood loss averaged 175 ml for the cases without vascular injury. We encountered no sympathetic dysfunction, sexual dysfunction, prolonged ileus, wound incompetence, DVT, pancreatitis, or bowel injuries, which have all been reported in series detailing complications of anterior approaches.[12]

CONCLUSION

With the appropriate training and experience in lateral transpsoas retroperitoneal surgery, surgeons may perform even complicated revision surgery of the lumbar spine safely and effectively with relatively low complication rates, as compared with the published literature for direct anterior revision spine surgery.

REFERENCES

1. Obenchain TE. Laparoscopic lumbar discectomy: case report. J Laparoendosc Surg 1:145-149, 1991.
2. Hannon JK, Faircloth WB, Lane DR, et al. Comparison of insufflation vs retractional technique for laparoscopic-assisted intervertebral fusion of the lumbar spine. Surg Endosc 14:300-304, 2000.
3. Baker JK, Reardon PR, Reardon MJ, et al. Vascular injury in anterior lumbar spine surgery. Spine 18:2227-2230, 1993.
4. Regan JJ, McAfee PC, Guyer RD, et al. Laparoscopic fusion of the lumbar spine in a multi-center series of the first 34 consecutive patients. Surg Laparosc Endosc 6:459-468, 1996.
5. Christensen FB, Bunger CE. Retrograde ejaculation after retroperitoneal lower lumbar interbody fusion. Int Orthop 21:176-180, 1997.
6. Flynn JC, Price CT. Sexual complications of anterior fusion of the lumbar spine. Spine 9:489-492, 1984.
7. Ozgur BM, Arayan HE, Pimenta L, et al. Extreme lateral interbody fusion (XLIF). A novel surgical technique for anterior lumbar interbody fusion. Spine J 6:435-443, 2006.
8. Bergey DL, Villavicencio AT, Goldstein T, et al. Endoscopic lateral transpsoas approach to the lumbar spine. Spine 29:1681-1688, 2004.
9. Nguyen HV, Akbania BA, van Dam BE, et al. Anterior exposure of the spine for removal of lumbar interbody device and implants. Spine 31:2449-2453, 2006.
10. Pimenta L, Diaz RC, Guerrero LG. Charité lumbar artificial disc retrieval: use of a lateral minimally invasive technique. Technical note. J Neurosurg Spine 5:556-561, 2006.
11. Pimenta L. Removal of a keeled TDR prosthesis via a lateral transpsoas retroperitoneal approach. Proceedings of the Twenty-Second Annual Meeting of the North American Spine Society (NASS), Austin, TX, Oct 2007.
12. Rajaraman V, Vingan R, Roth P, et al. Visceral and vascular complications resulting from anterior lumbar interbody fusion. J Neurosurg 91(1 Suppl):S60-S64, 1999.

18

Outpatient XLIF®

William D. Smith ▪ Kyle Malone

The success of lumbar microdiscectomy as an outpatient procedure was first reported in 1987.[1] Since then, a series of reports has confirmed the validity of this and other spine surgeries (including lumbar interbody fusion) performed as outpatient procedures.[2-10] The recent increase in the number of outpatient spine surgeries is largely the result of advances in minimally invasive techniques and technology, such as extreme lateral interbody fusion (XLIF, NuVasive®, Inc., San Diego, CA). These advances have allowed an increasing number of inpatient procedures to be performed safely and effectively as outpatient surgeries. These successes in outpatient spine surgery have also sparked the creation of several physician-owned surgery centers or ambulatory surgery centers which have reported impressive results in patient care and cost effectiveness.[3,5-10,11-14] However, the use of XLIF and other minimally invasive techniques in the outpatient setting is not yet universal, in part because of the historical precedent of inpatient open spine surgery in a general hospital setting. We believe that by integrating outpatient XLIF procedures in ambulatory surgery centers, surgeons have more environmental control than in an inpatient setting and can therefore provide the greatest benefits—and the least amount of risk—to their patients. XLIF appears to be the most reliable and effective approach for lumbar interbody fusion, allowing the greatest control of intraoperative complications with minimized negative postoperative outcomes.[15,16] Though other minimally invasive options for spine surgery are available, this chapter focuses on the efficacy of XLIF as an outpatient procedure and the inherent advantages of adopting this approach.

OPEN VERSUS MINIMALLY INVASIVE PROCEDURES

Minimally invasive spine surgeries (MISs) are increasing in prevalence, but remain only partially adopted in general hospitals. Currently, most spine procedures are performed via open techniques. These intensive procedures generally require extensive dissection, resulting in intraoperative trauma, prolonged postoperative hospitalization, and extended recovery time. Although prospective statistics on the surgical and postoperative efficacy of XLIF are being compiled, the retrospective results from our clinic, and the clinics of others, strongly suggest that XLIF has the benefits of decreased operating room time, decreased blood loss, a shorter time to postoperative ambulation, and a shorter hospital stay.[17-19] Why are XLIF and other MIS procedures not being adopted at higher rates if, in addition to the advantages listed previously, they offer the benefits of decreased postoperative pain, lower infection rates, and a faster return to functionality?

The reluctance to adopt these procedures—namely, endoscopic approaches—is attributed, in part, to the decreased reproducibility that results from the inherent procedural complexities of endoscopic approaches. In addition, intraoperative visualization is decreased with MIS procedures. Consequently, the surgeon must rely on fluoroscopy and technique, whereas procedures performed under direct visualization permit immediate troubleshooting. These reasons suggest that XLIF and other MIS procedures are associated with a higher learning curve and a slightly increased patient risk during a surgeon's early procedural use. In addition, MIS procedures lack the convention of open interbody fusion procedures, which have been performed for many decades. Over the past 10 years, innovations in open procedures have plateaued, necessitating a procedural "overhaul" and advancement to the next step of interbody fusion; XLIF seems to be that innovation.

WHY XLIF?

For thoracolumbar interbody fusions above L5-S1, XLIF is particularly well suited as an outpatient procedure (especially in ambulatory neurosurgery centers), because it drastically reduces the largest comorbid confounder of spine fusion: damage to the paraspinal muscle complex. The use of a lateral, blunt dissection, muscle-splitting technique through the psoas muscle decreases the operating room time and the overall cost by eliminating the need for an approach surgeon. The lateral transpsoas approach also avoids the vascular complications that are associated with anterior approaches. Instead, lateral approaches carry the potential for lumbar plexus injury. This can be mitigated, however, by incorporating real-time nerve monitoring (NeuroVision® JJB, NuVasive, Inc.), which tracks the location of nerves in the path of the approaching instruments. This added safeguard increases surgical efficacy and reliability and decreases surgical risks. In addition, the XLIF approach spares ligaments that are required to be dissected in open procedures. This preservation allows patients to maintain natural ligament stabilization during the healing process.

Results from our early XLIF surgeries support the use of XLIF as an outpatient procedure.[17] Seventy-two patients underwent XLIF procedures by a single surgeon (Smith) from June 2004 through May 2005 at a community hospital in Las Vegas, Nevada. Indications for surgery included failed-laminotomy syndrome, adjacent-level syndrome, internal disc disruption, disc herniation with instability, stenosis with instability, spondylolisthesis, and/or degenerative scoliosis. Posterior microdecompression was adjunctively performed in 26/72 cases (36%). The procedures included 99 levels: 52 single-level, 16 two-level, two three-level, one four-level, and one five-level procedure. Levels of operation included 39 at L4-5, 32 at L3-4, 23 at L2-3, three at L1-2, and two at T12-L1. Of the surgeries, 19% were stand-alone fusions, 22% used unilateral pedicle screws, and 59% used bilateral pedicle screws. The operating room times ranged from 20 to 130 minutes per level, with a 50-minute median time per level. On average, the XLIF procedure took 28 minutes, and posterior instrumentation took 35 minutes. The mean total operating room time was 66 minutes. The estimated blood loss ranged from 5 to 75 ml (median blood loss 20 ml). All patients ambulated within 8 hours of surgery, and the majority of patients were discharged from the hospital within 24 hours. Of the 100 patients treated as outpatients, the discharge range was 1 to 6.5 hours postoperatively (median discharge time 3.5 hours). The decision to treat on an inpatient basis was based mainly on the patient's age, significant comorbidities, and hospital policies. Complications included one retroperitoneal hematoma, one pseudarthrosis, and two cases of bone morphogenic protein (BMP)–related subsidence. No infections or neuropraxias occurred.

The complications in XLIFs performed by all participating surgeons in Las Vegas were compiled. More than 600 levels have been completed using the XLIF approach in Las Vegas, with seven pseudarthroses (1.2%), eight incidences of transient thigh weakness (1.3%), two cases of dysesthesia (0.3%), two peritoneal violations (0.3%), and no vascular injuries (0%).

CONCLUSION

Based on our data, the XLIF approach clearly facilitates shorter operating room times, lower risks, and better patient outcomes than similar open procedures. The use of XLIF as an outpatient procedure in ambulatory neurosurgery centers will further close the gap between MIS and open procedures in terms of patient outcome and surgical efficacy. The main goal of ambulatory neurosurgery centers and all specialty hospitals must be to determine which procedures are the safest and most reproducible, which procedures require minimal preoperative and postoperative care, and which procedures offer the greatest benefits to the patient. XLIF provides an excellent platform to further expand the scope of treatment options for surgeons at ASCs.

REFERENCES

1. Rogers LA. Outpatient microsurgical management of ruptured lumbar discs. N C Med J 48:117-120, 1987.
2. Asch HL, Lewis PJ, Moreland DB, et al. Prospective multiple outcomes study of outpatient lumbar microdiscectomy: should 75 to 80% success rates be the norm? J Neurosurg 96:34-44, 2002.
3. Bookwalter JW III, Busch MD, Nicely D. Ambulatory surgery is safe and effective in radicular disc disease. Spine 19:526-530, 1994.
4. Cares HL, Steinberg RS, Robertson ET, et al. Ambulatory microsurgery for ruptured lumbar discs: report of ten cases. Neurosurgery 22:523-526, 1988.

5. Silvers HR, Lewis PJ, Suddaby LS, et al. Day surgery for cervical microdiscectomy: is it safe and effective? J Spinal Disord 9:287-293, 1996.

6. Singhal A, Bernstein M. Outpatient lumbar microdiscectomy: a prospective study in 122 patients. Can J Neurol Sci 29:249-252, 2002.

7. Stieber JR, Brown K, Donald GD, et al. Anterior cervical decompression and fusion with plate fixation as an outpatient procedure. Spine J 5:503-507, 2005.

8. Wohns RNW, Robinett RD. Day surgery for lumbar microdiskectomy: experience with 60 cases. Ambul Surg 4:31-33, 1996.

9. Wohns RNW, Robinett RD. Outpatient anterior cervical microdiskectomy: experience with 106 cases. Ambul Surg 7:35-37, 1999.

10. Zahrawi F. Microlumbar discectomy. Is it safe as an outpatient procedure? Spine 19:1070-1074, 1994.

11. Cram P, Vaughan-Sarrazin MS, Wolf B, et al. A comparison of total hip and knee replacement in specialty and general hospitals. J Bone Joint Surg Am 89:1675-1684, 2007.

12. Greenwald L, Cromwell J, Adamache W, et al. Specialty versus community hospitals: referrals, quality, and community benefits. Health Aff (Millwood) 25:106-118, 2006.

13. Slotman GJ, Stein SC. Laparoscopic L5-S1 diskectomy: a cost-effective, minimally invasive general surgery–neurosurgery team alternative to laminectomy. Am Surg 62:64-68, 1996.

14. Vernooij F, Heintz P, Witteveen E, et al. The outcomes of ovarian cancer treatment are better when provided by gynecologic oncologists and in specialized hospitals: a systematic review. Gynecol Oncol 105:801-812, 2007.

15. Ozgur BM, Aryan HE, Pimenta L, et al. Extreme lateral interbody fusion (XLIF): a novel surgical technique for anterior lumbar interbody fusion. Spine J 6:435-443, 2006.

16. Pimenta L, Diaz RC, Guerrero LG. Charité lumbar artificial disc retrieval: use of a lateral minimally invasive technique. Technical note. J Neurosurg Spine 5:556-561, 2006.

17. Smith W, DeLappi J. XLIF: outpatient surgery. Presented at the Fourth International Meeting of the World Spine Society, Istanbul, Turkey, July 2007.

18. Wright N. eXtreme Lateral Interbody Fusion (XLIF): the United States experience 2003-2004. Presented at the Twelfth International Meeting on Advanced Spine Techniques, Banff, Alberta, Canada, July 2005.

19. Rodgers WB, Cox C, Gerber EJ. Experience and early results with a minimally invasive technique for anterior column support through eXtreme Lateral Interbody Fusion (XLIF). US Musculoskeletal Review 1:28-32, 2007.

19

XLIF® Thoracic Spine Surgery: The Minimal Answer to a Maximal Challenge

William R. Taylor

Historically, the technologic advancement of surgical methods of treatment for the thoracic spine has moved much more slowly than advancements for the cervical and lumbar spine. This discrepancy is probably the result of two major factors: the small numbers of non-trauma patients who become symptomatic from a disc in the thoracic region and the complexities surrounding the thoracic anatomy. Most significant traumatic spine injuries are treated in major metropolitan hospitals; thus many practicing spine surgeons have little experience with structures surrounding the thoracic spine, including the vasculature. Approach surgeons and assistant surgeons have even less familiarity with this region and may choose to undertake only the most common stabilization procedures. Additionally, because of the complexity of invasive, open thoracic procedures and the associated risks, symptomatic patients are often managed conservatively for longer periods and given significantly less encouragement to undergo surgery.

Because of recent innovations in thoracic minimally invasive spine surgery, surgeons can quickly and easily perform thoracic surgery or very complex minimal procedures without a thoracotomy. The instrumentation and technique have progressed in tandem, making the surgery less complicated and resulting in a procedure that is effective and less time consuming. Most importantly, however, XLIF (NuVasive®, Inc., San Diego, CA) makes surgery safer for the patient in even the most challenging cases.

The impetus to create truly minimally invasive spine surgery for the thoracic region began in the early 1990s with the development of the thoracoscopic sympathectomies, which were developed for patients with hyperhydrosis.[1-3] This building-block procedure eventually advanced to thoracic discectomies,[4,5] and complex corpectomies were undertaken to treat patients with thoracolumbar spinal trauma.[6,7] Although effective, these early procedures had an extremely steep learning curve, were exceptionally time consuming, and were very technologically demanding. If even the most minor portion of the necessary instrumentation was unavailable, it became nearly impossible to proceed with surgery.

Eventually, thoracoscopic and posterolateral approaches became more prevalent. Surgeons could choose to approach a lesion or fracture through an extrapleural,[8] retropleural,[9,10] or costotransversectomy incision.[11,12] Even a straight pediculotomy could be performed.[13,14] Although each of these access methods can be used to great effect, they do have limitations—longer access, dissection, and operative times, each of which exponentially increases the potential for blood loss and the risk of complications. None of these issues is minor, and all have a negative impact on the end result.

With the demand for a better procedure and the advent of truly minimally invasive instrumentation and methods, MAS® (NuVasive, Inc.) thoracotomy—using the extreme lateral interbody fusion (XLIF) thoracic technique—is rapidly gaining in scope and popularity. The MaXcess® Retractor (NuVasive, Inc.) can easily be deployed laterally between any level rib space or spaces T5-6 and below. Using the Retractor effectively creates a mild distraction, and a viable surgical corridor can be opened. This small but efficient dissection allows sufficient access to perform any surgical procedure in the thoracic spine in a minimally invasive fashion.

The thoracic XLIF procedure was adapted from the lumbar XLIF approach. Using similar instrumentation, the lumbar XLIF has been translated into the thoracic XLIF approach with a minimal need for changes in the technique and positioning. This approach can be used for any indication in the thoracic spine. Its advantages include that it provides open and direct visualization of the anatomy without the need to perform a complete thoracotomy. Lung deflation is unnecessary because the Retractors protect the lung. The access system includes an excellent lighting source, and a custom instrumentation package is incorporated, making it unnecessary to obtain specialized extra-long thoracic or extended anterior instruments from an outside provider before operative procedures can be performed.

SURGICAL CONSIDERATIONS

The XLIF thoracic procedure allows access to the thoracic spine through a direct lateral approach. The major anatomic landmarks to consider when preparing for this technique are the ribs, lung, diaphragm, aorta, and spinal anatomy.

The surgeon may choose to use double-lumen intubation to deflate the ipsilateral lung or may follow the described technique without deflating the lung. In the thoracic region, at least one direct lateral incision is necessary, depending on the number of spinal levels requiring treatment. Surgical access is either between the ribs, or, if necessary, a small section of rib is removed to expand access. Care should be taken to preserve the neurovascular bundle that lies under the inferior aspect of each rib.

Access is established by inserting an initial Dilator directed posteriorly along the interior chest wall and docking it, stopping at the junction of the rib head and vertebral body. After the Dilator and Retractor are placed, the Retractor is opened so the surgeon can visualize the pertinent anatomy; the Retractor is repositioned as needed. Preoperative magnetic resonance imaging (MRI) should be examined to identify the position of the aorta. In the midthoracic spine, especially in patients with scoliosis, the aorta tends to lie at the left lateral aspect of the vertebral body. In such cases, some surgeons approach from the opposite side to ensure that the instruments used to prepare the disc do not pass more than 2 mm through the contralateral anulus.

To successfully complete this technique, the following instruments are required:
- Radiolucent bendable surgical table
- C-arm
- Light source
- MaXcess III Access System
- MaXcess Articulating Arm
- MaXcess Disposable Kit
- XLIF thoracic instruments
- Anterior/lateral general instruments
- Interbody or vertebral body replacement (VBR) implants
- XLP™ Lateral Plating System (NuVasive, Inc.)
- NeuroVision® JJB System (NuVasive, Inc.)
- NeuroVision JJB Disposables

STEP 1: PLANNING, PATIENT POSITIONING, AND OPERATING ROOM SETUP

The patient is placed on a bendable surgical table in a direct lateral decubitus position (at a 90-degree angle), with the appropriate side elevated. Depending on the patient's anatomy, the approach may be from the left or right side. Particular care is needed in prescreening imaging to determine the approach side and to avoid major vascular structures. I recommend a preoperative MRI or computed tomography (CT), not so much to assess the pathologic condition, which is confirmed before surgery is scheduled, but to evaluate the internal anatomy surrounding the operative lesion. The surgeon should identify the descending aorta, vena cava, diaphragm, lung fields, bony anatomy, vascular structures, and/or other anatomic variances before beginning the procedure. It is most common to approach from the left side, because in most patients the diaphragm is lower in that location, allowing easier access to the thoracolumbar junction. However, if a lateral vessel is found, especially one that descends into the surgical field when the spine is rotated, it is best to approach from the opposite side.

If the surgery involves lumbar levels (for example, L4-5) as well as thoracic levels, the patient is positioned so that the table break is directly under the greater trochanter. If the surgery includes only thoracic levels, the patient is positioned with the table break under the midsurgical level. The patient is secured with tape at the following locations (Fig. 19-1):

1. Just below the iliac crest
2. Over the thoracic region, ensuring that the tape does not interfere with the surgical exposure of the level of interest
3. From the iliac crest to the knee, then secured to the table
4. From one side of the table to the knee, past the ankle, then secured to the other side of the table

Fluoroscopy is used to verify the location. The surgical table should be flexed to open the space between the ribs (Fig. 19-2, *A*). Once the patient is secured with tape, the table is adjusted so that true anteroposterior images are obtained when the C-arm is horizontal and true lateral images are obtained when the C-arm is vertical (Fig. 19-2, *B* and *C*). These real-time films should provide a three-dimensional picture, allowing the pedicles, endplates, and vertebral bodies to be aligned perfectly with the true orthogonal images (as with lumbar procedures). The table should be adjusted when accessing each level to maintain this relationship. The NeuroVision control unit should be placed opposite the surgeon to provide an unobstructed view (Fig. 19-2, *D*).

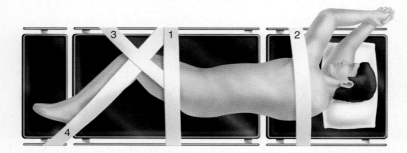

FIG. 19-1 The patient is positioned with the table break under the midsurgical level and secured with tape just below the iliac crest *(1);* over the thoracic region, ensuring that the tape does not interfere with the surgical exposure of the level of interest *(2);* from the iliac crest to the knee, then to the table *(3);* and from one side of the table to the knee, past the ankle, and to the other side of the table *(4).*

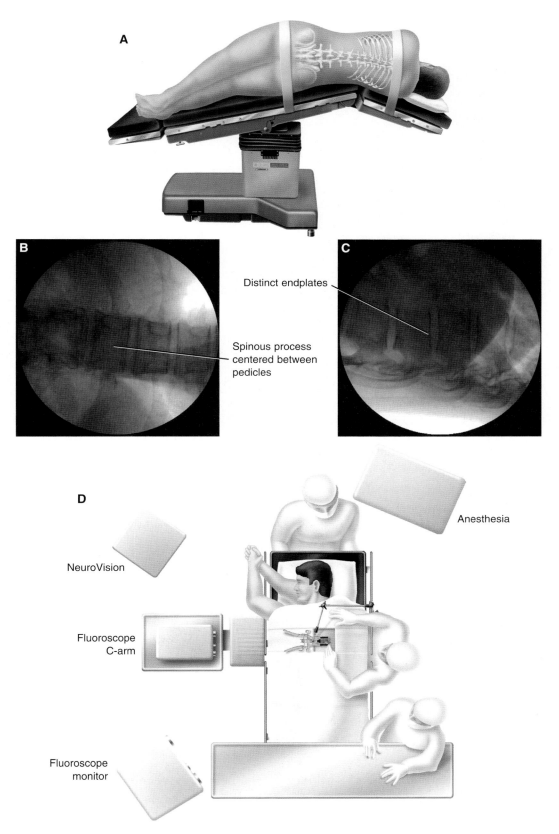

FIG. 19-2 **A,** The surgical table is flexed to open space between the ribs. **B** and **C,** True anteroposterior and lateral images show alignment of the pedicles, endplates, and vertebral bodies. **D,** The operating room setup allows an unobstructed view of the fluoroscopy monitor and NeuroVision screen.

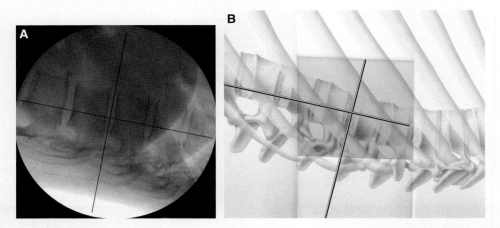

FIG. 19-3   **A,** The disc space is localized using lateral fluoroscopy. **B,** The predetermined access point at the intersection of the posterior and middle thirds of the disc space or vertebra is identified.

Step 2: Anatomic Landmark Identification and Initial Incisions

The surgical site is prepared aseptically, and the disc space is localized using lateral fluoroscopy. It may be necessary to count vertebral levels multiple times from above and below the surgical level to ensure that the correct level is targeted. When the correct level is aligned and identified, a single mark is made over the predetermined access point to the site of pathology at the intersection of the posterior and middle thirds of the disc space or vertebra (Fig. 19-3).

Step 3: Thoracic Access

An incision is made parallel to the ribs at the skin marking (Fig. 19-4, *A*). Dissection is performed through the subcutaneous tissue down to the ribs or intercostal space (Fig. 19-4, *B*). Two techniques are possible, depending on the desired size of exposure:

1. For a single-level discectomy, the rib-spreading technique is most commonly used. The standard technique involves dissection between the ribs, through the intercostal muscles, and down to the pleura. Pleural access is achieved by blunt hemostat dissection (Fig. 19-5).

2. As an alternative approach—with either a multilevel discectomy or corpectomy or when better visualization is necessary—a small portion of the rib (approximately 3 to 4 cm) can easily be resected at the beginning of the procedure. An incision is angled toward the rib with the midsection in the position of the access site incision. Thus the rib is exposed, identified, and stripped of the neurovascular bundle from su-

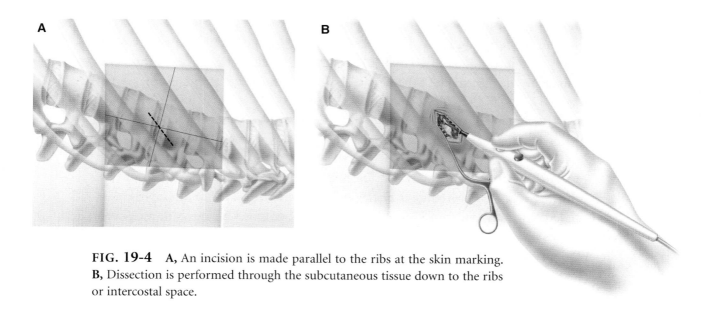

FIG. 19-4   A, An incision is made parallel to the ribs at the skin marking. **B,** Dissection is performed through the subcutaneous tissue down to the ribs or intercostal space.

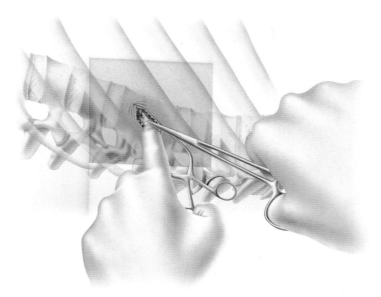

FIG. 19-5   In a single-level discectomy, the standard technique involves dissection between the ribs, through the intercostal muscles down to the pleura, which is then accessed by blunt hemostat dissection.

perior to inferior along its undersurface. A Rib Cutter, Kerrison, and/or Drill can be used to remove a portion of the chosen rib, which may be discarded or saved for bone graft material. With the rib dissection complete, a self-retaining Retractor is positioned, and after blunt or sharp dissection, the parietal pleura is identified and incised, and steps identical to those in the single-level procedure are completed. From this point, the remaining steps are the same for single-level and multilevel techniques.

Once the parietal pleura is incised, the surgeon uses an index finger to enter the pleural space and palpate the lung or diaphragm, displacing the structures anteriorly (Fig. 19-6, *A*). At this point, the lung can be seen in the field. When the chest wall is opened, a small diminution of lung volume caused by the loss of the internal vacuum occurs; this is just enough to allow safe placement of the Retractors without totally deflating the lung.

The initial (black) Dilator is introduced into the thoracic cavity and passed posteriorly along the ribs, down to the intersection of the rib head and the spine (Fig. 19-6, *B* and *C*).

The Retractor is placed in the cavity and the area is carefully examined for adhesions and other obstructions. This procedure is not typically recommended for or attempted in patients undergoing a revision procedure, who may have significant scarring in the access area. Once the absence of adhesions and obstructions is confirmed, a Dilator is placed laterally down the approach corridor.

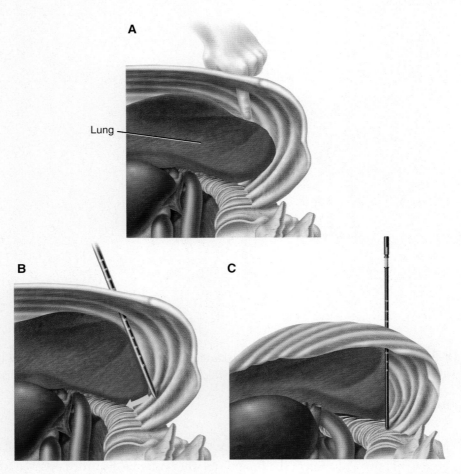

FIG. 19-6 **A,** Once the parietal pleura is incised, the index finger is used to enter the pleural space and palpate the lung or diaphragm and to displace the structures anteriorly. **B** and **C,** The initial (black) Dilator is introduced into the thoracic cavity and passed posteriorly along the ribs down to the intersection of the rib head and the spine.

Once the initial Dilator is on the spine, its position is verified with fluoroscopy. A lateral image is used to confirm that the Dilator is positioned in the posterior third of the disc space and parallel to the disc (Fig. 19-7, *A*). A cross-table anteroposterior image should confirm that the Dilator is positioned on, and in the plane of, the disc space (Fig. 19-7, *B*). Depth markings on the Dilator indicate the size of the appropriate length of the Blades to be attached to the MaXcess Access Driver (Fig. 19-8, *A*). The next two Dilators (magenta and blue) are then passed over the initial Dilator and down to the spine (Fig. 19-8, *B*).

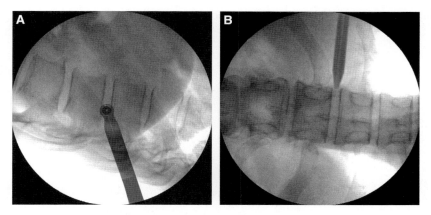

FIG. 19-7   **A,** A lateral image confirms that the Dilator is positioned in the posterior third of the disc space, parallel to the disc. **B,** A cross-table anteroposterior image confirms that the Dilator is placed on and in the plane of the disc space.

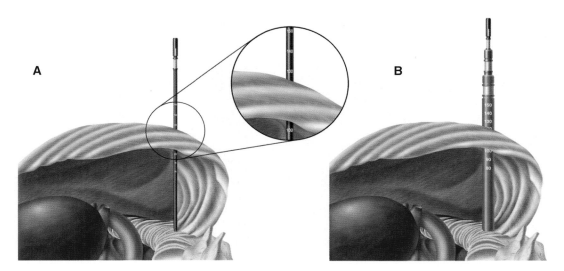

FIG. 19-8   **A,** Depth markings on the Dilator indicate the appropriate length of Blades to be attached to the MaXcess Access Driver. **B,** The next two Dilators, magenta and blue, are passed over the initial Dilator down to the spine.

TRANSITIONAL LEVEL (T12-L1) CONSIDERATIONS

Pleural access to the T12-L1 disc space and above may be established through the transthoracic approach, as previously described (Fig. 19-9, *A*). However, the T12-L1 level may also be accessed by passing between the ribs, through the diaphragmatic attachment at the ribs, and into the retroperitoneal space (Fig. 19-9, *B* and *C*). This method is most commonly employed when lumbar levels are also addressed. In such a scenario, the index finger is passed through the posterolateral incision made in the lumbar XLIF technique and into the retroperitoneal space to guide the initial Dilator down to the spine.

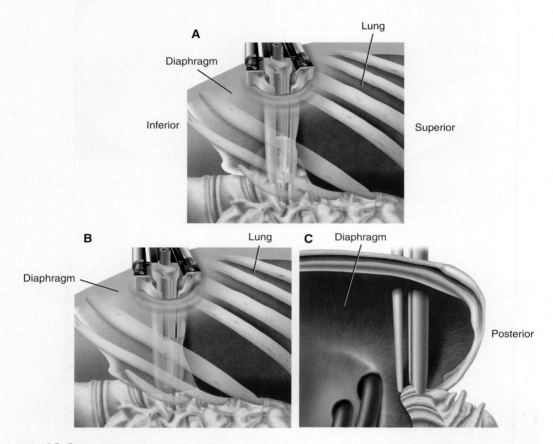

FIG. 19-9 **A,** Pleural access to the T12-L1 disc space and above may be established through the transthoracic approach. **B** and **C,** The T12-L1 level may also be accessed by passing between the ribs, through the diaphragmatic attachment at the ribs, and into the retroperitoneal space.

NEUROVISION MEP MONITORING

NeuroVision offers transcranial motor evoked potential (TcMEP) monitoring with clinically based alarm criteria and an easy-to-interpret user interface (Fig. 19-10, *A*). The NeuroVision MEP system provides unsurpassed efficiency in monitoring the safety and function of the descending motor pathways of the spinal cord, and it delivers critical patient information with more clarity than previous instruments.

MEP Manual Mode

MEP Manual mode provides a rapid and reliable method of confirming motor functionality throughout the procedure and includes the following features (Fig. 19-10, *B*):

- The system allows manual adjustment of the stimulation level for greater flexibility and speed.
- The interface correlates the amount of electrical stimulation with highly visible threshold response indicators of green or red, corresponding to muscle activity.

Working with the NeuroVision MEP Manual mode begins by setting the stimulation output dial to the desired level (in milliamperes). As the patient responds to this stimulation, the system communicates the presence or absence of a muscle response to the operating room staff: a green indicator lights when muscle activity is detected and with a red indicator when no muscle activity is found.

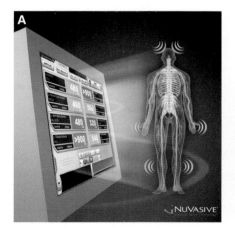
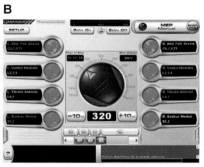

FIG. 19-10 **A,** NeuroVision provides transcranial motor evoked potential (TcMEP) monitoring with clinically based alarm criteria and an easy-to-interpret user interface. **B,** MEP Manual mode provides a rapid and reliable method of confirming motor functionality throughout the case.

Continued

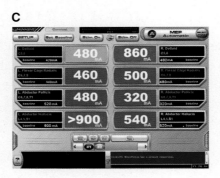

FIG. 19-10, cont'd   *C*, MEP Automatic mode provides clinically determined alarm criteria, rapid response thresholds, and easy-to-interpret results.

MEP Automatic Mode

NeuroVision MEP Automatic mode provides clinically determined alarm criteria and a simple, explicit interface (Fig. 19-10, *C*). The following features make this technology a valuable tool:

- Automation delivers threshold criteria that allow precise, repeatable coupling of the stimulation and response.
- Threshold responses can be quickly identified for multiple responding myotomes.
- Data are communicated at a higher speed than can be obtained manually.
- Changes in thresholds can be more closely tracked over time.
- All monitoring results are automatically recorded to a patient report.
- The threshold determination algorithm delivers the lowest stimulation required to elicit a response, maximizing patient safety.

STEP 4: EXPOSURE

The Access Driver is introduced over the third Dilator, with the handles pointing anteriorly (Fig. 19-11, *A*). Cross-table anteroposterior fluoroscopy is used to confirm the correct position of the Access Driver Blades on the spine and to ensure that the Blades are parallel to the disc space (Fig. 19-11, *B* and *C*).

With the Retractor Blades in position, an Articulating Arm is connected to the posterior arm attachment point (Fig. 19-11, *D*), which affixes the body of the Access Driver to the table. When the Retractor is opened, the center Blade moves anteriorly to retract the lung and/or diaphragm and expose the spine (Fig. 19-11, *E*). The Retractor can be turned slightly so that the spreading is done not against the ribs, but in the superior and inferior planes for a single level. With the Retractor in place, the surrounding structures are identified.

Gentle intercostal distraction is performed, and clear plastic Shims are placed in the single center Blade and in the cephalocaudal Blades (Fig. 19-11, *F*). These can be doubled toward

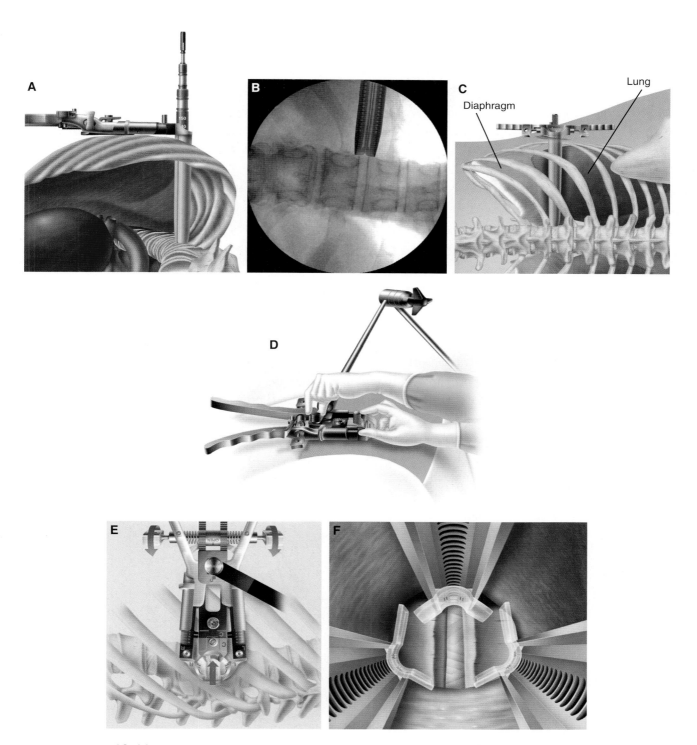

FIG. 19-11 **A,** The Access Driver is introduced over the third Dilator, with the handles pointing anteriorly. **B** and **C,** Cross-table anteroposterior fluoroscopy is used to confirm the correct position of the Access Driver Blades on the spine and to ensure that the Blades are parallel to the disc space. **D,** With the Retractor Blades in position, an Articulating Arm is attached to the posterior arm attachment site. **E,** When the Retractor is opened, the center Blade moves anteriorly to retract the lung and/or diaphragm and expose the spine. **F,** The Retractor is placed, gentle intercostal distraction is performed, and clear plastic Shims are placed in the single center Blade and in the cephalocaudal Blades.

the Retractor opening if the lung and/or diaphragm extend into the operative field. A lap sponge can be placed to further retract the lung if necessary.

In this way, access can be obtained from L1-2 to approximately the T5-6 level. Inferiorly, the diaphragm extends over that area, allowing access to the inferior levels from the retroperitoneal space. Superiorly, the intercostal spaces become smaller, which, along with the location of the scapula and the angle of the chest, makes access above the T5-6 location difficult.

If necessary, one or both of the cephalocaudal Blades can be rotated to expand the exposure in either direction to permit optimal access to the site of pathology. Care should be taken when expanding the Blades near the midvertebral body to minimize the risk of injury to segmental vessels.

STEP 5: ANULOTOMY AND DISC SPACE PREPARATION

The parietal pleura covers the surface of the spine and is incised to gain access to the disc space. An anulotomy approximately 16 mm in length (anterior to posterior) is created with an Anulotomy Knife. A Cobb Elevator may be passed along both endplates to release the disc and cartilage from the subchondral bone. The surgeon must be careful to avoid damaging structures deep to the contralateral anulus, as indicated on the preoperative MRI. Pituitaries, Curettes, Disc Cutters, Endplate Scrapers, and other disc preparation instruments can be used to thoroughly evacuate the disc and prepare the endplates for fusion (Fig. 19-12).

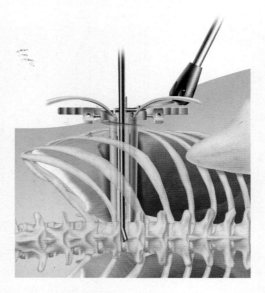

FIG. 19-12   Pituitaries, Curettes, Disc Cutters, Endplate Scrapers, and other disc preparation instruments are used to thoroughly evacuate the disc and prepare the endplates for fusion.

STEP 6: IMPLANT SIZING AND PLACEMENT

Paddle Sizers may be used to distract the space, and the appropriately sized Trial is gauged. Under anteroposterior fluoroscopy, the Trial is gently impacted into the space until the distal end reaches the contralateral margin of the disc space. The proper anteroposterior position is verified using lateral fluoroscopy. Sequentially larger Trials are used until the desired fit and placement are achieved.

The corresponding implant is selected, filled with graft material, and gently impacted into the space while anteroposterior fluoroscopic monitoring is used to check placement. The ideally placed implant is centered across the space from a mediolateral perspective and in the center of the space from an anteroposterior perspective (Fig. 19-13, *A*). A segmental lateral Plate (XLP) can be placed to add stability to the construct as needed (Fig. 19-13, *B*).

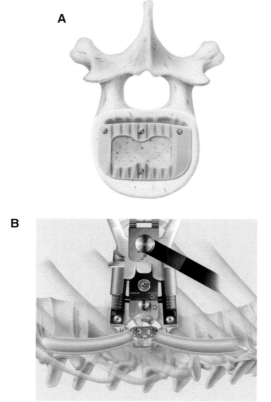

FIG. 19-13   A, The ideally placed implant is centered across the disc space from a medial/lateral perspective and in the center of the space from an anterior/posterior perspective. **B,** A segmental lateral Plate (XLP) can be used to add stability to the construct as needed.

STEP 7: CLOSURE

When the procedure is completed, the Retractor is removed under direct visualization to verify that there is no significant bleeding. A chest tube may be placed and the wound closed by layer. Alternatively, a red rubber catheter can be inserted and the pleural space aspirated with suction to remove air from the pleural cavity as the lung is inflated by the anesthesiologist. A chest radiograph should be obtained postoperatively. The skin is closed using standard subcuticular suture.

INDICATION-SPECIFIC TECHNIQUES

CORPECTOMY

Corpectomy is the most common procedure in the thoracic spine. In the inferiormost aspect of the dissection cavity, an L1 or a T12 corpectomy can easily be performed to treat a thoracolumbar fracture. In this location, when the Retractor is open, the superior leaflets of the diaphragm often extend over the vertebral body, obscuring its posterior and anterior aspects. With fluoroscopic guidance, the vertebral body is mapped out on the skin and over the course of the diaphragm in that location. The surgeon carefully continues the dissection down to the disc space at the first level within the midportion of the disc. Straying between the disc spaces will bring the dissection down on top of the segmental vessels, which often cannot be seen through the muscle of the diaphragm.

With the vertebral body mapped out over the diaphragm muscles, the muscle can be incised with a Bovie electrosurgical unit over the disc space. Quite often, an ultrasonic scalpel and/or a Bovie can be used to extend this incision superiorly over the entire body of L1 and/or T12. In these locations the vessels and neurovascular bundle are clipped and/or ligated using bipolar coagulation, as needed. The intervening vessels are controlled with a careful dissection. The corpectomy is completed and the superior half of the body of L2 can be easily identified for placement of inferior lateral instrumentation; alternatively, percutaneous pedicle screws can be placed posteriorly.

DISCECTOMY/FUSION

The second most common procedure in the midthoracic spine is discectomy. Herniation can occur anywhere from T5-6 to T11-12, but it occurs most commonly in the midthoracic curve at approximately T8-9 to T9-10. The diaphragm does not overlie this area, and the extent of the vertebral body is easily seen. Starting at approximately T10 and moving superiorly, the rib head covers the posterior half of the disc space and must be removed to adequately expose the posterior half and to decompress the dural sleeve. The rib head is removed quite simply by cutting the costotransverse ligaments and the remaining attachments with a sharp Cobb Curette. The rib is removed superiorly and taken out as a single piece. Alternatively, a high-speed Drill is used to remove the portion of rib. With the rib head removed, both pedicles and the foramen are easily identified, and a complete discectomy can be performed. Commonly, the disc is decompressed from the midportion to the anterior portion of the body, and then the space created allows the disc to be delivered anteriorly by using an angled Curette. In the midportion of the body in a large, barrel-chested person, the Retractors need to be as long as possible to perform this dissection. With the rib head removed, the discectomy is performed at the primary site, and, if necessary, the procedure is repeated at each additional location. Intervertebral fusion cages, bone grafts, and lateral Plates may be used as fixation requirements demand.

CONCLUSION

The minimally invasive XLIF thoracic procedure offers an excellent alternative to an open thoracotomy or a video-assisted thoracoscopic discectomy. The lung is easily controlled without deflation, and access all the way to lower portions of the spine is possible, using the diaphragm as a boundary. If necessary, a rib section can be removed for greater access at a single level or for multiple-level procedures. Alternatively, the intervals between the ribs can be accessed without removing a rib section. In addition, the Retractor is easily adapted to multiple thoracic pathologies, and the complications and difficulties of an open procedure are avoided. Closure is performed in the standard, layered manner and a chest tube can be placed to allow air, blood, and other debris to be removed from the pleural cavity.

Through a minimal corridor, complex corpectomies can be performed at most levels, allowing an approach for elective decompressive procedures and traumatic repair. We have successfully used this method to treat patients with traumatic spine injuries, metastatic tumor disease, thoracic disc disease, and to correct deformities. We have encountered no significant postoperative pulmonary problems, because we avoid dropping the lung during the procedure. We have also seen no evidence of pulmonary contusions. The skin can be closed and the remainder of the procedure conducted in the normal fashion, and a chest tube can be placed to release air from the cavity or to drain blood and other debris, if necessary. The Retractor is easily adaptable to the treatments of various thoracic pathologic conditions and avoids the complications and difficulties associated with an open procedure.

Thoracic XLIF surgery encompasses all of the positive aspects of a standard open procedure, with fewer significant risks. As this technology continues to develop, it is expected to become the preferred technique.

REFERENCES

1. Lin CC. A new method of thoracoscopic sympathectomy in hyperhidrosis palmaris. Surg Endosc 4:224-226, 1990.
2. Lin CC. Extended thoracoscopic T2-sympathectomy in treatment of hyperhidrosis: experience with 130 consecutive cases. J Laparoendosc Surg 2:1-6, 1992.
3. Chou SH, Lee SH, Kao EL. Thoracic endoscopic T2-T3 sympathectomy in palmar hyperhidrosis: experience of 112 cases. Surg Today 23:105-107, 1993.
4. Horowitz MB, Moossy JJ, Julian T, et al. Thoracic discectomy using video assisted thoracoscopy. Spine 19:1082-1086, 1994.
5. Regan JJ, Mack MJ, Picetti GD. A technical report on video-assisted thoracoscopy in thoracic spinal surgery. Preliminary description. Spine 20:831-837, 1995.
6. Hertlein H, Hartl WH, Dienemann H, et al. Thoracoscopic repair of thoracic spine trauma. Eur Spine J 4:302-307, 1995.
7. McAfee PC, Regan JR, Fedder IL, et al. Anterior thoracic corpectomy for spinal cord decompression performed endoscopically. Surg Laparosc Endosc 5:339-348, 1995.
8. Islam S, Hresko MT, Fishman SJ. Extrapleural thoracoscopic anterior spinal fusion: a modified video-assisted thoracoscopic surgery approach to the pediatric spine. JSLS 5:187-189, 2001.
9. Angevin PD, McCormick PC. Retropleural thoracotomy. Technical note. Neurosurg Focus 10:ecp1, 2001.
10. McCormick PC. Retropleural approach to the thoracic and thoracolumbar spine. Neurosurgery 37:908-914, 1995.
11. Kim KD, Babbitz JD, Mimbs J. Imaging-guided costotransversectomy for thoracic disc herniation. Neurosurg Focus 9:e7, 2000.
12. Smith JT, Gollogly S, Dunn HK. Simultaneous anterior-posterior approach through a costotransversectomy for the treatment of congenital kyphosis and acquired kyphoscoliotic deformities. J Bone Joint Surg Am 87:2281-2289, 2005.
13. Bilsky MH. Transpedicular approach for thoracic disc herniations. Neurosurg Focus 9:e3, 2000.
14. Jho HD. Endoscopic microscopic transpedicular thoracic discectomy. Technical note. Neurosurg Focus 4:e7, 1998.

20

Thoracic Disc Herniation: Extreme Lateral Approach

Vedat Deviren ▪ Murat Pekmezci ▪ Bobby Tay

Thoracic disc herniation is a relatively uncommon spinal condition that can cause severe functional disability. Unfortunately, there is no characteristic clinical presentation. Signs and symptoms can vary from obscure thoracic or abdominal pain to bowel/bladder dysfunction with severe myelopathy. However, magnetic resonance imaging (MRI) has revolutionized the detection and diagnosis of this problem. Because the natural history of the disease is also not well defined, indications for surgery—as well as the type of surgery that is optimal—are controversial. Surgical treatment is indicated for patients with frank myelopathy or severe radiculopathy, but the role of surgery for axial pain is still controversial. The optimal method of decompression is another topic for which a consensus has not been reached. There are several approaches to decompression, each with its own advantages and disadvantages. This chapter focuses on the general aspects of thoracic disc disease and treatment options, with an emphasis on a novel mini-incision, anterolateral, transthoracic, transpleural approach.

INCIDENCE

Thoracic disc disease is a rare affliction, with an incidence of one case per million per year.[1] However, the incidence and prevalence of thoracic disc disease complicated by radiculopathy and/or myelopathy are unknown. Asymptomatic thoracic disc herniation may exist in up to 15% to 37% of the population in the United States.[2,3] Thoracic disc herniation is responsible for the symptoms in 0.2% of patients with back pain.[4] Surgery for thoracic disc herniation composes 0.15% to 1.8% of surgeries performed for all disc herniations.[5,6]

ETIOLOGIC FACTORS AND PATHOGENESIS

In most cases, thoracic disc disease is a consequence of a degenerative process with or without coincident trauma. This observation is supported by the fact that most thoracic disc herniations are found in the lower thoracic spine, where degenerative changes are more prevalent.[7-9] Seventy-five percent of thoracic disc herniations occur below T8, and the most commonly affected level is T11-12.[10] This is attributed to the relative increased mobility of the lower thoracic spine and the relative weakness of the posterior longitudinal ligament in that area.

The thoracic spine and spinal cord have several unique features that make them vulnerable to injury.[11] The development of clinical symptoms is attributed to local vascular compromise leading to spinal cord dysfunction.[4,12,13] Doppman and Girton[14] demonstrated in an experimental animal model that neurologic deficits can recover—even in the presence of spinal cord distortion—if normal circulation is restored, whereas deficits usually persist if normal hemodynamics cannot be restored. These experimental results are supported by clinical observations that demonstrate both the persistence of neurologic deficits at several levels above the affected site and the lack of functional recovery even after an adequate decompression.[4,12,15]

Several anatomic structures and relationships predispose the thoracic spinal cord to anterior compression. The thoracic spine is normally kyphotic, and the spinal cord runs close to the posterior aspect of the vertebral bodies. Additionally, the dentate ligaments tether the spinal cord—limiting the cord's ability to drift away from anterior impingement.[16] The ratio of the spinal cord diameter to canal diameter is higher in the thoracic spine than in the cervical and lumbar areas, leaving less room for the spinal cord in case of stenosis.[11] Finally, the thoracic spinal cord is vulnerable to ischemic injury because of the presence of an anatomic area of poor blood supply called the *watershed zone.*[17] Unlike cervical and lumbar disc herniations, thoracic disc herniations are more frequently centrally located and are more likely to calcify.[18] They may be adherent to—and may even erode through—the dural sac over time. These characteristics of the thoracic spine and spinal cord are important for understanding the pathophysiology and treatment approaches for symptomatic thoracic disc disease.

NATURAL HISTORY

There is limited information on the natural history of thoracic disc disease. Wood et al[6] studied 20 asymptomatic patients with thoracic disc disease and reported that after 26 months of follow-up, all patients remained asymptomatic. In addition, 35 of the 48 disc herniations did not demonstrate any measurable change in size at the final follow-up. Brown et al[20] reviewed 55 patients who presented with symptomatic protrusions. Of these patients, 73% (40) were treated conservatively; 77% of those who were treated conservatively returned to their previous level of activity. Limited studies have concluded that patients with both axial pain and radiculopathy often respond to conservative treatment.

Natural history also differs among patients depending on symptoms. Patients with lower extremity symptoms tend to progress—the initial complaint of lower extremity pain is often followed by sensory disturbances, sphincter dysfunction, and myelopathy.[20,21] Rapid development of myelopathy is more common in younger patients who have a history of trauma. In the middle-aged population with degenerative disc disease and no significant trauma, the development of myelopathy occurs at a significantly slower pace.[12] Spontaneous recovery is not expected in patients with frank myelopathy, and surgical decompression is usually recommended.

CLINICAL PRESENTATION

Thoracic disc herniation affects males and females equally and occurs more commonly during the third, fourth, and fifth decades of life.[4,12,22-25] Clinical presentation varies depending on the location and severity of the herniation. There is a wide variety of clinical presentations; back pain is usually the most common initial presentation, often described as a "burning" or "shooting" sensation that can be intermittent or constant.[26,27] Patients usually describe a pain that "bores right through the chest" or a band-like pain that radiates through the chest wall or flank. Depending on the neurologic level of involvement, patients may experience flank, abdominal, or groin pain. Because of this wide variation in the pain pattern, it is not uncommon for patients to be misdiagnosed with gallbladder disease, gastritis, and renal calculi.[25,27-31] Arce and Dohrmann,[10] in their review of the literature, reported that of 179 patients, 57% reported pain, 24% reported sensory disturbance, 17% reported motor weakness, and 2% described sphincter dysfunction. Most patients have signs and symptoms of cord compression at initial presentation.

Progression of spinal cord compression can result in bowel and bladder dysfunction, gait disturbance, variable sensory and/or motor dysfunction in the lower extremities, and paraplegia. Lesions between T11 and L1 can compress the conus medullaris and the cauda equina, resulting in lower extremity radiculopathy and sphincter disturbance. Patients who have compression above the conus medullaris usually present with long-tract signs such as gait disturbance, weakness, spasticity, and/or bowel and bladder dysfunction (retention, frequency, incomplete evacuation, or incontinence). Patients who have thoracic disc disease should have normal upper extremity function. If there are neurologic symptoms in the upper extremities, one should search for coexisting cervical stenosis, cranial pathology, or a systemic neurologic disease process.

DIAGNOSIS

Evaluating thoracic disc herniation includes correlating the patient's symptoms with a detailed neurologic evaluation and a neuroradiologic evaluation. If a patient has long-tract signs and upper extremity involvement, the cervical spine should be examined to rule out cervical cord compression. In the absence of myelopathy, it is easy to overlook thoracic pathology and blame the often coexisting lumbar degenerative process for the patient's symptoms. Allowing patients to localize their back pain may help the clinician to reach the correct diagnosis.

MRI is becoming the gold standard for confirming diagnoses and localizing pathology in patients suspected to have thoracic disc disease (Fig. 20-1, *A*). It can help to differentiate among infectious, neoplastic, congenital, and degenerative processes.[8,32-34] Computed tomography (CT)-myelography also provides valuable information, because it can better delineate the degree of compression as well as diagnose ossification of the posterior longitudinal ligament or the ligamentum flavum (Fig. 20-1, *B*). Both imaging modalities provide valuable information and should be routine for evaluating patients with suspected thoracic disc disease.[10,32,33]

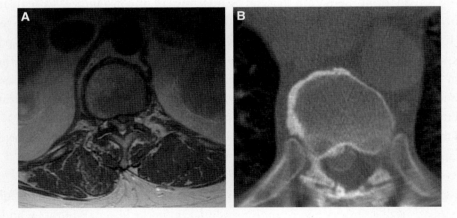

FIG. 20-1 A, Axial T-2 weighted MRI image of a patient who presented with worsening lower extremity spasticity and gait disturbance caused by a large central-paracentral thoracic disc herniation. **B,** Axial CT scan that demonstrates the large herniation compressing upon the thoracic spinal cord.

TREATMENT

Patients with thoracic disc disease can be divided into three groups. The first group includes patients who have myelopathy, with or without associated back pain or radicular symptoms. The second group consists of patients with lower extremity weakness or paralysis. The third group includes patients who present with back pain and radiculopathy without myelopathy. Surgical decompression is clearly indicated for the first and second groups, whereas the patients in the third group may benefit from conservative treatment. Surgery in the third group of patients is usually performed when there are persistent disabling symptoms despite optimal conservative care. Conservative treatment options include drug therapy with nonsteroidal antiinflammatory drugs, narcotics, and third generation pain medications such as tricyclics and serotonin-reuptake inhibitors; physical therapy; and intercostal nerve blocks.

When a surgical treatment is chosen, the affected level(s) should be confirmed with MRI. Several approaches have been reported in the literature for treating thoracic disc herniations. There is no gold standard approach, and each technique has advantages and disadvantages. There are several possible approaches—anterior, lateral, posterolateral, and posterior (Box 20-1). The posterior approach is laminectomy. Posterolateral approaches include transpedicular (with or without endoscopy) and transfacet, pedicle-sparing approaches. The lateral approach is costotransversectomy (lateral extracavitary approach). Anterior decompression can be achieved through either the transthoracic or the thoracoscopic approach.

POSTERIOR APPROACH
Laminectomy

Simple laminectomy with or without discectomy was the first technique used to treat thoracic disc herniations.[4,13,21,35] However, it is difficult to eliminate the anterior compressive forces over the thoracic spinal cord with this technique.[14,15] Excising the disc material using

---

BOX 20-1   Surgical Approaches for Treating Thoracic Disc Disease

Anterior (Anterolateral) Approaches
- Transthoracic extrapleural
- Transthoracic transpleural
- VATS

Posterolateral Approaches
- Lateral extracavitary
- Transpedicular
- Transpedicular facet sparing

Posterior Approaches
- Laminectomy

laminectomy is associated with significant morbidity and mortality.[4,21,35,36] In addition, it can further destabilize the posterior tension band, resulting in increased kyphosis and progression of compression. Perot and Munro[36] reviewed the literature to evaluate the safety and efficacy of laminectomy and discectomy to treat thoracic disc herniation. Of the 91 patients in the review, 40 had no improvement, and 16 became paraplegic. Some patients became paraplegic following simple laminectomy without any attempt to remove the herniated disc. Of note, 15 of the 16 patients who developed paraplegia had centrally located discs, which confirms the limited access to central discs with this approach. Laminectomy for thoracic disc disease is no longer used.

POSTEROLATERAL APPROACHES
Transpedicular Approach

The transpedicular approach was first described by Patterson and Arbit.[11] The major advantage of this approach is that it is less extensive, requiring less soft tissue dissection. Thus there are potential advantages, including decreased operation time, less blood loss, a shortened hospital stay, and a shorter period of rehabilitation. Posterolateral approaches allow better visualization of the herniated disc than posterior approaches and can be performed at any level. However, these approaches still limit visualization of the anterior spinal canal. Decompression of a central or centrolateral disc fragment is done blindly. It is also difficult to manage calcified discs or osteophytes. This problem can be alleviated either by using intraoperative ultrasound to assess the adequacy of decompression or by rotating the patient 15 to 20 degrees away from the surgeon. This modified transpedicular approach requires subtotal removal of the facet and pedicle. When performed unilaterally at one level, iatrogenic instability is uncommon. However, if more extensive pedicle and facet resection are required, posterior fusion and stabilization may be needed to prevent late kyphosis or olisthesis. Patterson and Arbit[11] reported on three patients who had thoracic disc herniation with myelopathy. The entire pedicle and facet were removed to achieve decompression. Two patients were cured, and one improved. However, this was an aggressive approach that created instability, and the procedure was modified to preserve as much of the facet and pedicle as possible. Le Roux et al[37] reported significant improvement in 20 patients who underwent decompression of their thoracic disc herniations using the transpedicular approach. Stillerman et al[38] described the transfacet pedicle-sparing approach in 1995. However, this approach still does not allow adequate viewing of central lesions, and the extent of decompression is difficult to evaluate.

Lateral Extracavitary Approach

The lateral extracavitary approach popularized by Larson et al[39] in 1976 evolved from early attempts at surgical treatment of Pott's disease of the spine.[40] Some earlier versions of the approach have been known as costotransversectomy, supradiaphragmatic splanchnicectomy, or lateral rachotomy.[41-43] In 1991, Fessler et al[44] reported a modification of the lateral extracavitary approach that extended its exposure up to the inferior aspect of C7. This technique is the lateral parascapular extrapleural approach and is most appropriate for anterior lesions from C7 to T6.

This approach provides access to every level of thoracolumbar spine, achieving a combined anterior-posterior procedure through the same incision. It provides excellent simultaneous exposure of the anterior, lateral, and posterior spine elements. It also allows simultaneous exposure of multiple segments between the inferior aspects of C7 down to L5. However, it is not useful for central or intradural disc herniations, because it provides poor exposure across the entire spinal canal.

The ideal patient for this approach is one with posterolateral disc herniation and significant comorbidities who may not tolerate a thoracotomy. In general, any disease process that causes myelopathy from anterior spinal cord compression or anterior spinal instability can be effectively treated using this approach. The procedure is performed with the patient in the prone or lateral decubitus position. The posterior portion of each rib on the side of the herniated disc is excised, and the pleura is mobilized and reflected anterolaterally. The transverse processes and remaining head and neck of each excised rib are then removed. The intervertebral foramen is enlarged by partial removal of the corresponding pedicles, and the dural sac is exposed. A cavity is created in the posterior aspect of the bodies and disc, allowing removal of disc fragments through the defect without manipulation of the spinal cord. The reported average clinical improvement is 85%, with a range of 71% to 91%.[45-47] Although radicular pain usually resolves, many patients continue to complain of intermittent back pain.[23,46]

ANTERIOR (ANTEROLATERAL) TRANSTHORACIC APPROACHES

Although lateral extracavitary and transpedicular approaches can provide good exposure of paracentral lesions, they are still inferior to the anterior approach for lesions that are directly ventral to the spinal cord. Furthermore, these approaches are less useful when there is intradural extension of a disc fragment or when there are significant adhesions between a disc and the dura.

There are several advantages to the transthoracic approach. It allows access to all herniations below T4. It provides direct exposure for all types of thoracic disc herniations (central, paracentral, and lateral). It enables access to both soft and hard discs and is especially helpful when decompressing calcified central herniations. It allows easy access to adjoining levels for multiple disc herniations. Finally, it permits excellent exposure and access for performing interbody fusion after the removal of a disc.

There are several drawbacks to the transthoracic approach. Pulmonary atelectasis often occurs postoperatively. If the diaphragm is released, a diaphragmatic hernia can occur. The great arterial and venous vessels can be damaged. Patients may develop persistent pain. There is a risk to the artery of Adamkiewicz during a left-sided approach, which can lead to spinal cord infarction. Some authors recommend using angiography to identify this major segmental vessel so that the exposure can be modified accordingly. Conversely, there is abundant collateral circulation in the region of the neural foramina that can provide blood flow to the cord, even with ligation of the artery of Adamkiewicz.[17,48,49] As long as electrocautery is used with caution when coagulating the vessels near the foramen, the risk to the vessel is small.[50]

Anterior Video-Assisted Thoracoscopic Surgery

Thoracoscopic spine surgery has found increased use over the past decade, and thoracic discectomy has become one of the common indications for the procedure.[51-55] Regan et al[55] reported on 29 patients who had thoracic discectomy with video-assisted thoracoscopic surgery (VATS); 76% of the patients reported satisfactory results. The advantages of VATS include reduced perioperative morbidity from minimal surgical dissection, avoidance of rib resection or spreading, enhanced visualization for the operating surgeons and support team, reduced postoperative pain with improved ventilatory excursion, shorter hospitalization and rehabilitation, and consequent decreased overall cost of care. In addition, because the ribs do not need to be retracted, the incidence of intercostal neuralgia is decreased. The main disadvantage of thoracoscopy is the technique itself. The procedure is performed with endoscopic visualization, which is very dependent on accurate portal placement. The average spine surgeon requires additional training to effectively perform the procedure, and the learning curve initially may result in prolonged operating times and an occasional conversion to open thoracotomy. In addition, the ipsilateral lung should be deflated during the procedure, which increases the risk for pulmonary complications such as pleural effusion, atelectasis, pneumonia, and pneumothorax. Anand and Regan[51] reported a 21% complication rate in a series of 100 patients. Of the complications, 15% were pulmonary in nature. McAfee et al[54] reported perioperative complications in 78 patients who had VATS (41 for thoracic disc herniation); the most common complications were intercostal neuralgia (8%) and atelectasis sufficient to delay discharge (6%). Although VATS has advantages, there are no studies in the literature that compare open thoracotomy with VATS in myelopathic patients with thoracic disc disease.

Anterior Transthoracic Transpleural Approach

An anterior transthoracic approach provides an excellent view of the dura-disc interval and allows decompression of the canal with the least manipulation of the neural structures. The anterior approach using a thoracotomy was described in 1969 by Perot and Munro,[36] and again in 1988 by Bohlman and Zdeblick.[2] Thoracotomy has been associated with significant perioperative discomfort and pulmonary complications. It usually involves resection of a rib, deflation of the ipsilateral lung, and insertion of a chest tube. Each of these maneuvers contributes to increased postoperative pain levels and pulmonary complications such as atelectasis and pneumonia. Depending on the extent of the decompression, an anterior fusion may be performed to prevent instability or deformity. Bohlman and Zdeblick[2] reported on 19 patients and concluded that the transthoracic approach, with its superior exposure, was preferred over costotransversectomy. Mulier and Debois's review[56] revealed superior neurologic recovery rates with anterior approaches compared with lateral and posterolateral approaches, at the expense of higher pulmonary complication rates. Otani et al[57] described a transthoracic extrapleural approach with the primary goal of decreasing pulmonary complications. They reported on 23 patients, and the results were similar to those in other series of transthoracic decompressions with no pulmonary complications.

MINIMALLY INVASIVE ANTEROLATERAL TRANSTHORACIC TRANSPLEURAL APPROACH

The lead author's (V.D.) preferred approach is the minimally invasive anterolateral transthoracic transpleural approach (XLIF-thoracic approach using the MaXcess® Access [NuVasive®, Inc., San Diego, CA] system), or a modification of a mini-thoracotomy approach. As with the lumbar XLIF procedure, the objective is to perform conventional surgery while avoiding collateral approach-related trauma. The XLIF technique allows surgeons to perform standard anterior discectomy and fusion with instrumentation through a minimally invasive approach. The advantages of this approach in the thoracic region include avoiding rib resection, performing the procedure under direct vision, and less perioperative morbidity. Because it allows for direct vision and conventional surgical techniques, the learning curve is much less than those for previously discussed minimally invasive options.

The MaXcess Retractor system eliminates the need to deflate the ipsilateral lung, theoretically decreasing the risk of postoperative atelectasis and pulmonary complications. We did not experience any pulmonary complications in the first 8 patients on whom we performed this procedure. We entered the thoracic cavity at the superior margin of the inferior rib to avoid the neurovascular bundle. Despite this, we had one patient with postoperative intercostal neuralgia. We believe this was caused by the use of a rigid retractor system. This technique does not necessarily eliminate chest tube placement after surgery, which is often a routine part of the conventional thoracotomy and thoracoscopy.

Surgical Technique

The procedure is performed under general endotracheal anesthesia. Because a very small area of the thoracic cavity is needed to perform the procedure, a regular endotracheal tube rather than a double lumen tube is used. Neuromonitoring is a standard part of the procedure and includes somatosensory evoked potentials (SSEPs), motor evoked potentials

(MEPs), and electromyogram (EMG) for the lower thoracic segments (T8-T12). A standard reversed operative table is used, and the patient is placed in the left lateral decubitus position so that the affected level lies at the break in the table. All the bony prominences are carefully padded. The patient is fixed to the table with 4-inch tape, and the table is flexed to open the affected level (Fig. 20-2, *A* and *B*).

The surgical field is widely prepared so the incision can be extended to a regular thoracotomy if necessary. The junction between the posterior and middle thirds of the disc space is marked on the skin using fluoroscopy (Fig. 20-2, *C* through *E*). A 4 to 5 cm incision is centered over the mark. The subcutaneous tissue and the intercostal muscles are divided using electrocautery. We prefer to enter the thoracic cavity through the superior edge of the rib that is overlying the disc space to avoid the neurovascular bundle at the superior aspect of the intercostal space. The level is verified with the C-arm, and Dilators are placed over the affected disc space (Fig. 20-2, *F* through *I*). Then the NuVasive MaXcess Retractor is introduced into the thoracic cavity (Fig. 20-2, *J* through *M*).

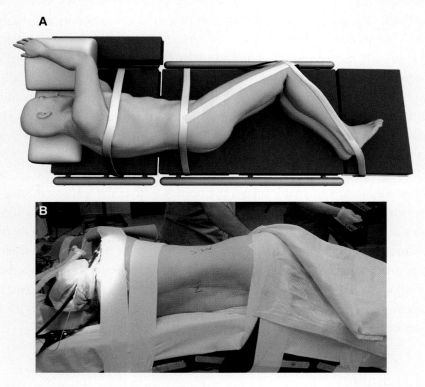

FIG. 20-2   **A,** An overhead view of a patient in the lateral decubitus position. The patient is secured to the operative table with 4-inch tape, with the lumbosacral spine at the break in the table to facilitate exposure. **B,** An intraoperative photograph of a patient in the lateral decubitus position, with the table flexed to facilitate exposure.

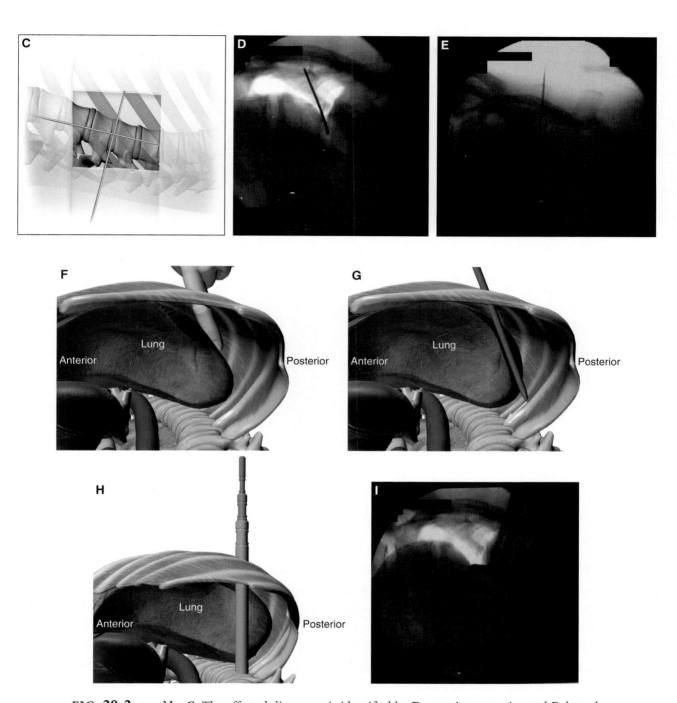

FIG. 20-2, cont'd   C, The affected disc space is identified by **D,** anterior-posterior and **E,** lateral fluoroscopic imaging using a long guidewire placed on the skin to direct the location of the skin incision. **F-I,** The chest is entered through a 4-cm intercostal incision centered over the affected disc space. The first Dilator is placed through the incision to rest on the lateral aspect of the affected disc space, centered on the disc space in the lateral plane and in line with the disc space in the anterior-posterior plane.   *Continued*

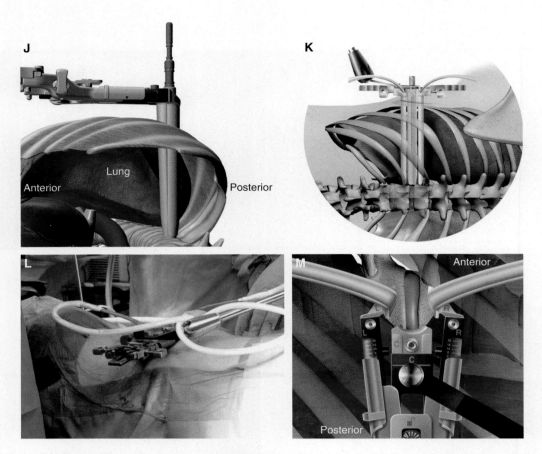

FIG. 20-2, cont'd   J-M, An XLIF Retractor is placed over the final Dilator and docked onto the center of the disc space with the third Blade placed anteriorly (in contrast to the lumbar spine where the third Blade is positioned posteriorly).

This Retractor is specially designed for minimally invasive lateral and posterior lumbar procedures. It has three Blades for retracting soft tissue—a center Blade and two lateral Blades. The lateral Blades can be angled up to 25 degrees. Using the traditional approach, the middle Blade is fixed to the posterior third of the disc space with a Shim, and the two lateral Blades can be distracted to improve the operative field. Additional Shims in varying sizes can be attached to the Blades to prevent protrusion of soft tissues (such as the lung and diaphragm) to the field. During anterior thoracic discectomy, the Retractor is reversed to provide a better exposure (Fig. 20-3, *A* through *C*). Wet lap sponges are used behind the proximal Blade to retract the lung. Then a longitudinal incision is made over the parietal pleura. After blunt dissection of the pleura, the segmental vessels above and below the disc space are identified and clipped. The rib head overlying the posterolateral corner of the disc is identified and osteotomized (Fig. 20-3, *D*), which helps identify the posterolateral corner of the disc and the vertebral body. The disc is cut with a disc knife, and a standard discectomy is performed (Fig. 20-3, *E*). The anterior and posterior anulus is left intact. The posteroinferior corner of the vertebra above and the posterosuperior corner of the vertebra below are excised with a

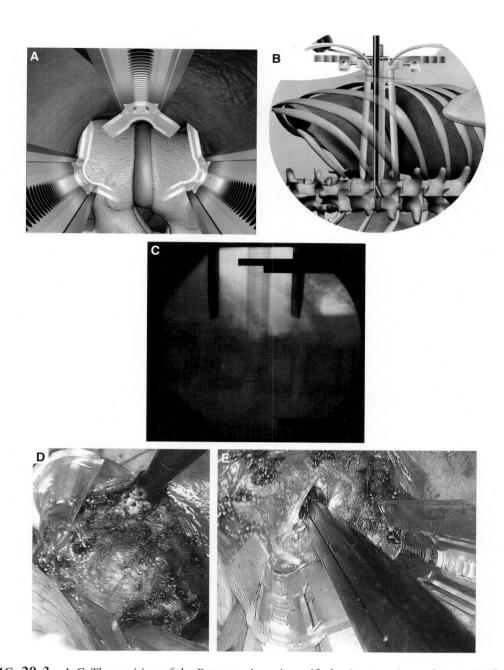

FIG. 20-3   **A-C,** The position of the Retractor is again verified using anterior and posterior fluoroscopy after the Retractor is expanded. **D,** The rib head is identified and removed with an osteotome to expose the pedicle. The bone is saved for use in the fusion. **E,** Disc material is removed with a Pituitary Rongeur to partially decompress the middle portion of the disc space to allow safer decompression of the spinal canal.

Continued

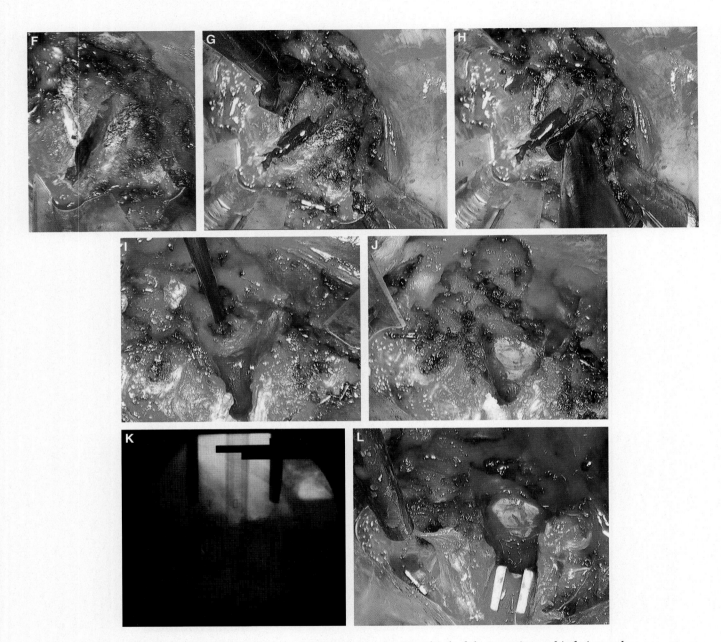

FIG. 20-3, cont'd   F-H, Partial osteotomy of the posterior third of the superior and inferior end-plates allows better visualization and decompression of the neural elements. **I** and **J,** The posterior longitudinal ligament is dissected away from the dura with a Penfield Dissector and is then cut transversely with a knife; the Penfield is used to protect the dura and spinal cord. **K** and **L,** Following decompression, the disc space is prepared with Rasps and reconstructed with a thoracic XLIF cage filled with local bone and bone morphogenic protein.

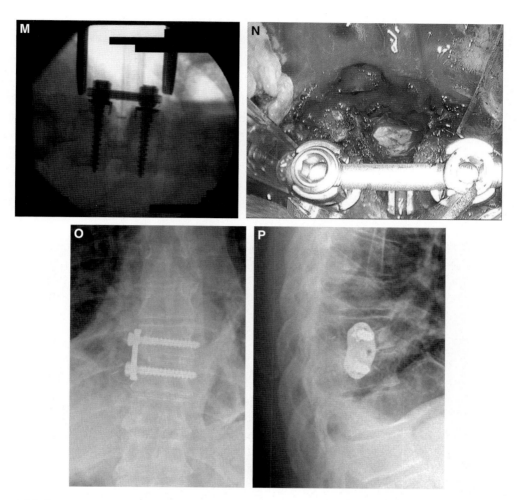

FIG. 20-3, cont'd **M** and **N**, The interspace is further stabilized with a lateral single-rod construct, as evidenced on the radiographs and intraoperative views of the construct. **O** and **P**, AP and lateral radiographs showing thoracic decompression with fusion and use of lateral plating (XLP®, NuVasive, Inc.).

straight osteotome to facilitate decompression (Fig. 20-3, *F* through *H*). I prefer using an osteotome to preserve local bone, which can be used as a bone graft during anterior fusion. The posterior border of the posterior anulus and posterior longitudinal ligament is identified and dissected off the dura using a Penfield Dissector. The posterior longitudinal ligament (PLL) is then dissected and removed using Curettes and Pituitary Rongeurs. The decompression is extended to the level of the contralateral pedicle (Fig. 20-3, *I* and *J*).

Following decompression of the spinal cord, a cage filled with local bone is placed into the disc space (Fig. 20-3, *K* and *L*). The affected level is stabilized with anterior instrumentation using either a screw-rod construct or a plate (Fig. 20-3, *M* through *P*).

The incision is closed in a standard fashion. A chest tube is placed, and it is removed on postoperative day 1 or 2, depending on the output. All patients are braced with a thoracolumbosacral orthosis (TLSO) for 6 weeks before they are allowed to move as tolerated.

CASE EXAMPLE

A 20-year-old woman presented with a primary complaint of worsening bilateral lower extremity pain, urinary retention, and fecal incontinence. An MRI examination revealed a T12-L1 disc herniation (Fig. 20-4, *A* and *B*). She was treated with anterior transthoracic transpleural discectomy and fusion (Fig. 20-4, *C* and *D*). Following surgery her lower extremity and bowel/bladder symptoms improved significantly. Her incision healed uneventfully (Fig. 20-4, *E*).

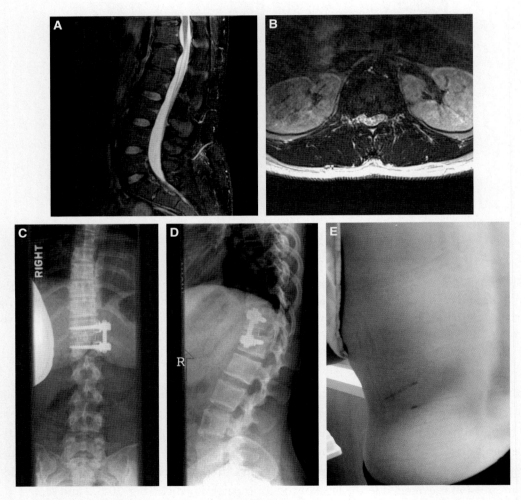

FIG. 20-4   A, Sagittal and **B,** axial T2-weighted MRI of a 20-year-old woman who presented with worsening bilateral lower extremity pain, urinary retention, and fecal incontinence. The MRI demonstrates a T12-L1 central disc herniation. **C,** Anteroposterior and **D,** lateral radiographs of this patient after treatment with thoracic disc excision and interbody fusion with lateral instrumentation. **E,** The minimal postoperative scar 1 month after the procedure.

CONCLUSION

Thoracic disc herniation is clinically challenging. Because it is rare—and because patients present with a variety of symptoms—diagnosis is often delayed or patients receive inappropriate treatment because of an incorrect diagnosis. Surgical treatment is indicated for patients with neurologic deficits or persistent pain that is refractory to conservative treatment. Appropriate surgical treatment provides both motor and gait improvement, with pain relief in approximately 80% to 90% of patients. Patients with risk factors such as coexistent neurologic disease, advanced age, long illness, and severe myelopathy often have less postoperative improvement than typical patients.[37]

There are several different approaches for treating thoracic disc herniation. Although there is no gold standard treatment, most surgeons agree that anterior decompression using a transthoracic, transpleural approach provides the best exposure and the most consistent decompression. Although VATS may provide less morbidity, it has a steep learning curve. We use a new minimally invasive, transthoracic, transpleural decompression technique that can be performed by spine surgeons without extensive training. The proposed advantages are less dissection (resulting in less perioperative morbidity), along with the advantages of conventional thoracotomy. However, long-term follow-up results remain to be documented.

REFERENCES

1. Russell T. Thoracic intervertebral disc protrusion: experience of 67 cases and review of the literature. Br J Neurosurg 3:153-160, 1989.
2. Bohlman HH, Zdeblick TA. Anterior excision of herniated thoracic discs. J Bone Joint Surg Am 70:1038-1047, 1988.
3. Otani K, Nakai S, Fujimura Y, et al. Surgical treatment of thoracic disc herniation using the anterior approach. J Bone Joint Surg Br 64:340-343, 1982.
4. Love JG, Kiefer EJ. Root pain and paraplegia due to protrusions of thoracic intervertebral disks. J Neurosurg 7:62-69, 1950.
5. Awwad EE, Martin DS, Smith KR, et al. Asymptomatic versus symptomatic herniated thoracic discs: their frequency and characteristics as detected by computed tomography after myelography. Neurosurgery 28:180-186, 1991.
6. Wood KB, Blair JM, Aepple DM, et al. The natural history of asymptomatic thoracic disc herniations. Spine 22:525-529; discussion 529-530, 1997.
7. Tahmouresie A. Herniated thoracic intervertebral disc—an unusual presentation: case report. Neurosurgery 7:623-625, 1980.
8. Blumenkopf B. Thoracic intervertebral disc herniations: diagnostic value of magnetic resonance imaging. Neurosurgery 23:36-40, 1988.
9. Videman T, Battié MC, Gill K, et al. Magnetic resonance imaging findings and their relationships in the thoracic and lumbar spine. Insights into the etiopathogenesis of spinal degeneration. Spine 20:928-935, 1995.
10. Arce CA, Dohrmann GJ. Thoracic disc herniation. Improved diagnosis with computed tomographic scanning and a review of the literature. Surg Neurol 23:356-361, 1985.

11. Patterson RH Jr, Arbit E. A surgical approach through the pedicle to protruded thoracic discs. J Neurosurg 48:768-772, 1978.

12. Arseni C, Nash F. Thoracic intervertebral disc protrusion: a clinical study. J Neurosurg 17:418-430, 1960.

13. Logue V. Thoracic intervertebral disc prolapse with spinal cord compression. J Neurol Neurosurg Psychiatry 15:227-241, 1952.

14. Doppman JL, Girton M. Angiographic study of the effect of laminectomy in the presence of acute anterior epidural masses. J Neurosurg 45:195-202, 1976.

15. Bennett MH, McCallum JE. Experimental decompression of spinal cord. Surg Neurol 8: 63-67, 1977.

16. Kahn EA. The role of dentate ligaments in spinal cord compression and the syndrome of lateral sclerosis. J Neurosurg 4:191-199, 1947.

17. Dommisse GF. The blood supply of the spinal cord. A critical vascular zone in spinal surgery. J Bone Joint Surg Br 56:225-235, 1974.

18. Severi P, Ruelle A, Andrioli G. Multiple calcified thoracic disc herniations. A case report. Spine 17:449-451, 1992.

19. Brown CW, Deffer PA Jr, Akmakjian J, et al. The natural history of thoracic disc herniation. Spine 17(6 Suppl):S97-S102, 1992.

20. Campbell E, Kite WC Jr, Whitfield RD. The thoracic herniated intervertebral disc syndrome. J Neurosurg 14:61-67, 1957.

21. Tovi D, Strang RR. Thoracic intervertebral disk protrusions. Acta Chir Scand Suppl Suppl 267: 1-41, 1960.

22. Abbott KH, Retter RH. Protrusions of thoracic intervertebral disks. Neurology 6:1-10, 1956.

23. Arce CA, Dohrmann GJ. Herniated thoracic disks. Neurol Clin 3:383-392, 1985.

24. Albrand OW, Corkill G. Thoracic disc herniation. Treatment and prognosis. Spine 4:41-46, 1979.

25. Benson MK, Byrnes DP. The clinical syndromes and surgical treatment of thoracic intervertebral disc prolapse. J Bone Joint Surg Br 57:471-477, 1975.

26. Wood KB, Garvey TA, Gundry C, et al. Magnetic resonance imaging of the thoracic spine. Evaluation of asymptomatic individuals. J Bone Joint Surg Am 77:1631-1638, 1995.

27. Xiong Y, Lachmann E, Marini S, et al. Thoracic disk herniation presenting as abdominal and pelvic pain: a case report. Arch Phys Med Rehabil 82:1142-1144, 2001.

28. Lyu RK, Chang HS, Tang LM, et al. Thoracic disc herniation mimicking acute lumbar disc disease. Spine 24:416-418, 1999.

29. Eleraky MA, Apostolides PJ, Dickman CA, et al. Herniated thoracic discs mimic cardiac disease: three case reports. Acta Neurochir (Wien) 140:643-646, 1998.

30. Ozturk C, Tezer M, Sirvanci M, et al. Far lateral thoracic disc herniation presenting with flank pain. Spine J 6:201-203, 2006.

31. Whitcomb DC, Martin SP, Schoen RE, et al. Chronic abdominal pain caused by thoracic disc herniation. Am J Gastroenterol 90:835-837, 1995.

32. Alvarez O, Roque CT, Pampati M. Multilevel thoracic disk herniations: CT and MR studies. J Comput Assist Tomogr 12:649-652, 1988.

33. Chambers AA. Thoracic disk herniation. Semin Roentgenol 23:111-117, 1988.

34. Francavilla TL, Powers A, Dina T, et al. MR imaging of thoracic disk herniations. J Comput Assist Tomogr 11:1062-1065, 1987.

35. Epstein JA. The syndrome of herniation of the lower thoracic intervertebral discs with nerve root and spinal cord compression. J Neurosurg 11:525-538, 1954.

36. Perot PL Jr, Munro DD. Transthoracic removal of midline thoracic disc protrusions causing spinal cord compression. J Neurosurg 31:452-458, 1969.

37. Le Roux PD, Haglund MM, Harris AB. Thoracic disc disease: experience with the transpedicular approach in twenty consecutive patients. Neurosurgery 33:58-66, 1993.
38. Stillerman CB, Chen TC, Day JD, et al. The transfacet pedicle-sparing approach for thoracic disc removal: cadaveric morphometric analysis and preliminary clinical experience. J Neurosurg 83: 971-976, 1995.
39. Larson SJ, Holst RA, Hemmy DC, et al. Lateral extracavitary approach to traumatic lesions of the thoracic and lumbar spine. J Neurosurg 45:628-637, 1976.
40. Menard V. Causes de la paraplegia dans la maladie de Pott, son traitement chirurgical par l'ouverture directe du foyer tuberculeaux des vertebras. Rev Orthop 5:47-64, 1894.
41. Alexander GL. Neurological complications of spinal tuberculosis. Proc R Soc Med 39:730-734, 1946.
42. Armour D. Lettsomian lecture on the surgery of the spinal cord and its membranes. Lancet 1:423-430, 1927.
43. Capener N. The evolution of lateral rhachotomy. J Bone Joint Surg Br 36:173-179, 1954.
44. Fessler RG, Dietze DD JR, Millan MM, et al. Lateral parascapular extrapleural approach to the upper thoracic spine. J Neurosurg 75:349-355, 1991.
45. Dietze DD Jr, Fessler RG. Thoracic disc herniations. Neurosurg Clin N Am 4:75-90, 1993.
46. Maiman DJ, Larson SJ, Luck E, et al. Lateral extracavitary approach to the spine for thoracic disc herniation: report of 23 cases. Neurosurgery 14:178-182, 1984.
47. Stillerman CB, Chen TC, Couldwell WT, et al. Experience in the surgical management of 82 symptomatic herniated thoracic discs and review of the literature. J Neurosurg 88:623-633, 1998.
48. Di Chiro G, Fried LC, Doppman JL. Experimental spinal cord angiography. Br J Radiol 43:19-30, 1970.
49. Currier BL, Eismont FJ, Green BA. Transthoracic disc excision and fusion for herniated thoracic discs. Spine 19:323-328, 1994.
50. Connolly E, moderator. Treatment of thoracic disc herniation with myelopathy: thoracotomy vs. costotransversectomy vs. the lateral extracavitary approach. In Al-Mefty O, Origitano TC, Harkey HL, eds. Controversies in Neurosurgery. New York: Thieme Medical Publishers, 1996, 246-250.
51. Anand N, Regan JJ. Video-assisted thoracoscopic surgery for thoracic disc disease: classification and outcome study of 100 consecutive cases with a 2-year minimum follow-up period. Spine 27:871-879, 2002.
52. Horowitz MB, Moossy JJ, Julian T, et al. Thoracic discectomy using video assisted thoracoscopy. Spine 19:1082-1086, 1994.
53. Mack MJ, Regan JJ, McAfee PC, et al. Video-assisted thoracic surgery for the anterior approach to the thoracic spine. Ann Thorac Surg 59:1100-1106, 1995.
54. McAfee PC, Regan JR, Zdeblick T, et al. The incidence of complications in endoscopic anterior thoracolumbar spinal reconstructive surgery. A prospective multicenter study comprising the first 100 consecutive cases. Spine 20:1624-1632, 1995.
55. Regan JJ, Ben-Yishay A, Mack MJ. Video-assisted thoracoscopic excision of herniated thoracic disc: description of technique and preliminary experience in the first 29 cases. J Spinal Disord 11:183-191, 1998.
56. Mulier S, Debois V. Thoracic disc herniations: transthoracic, lateral, or posterolateral approach? A review. Surg Neurol 49:599-606; discussion 606-608, 1998.
57. Otani K, Yoshida M, Fujii E, et al. Thoracic disc herniation. Surgical treatment in 23 patients. Spine 13:1262-1267, 1988.

21

XLIF® Corpectomy

William D. Smith • John A. Anson
Stuart S. Kaplan • Kyle Malone

Thoracolumbar corpectomies have traditionally been performed via an open anterior approach. This open procedure allows resectioning of the anterior, load-bearing column to treat tumors,[1] vertebral burst fractures,[2-6] or vertebral osteomyelitis[7] and can be readily paired with anterolateral or posterior fixation.[8-12] The benefits of this procedure include a large, anterior working space, a relatively low learning curve (standard techniques for corpectomy), and relative ease of handling intraoperative complications. The surgical disadvantages to this procedure, however, include a large wound field (Fig. 21-1), which results in an increased infection rate; an increased recovery time; and an increased likelihood for intraoperative complications. In addition, working anterior to posterior increases the potential for spinal cord injuries by the posterior migration of retropulsed fragments.[10,13] These

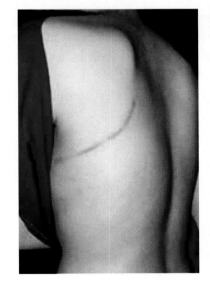

FIG. 21-1   This patient shows a thoracotomy incision.

artifacts of open techniques result in high complication rates—namely, intercostal neuralgia and postthoracotomy pain[14-17]—and the use of dual-lumen intubation for ipsilateral lung deflation requires the placement of a chest tube postoperatively and greatly increases the risk for atelectasis and pneumonia. The open approach requires an approach surgeon whose scheduling conflicts can delay immediate decompression for patients with traumatic injuries, which may increase the likelihood for permanent disability.[18-20]

The use of endoscopic (thoracoscopic and laparoscopic) techniques for anterior thoracolumbar reconstruction began in the second half of the 1990s,[17,21-28] and has not been widely adopted because of the extended surgical times, steep learning curves, expensive equipment, and a relative inability to control intraoperative complications.[16,29-31] Recently, mini-open techniques have been introduced to control these intraoperative issues without the postoperative complications common to the historical wide-open procedures.[8,9,11,12,32]

This chapter introduces a novel technique for thoracolumbar corpectomies using extreme lateral interbody fusion (XLIF; NuVasive®, Inc., San Diego, CA), which has many advantages, including a direct, mini-open corridor to the pathology, decreased tissue disruption, a decreased infection rate (because of the small wound field), decreased operative time, decreased postoperative pain, and decreased recovery time. In addition, XLIF provides an increased ability to manage intraoperative complications compared with endoscopic techniques, allows the surgeon to use familiar general surgical techniques similar to open procedures (moderated learning curves), and gives the surgeon the opportunity for immediate decompression (because an approach surgeon is not needed). As a result, there is a decrease in the overall cost and resources used.

CLINICAL EXPERIENCE

Between February 2007 and February 2008, 19 patients underwent corpectomies via an XLIF approach by three neurosurgeons in one private neurosurgical practice in Las Vegas, Nevada (Box 21-1). Four patients underwent posterior transpedicular fixation from one level above to one level below the corpectomized level. The remaining 15 patients received lateral plating without posterior fixation.

BOX 21-1   Treatment Demographics

Sex	*Levels*
Male: 9	T8: 3
Female: 10	T9: 2
	T10: 2
Pathology	T12: 3
Trauma: 7	L1: 4
Compression fracture: degenerative scoliosis: 3	L2: 3
Tumor: 6	L3: 1
Infection: 3	L4: 1

Mean age: 44.7 years. Age range: 18 to 72 years.

SURGICAL TECHNIQUE

In our clinic, we have found the XLIF approach for corpectomies to be safe and reproducible from T8 to L4. Thoracic corpectomies are approached by following the access techniques described for thoracic XLIF disc procedures, but require rib resectioning for retractor access. Lumbar corpectomies use the approach techniques of lumbar XLIF but are generally more difficult because of the thick psoas muscle in this area. Corpectomies in and around the thoracolumbar junction require navigational considerations around the diaphragm. All operations have been performed by a single neurosurgeon without an approach surgeon. For thoracic levels, normal single-lumen ventilation is used, and patients are placed in the lateral decubitus position. All patients are administered preoperative antibiotic agents and steroids. Intraoperative localization is accomplished using direct visualization with biplanar fluoroscopy—the treatment levels are identified and the vertebral bodies are marked (Fig. 21-2, *A* and *B*).

An oblique incision approximately 4 cm long is made 90 degrees directly lateral to the anterior axis of the vertebral column. Variable lengths of rib are resected to allow the MaXcess® III Retractor System (NuVasive, Inc.) to be inserted and expanded (Fig. 21-2, *C* and *D*). Using normal ventilation, the lung is deflected using the MaXcess Dilators, which are incrementally increased in diameter until the Retractor is inserted (Fig. 21-2, *E* through *G*). For lumbar levels, motor evoked potentials are monitored using the NeuroVision® monitoring system (NuVasive, Inc.).

Dilators are used to identify and localize nervous tissue disruption. The locations are confirmed with fluoroscopy, and the Retractor is carefully inserted, bordering the lung (Fig. 21-2, *H* through *J*). The fourth Blade was added to the MaXcess Retractor to define the working space for vertebral body removal. Working from the patient's posterior aspect, the three standard Blades of the Retractor outline the anterior border of the thecal sac and the superior/inferior aspects of the adjacent discs (see Fig. 21-2, *H* through *J*). As seen in Fig. 21-2 *K*, the incision required for the XLIF procedure is minimal.

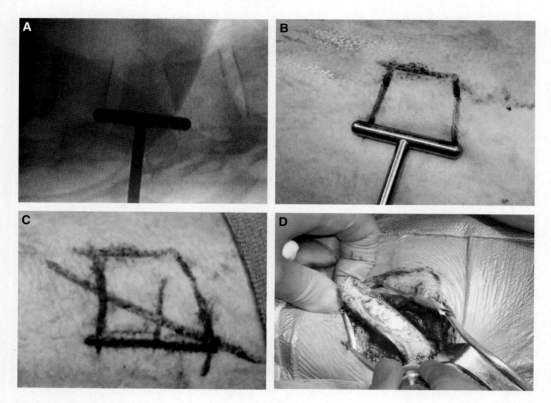

FIG. 21-2   A, Localization for a traumatic L1 burst fracture is seen on the lateral intraoperative fluoroscopic view. **B,** The location of the vertebral body is mapped on the skin for corpectomy. **C,** A rib and vertebra are mapped on the skin preoperatively. **D,** A portion of a rib is resected for greater access.

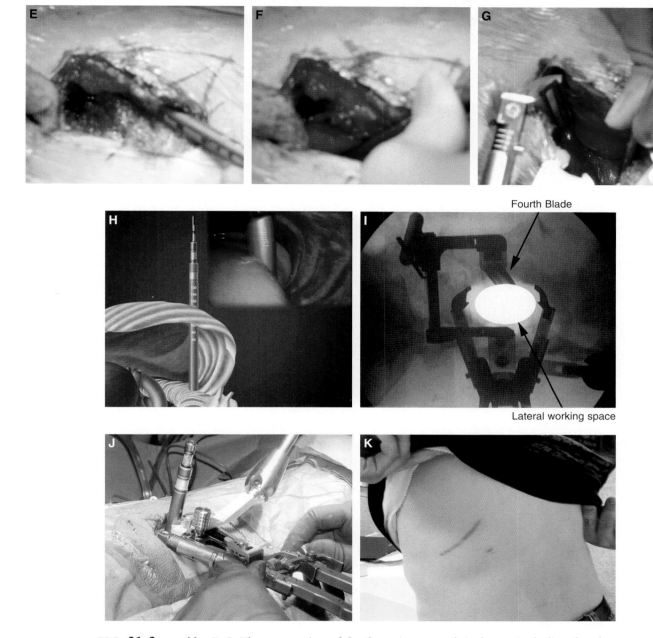

FIG. 21-2, cont'd   E-G, The progression of the thoracic approach is shown, including the placement of a sequential Dilator and subsequent Retractor advancement and expansion. **H** and **I,** The MaXcess Dilators and Retractor (with the fourth Blade attached) are placed in the thorax. In **J,** the lateral working space is defined by the borders of the Retractor Blades, with the border of the thecal sac on the posterior aspect. **K,** The incision for XLIF is minimal.

After achieving sufficient exposure, the standard technique for corpectomy is used, beginning with the vertebral body and adjacent disc removal. The anterior segment is removed, and the corpectomized segments replaced with corpectomy cages (Fig. 21-3, *A* through *F*). In four of the 19 patients treated in this manner at our institution, posterior transpedicular fixation and scaffolding were used to increase structural salience. In the remaining 15 patients, lateral plating was used for anterior column stabilization.

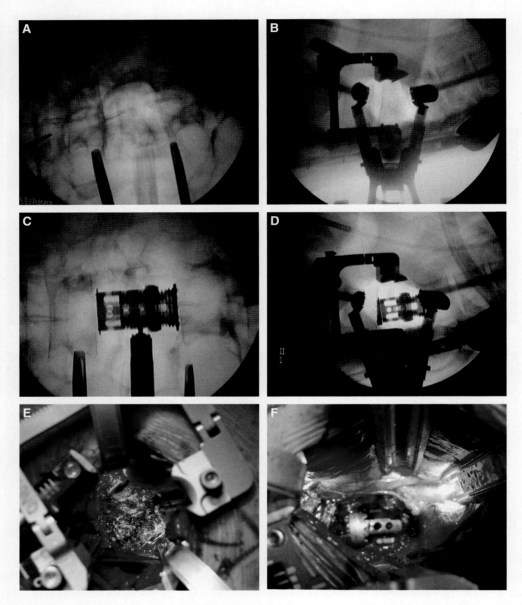

FIG. 21-3   A-F, These progressive intraoperative images show vertebral body targeting and cage placement using the MaXcess Retractor with the fourth Blade attached.

BOX 21-2   Intraoperative Series Statistics (19 Patients)

Operating Room Time

Mean: 136 minutes

Range: 35 to 394 minutes

Estimated Blood Loss

Median: 220 milliters

Range: 50 to 2200 milliters

CLINICAL RESULTS

As of this writing, 12-month follow-up is available for only two patients. No serious intraoperative or postoperative complications have been reported, and no revisions have been performed. Box 21-2 lists operating room times and estimated blood loss (EBL) as obtained via retrospective chart review. The largest volume of EBL was the result of severe trauma rather than surgical manipulation. Because the majority of the patients in the study were admitted to the emergency room for acute trauma, pain surveys were not obtained before surgery for 10 of the 19 patients. The following three case studies are from this series.

CASE EXAMPLES

CASE ONE

An 18-year-old woman was involved in a 90 mph motor vehicle accident that caused her vehicle to roll over. She presented to the emergency room with complete motor paraplegia caused by an L1 burst fracture (Fig. 21-4, *A* through *C*). The neurosurgeon on call was available, but no approach surgeon could arrive until the following morning. The surgery began approximately 45 minutes after the patient arrived at the emergency room. The patient underwent a complete L1 corpectomy via an XLIF approach, facilitated by the MaXcess Retractor with the fourth Blade attached (Fig. 21-4, *D* through *F*).

Partial corpectomies were performed at T12 and L2, and the L1 space was fitted with an expandable titanium cage. Because of the extreme nature of the fracture, bilateral transpedicular screws were used at T12 and L2 (Fig. 21-4, *G* and *H*). The operating room time was 158 minutes and the EBL was 220 ml. The patient was discharged (ambulatory) 5 days postoperatively.

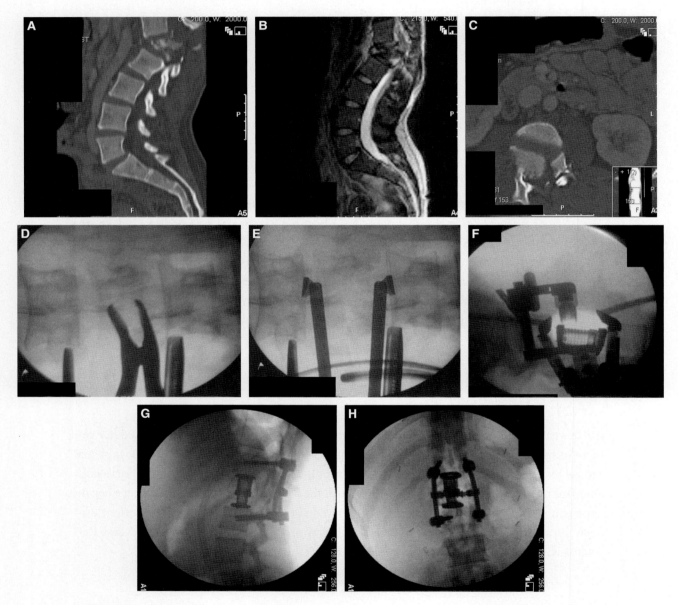

FIG. 21-4   A-C, This 18-year-old woman was in a motor vehicle accident. Preoperative computed tomography (CT) and magnetic resonance imaging (MRI) showed an L1 burst fracture. **D-H.** These intraoperative fluoroscopic images show the lateral corpectomy procedure and final construct.

CASE TWO

A 75-year-old woman presented with a 20-year history of increasingly severe intractable back pain and bilateral leg symptoms. She was not able to ambulate independently and received minimal relief from recumbency. Conservative treatment, including physical therapy and injections, was unsuccessful. She had obtained two previous surgical consultations—one surgeon suggested immediate surgical intervention, and the second deemed the case too severe to operate. She had surgery on her lower back in 1989 and a 20-year history of smoking. The physical examination revealed an obvious scoliotic deformity; a patchy, diminished sensation in a stocking distribution in her lower extremities; and a Lasègue maneuver bilaterally, with flexion and extension limited to approximately 25% of normal. MRI and CT scans revealed a compression fracture with cord compression at L1 and a retropulsed fragment in the T12-L1 and L1-2 region. She also had a scoliotic deformity at L3-4 and L4-5 with a Knudson phenomenon. The surgical strategy was to perform an L1 corpectomy via an XLIF approach and fusion using an expandable cage and lateral plating. Because this addressed only the burst fracture and not the scoliotic deformity, minimally invasive L3-5 interbody fusion using the XLIF procedure was also planned. The patient underwent complete discectomies at L3-4 and L4-5 with an XLIF approach. A poly-ether-ether-ketone (PEEK) implant (CoRoent® XL, NuVasive, Inc.) with bone from a local source and bone morphogenic protein (BMP) was placed, with lateral Plates (XLP™, NuVasive, Inc.) at L3-4 and L4-5. Through a separate fascial incision, a complete corpectomy was performed at L1, with complete discectomies at L1-2 and L2-3. An expandable cage was implanted at L1 with bone from a local source, BMP, and rib for structural purposes, and anterolateral plating was placed from T12 through L2 (Fig. 21-5, *A* through *G*). Table 21-1 shows the time and EBL for each procedure. The patient was discharged 4 days postoperatively, ambulating with assistance.

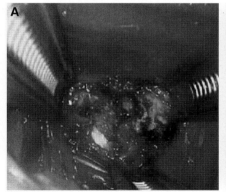 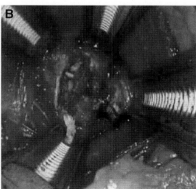 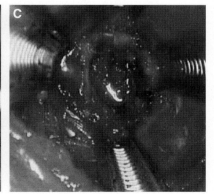

FIG. 21-5 This 75-year-old woman had a 20-year history of increasingly severe back pain and bilateral leg symptoms. A lateral corpectomy was performed to treat an L1 burst fracture with retropulsed fragments, in addition to an L3-5 XLIF for correction of scoliosis. **A,** L1 was exposed. **B** and **C,** The vertebral body was extravasated.   *Continued*

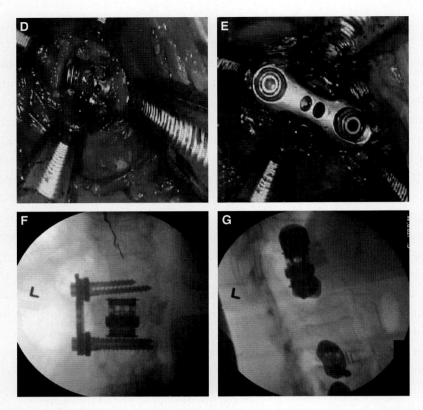

FIG. 21-5, cont'd   D, An expandable cage was placed. **E,** The lateral Plate is placed. **F** and **G,** Antero-posterior and lateral fluoroscopic images of the final constructs were obtained.

TABLE 21-1   Results for L1 Corpectomy Through an XLIF Approach With L3-5 XLIF to Correct Scoliotic Deformity

Level	Procedure	Time (minutes)	Estimated Blood Loss (ml)
L1	Corpectomy	55	150
L3-4	XLIF	10	10
	XLP	10	5
L4-5	XLIF	10	15
	XLP	10	5
TOTAL		95	185

XLIF, extreme lateral interbody fusion; *XLP,* lateral Plate.

CASE THREE

A 30-year-old woman presented with a 4-week history of paraparesis. She was unable to stand or walk independently. She had urinary incontinence 2 days before admission. Imaging revealed a very large intradural tumor that was confirmed by pathology to be a neurofibroma described as an intradural, extramedullary spinal cord tumor at T9-10 with severe cord compression and injury (Fig. 21-6, *A* and *B*). The surgical plan was to perform a complete corpectomy at T9 with a partial corpectomy at T10 via a transthoracic XLIF approach, with rib harvesting through a separate fascial incision. Discectomies were to be completed at T8-9 and T9-10, with intradural exploration for complete excision of meningioma. A lumbar drain was inserted before surgery for cerebrospinal fluid (CSF) drainage. Interbody fusion was carried out using an expandable titanium cage with anterolateral plating (Fig. 21-6, *C* through *J*). The surgery was performed without complications, and a separate chest tube was placed postoperatively. The operating room time was 156 minutes and the EBL was 220 ml. The chest tube and lumbar drain were removed 12 hours and 48 hours after surgery, respectively. The patient was discharged, ambulatory, 72 hours postoperatively. At the 6-month follow-up, she is fully functional and asymptomatic. She does have headaches; these are probably spinal headaches caused by CSF leakage.

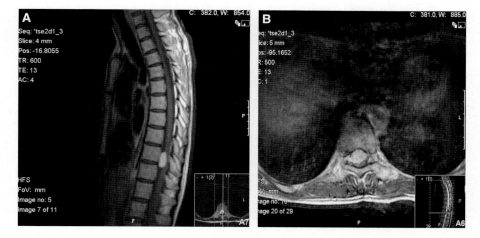

FIG. 21-6   This 30-year-old woman had a 4-week history of paraparesis and was unable to stand or walk independently. **A** and **B,** Preoperative MRIs showed a very large intradural, extramedullary spinal cord tumor at T9-10, with severe cord compression and injury.   *Continued*

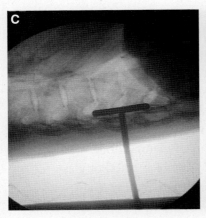

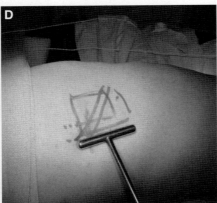

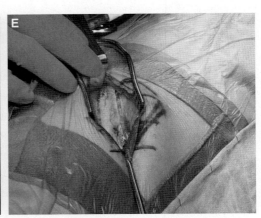

Intradural, extramedullary
spinal cord tumor

Tumor

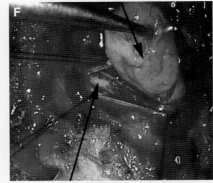

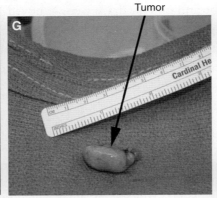

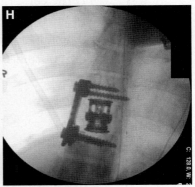

Spinal cord

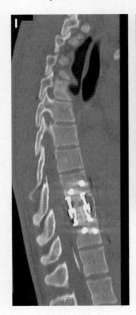

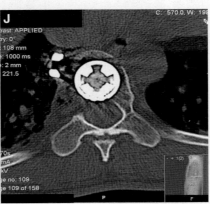

FIG. 21-6, cont'd   C-G, Intraoperative images show the approach for spinal cord tumor removal via transthoracic XLIF. **H,** Intraoperative fluoroscopic view. **I** and **J,** Postoperative CT views of the T9 corpectomy with an expandable cage and lateral instrumentation.

COMPLICATIONS AND BENEFITS OF THE XLIF APPROACH

Major concerns when performing thoracolumbar corpectomies to treat patients with traumatic injuries are immediate decompression,[18-20] the manipulation of retropulsed fragments, and the stabilization of the anterior load-bearing column.[8,9,11,12,32] The XLIF approach for corpectomy does not require an approach surgeon, which is important because most extreme trauma cases require urgent intervention.

In an anterior approach, retropulsed fragments have a high risk of posterior migration during extravasation of the vertebral body. Using an XLIF approach and working within the borders of the retractor system allows a clean, 90-degree environment that borders the adjacent vertebral segments and the thecal sac posteriorly. This arrangement decreases the likelihood of posterior fragment migration. In our series, no spinal cord damage resulted from migrating retropulsed fragments. In addition, localizing the retractor allows anatomic definition in cases that lack regular anatomic landmarks because of injury.

Finally, our series shows that the working space created using a true lateral, mini-open approach is sufficient to safely and reproducibly perform corpectomies. Although no intraoperative complications occurred in our series, we believe that they would be easily contained because of the robust exposure at the site, regardless of the relatively small incision.

CONCLUSION

The results of our series of 19 patients who underwent lateral thoracolumbar corpectomies suggest that these procedures can be performed safely and reproducibly without an access surgeon. The mini-open approach causes less soft tissue disruption and provides a direct corridor to the pathology. The MaXcess Retractor system, with the fourth Blade attached, allows the anatomy to be localized and defined and protects the spinal cord from retropulsed fragments. Most importantly, this approach does not have the steep learning curve associated with endoscopic techniques. This system involves the same general principles and procedures as corpectomy via an open approach, but with fewer operative morbidities.

ACKNOWLEDGMENTS

This research was funded, in part, by grants from the Western Regional Center for Brain and Spine Surgery and the Nevada Neurosciences Institute Research Foundation.

REFERENCES

1. Fourney DR, Gokaslan ZL. Anterior approaches for thoracolumbar metastatic spine tumors. Neurosurg Clin N Am 15:443-451, 2004.

2. Oskouian RJ Jr, Shaffrey CI, Whitehill R, et al. Anterior stabilization of three-column thoracolumbar spinal trauma. J Neurosurg Spine 5:18-25, 2006.

3. Payer M. Immediate open anterior reduction and antero-posterior fixation/fusion for bilateral cervical locked facets. Acta Neurochir (Wien) 147:509-513; discussion 513-514, 2005.

4. Payer M. Unstable burst fractures of the thoraco-lumbar junction: treatment by posterior bisegmental correction/fixation and staged anterior corpectomy and titanium cage implantation. Acta Neurochir (Wien) 148:299-306; discussion 306, 2006. Epub Nov 28, 2005.

5. Sasso RC, Renkens K, Hanson D, et al. Unstable thoracolumbar burst fractures: anterior-only versus short-segment posterior fixation. J Spinal Disord Tech 19:242-248, 2006.

6. Schultheiss M, Kinzl L, Claes L, et al. Minimally invasive ventral spondylodesis for thoracolumbar fracture treatment: surgical technique and first clinical outcome. Eur Spine J 12:618-624, 2003.

7. Pappou IP, Papadopoulos EC, Swanson AN, et al. Pott disease in the thoracolumbar spine with marked kyphosis and progressive paraplegia necessitating posterior vertebral column resection and anterior reconstruction with a cage. Spine 31:E123-E127, 2006.

8. Muhlbauer M, Pfisterer W, Eyb R, et al. Minimally invasive retroperitoneal approach for lumbar corpectomy and anterior reconstruction. Technical note. J Neurosurg 93:161-167, 2000.

9. Muhlbauer M, Pfisterer W, Eyb R, et al. Minimally invasive retroperitoneal approach for lumbar corpectomy and reconstruction. Technical note. Neurosurg Focus 7:e4, 1999.

10. Naunheim KS, Barnett MG, Crandall DG, et al. Anterior exposure of the thoracic spine. Ann Thorac Surg 57:1436-1439, 1994.

11. Payer M, Sottas C. Mini-open anterior approach for corpectomy in the thoracolumbar spine. Surg Neurol 69:25-31; discussion 31-32, 2008.

12. Pflugmacher R, Schleicher P, Schaefer J, et al. Biomechanical comparison of expandable cages for vertebral body replacement in the thoracolumbar spine. Spine 29:1413-1419, 2004.

13. Korovessis P, Petsinis G, Koureas G, et al. Anterior surgery with insertion of titanium mesh cage and posterior instrumented fusion performed sequentially on the same day under one anesthesia for septic spondylitis of thoracolumbar spine: is the use of titanium mesh cages safe? Spine 31:1014-1019, 2006.

14. Dajczman E, Gordon A, Kreisman H, et al. Long-term postthoracotomy pain. Chest 99:270-274, 1991.

15. Faciszewski T, Winter RB, Lonstein JE, et al. The surgical and medical perioperative complications of anterior spinal fusion surgery in the thoracic and lumbar spine in adults. A review of 1223 procedures. Spine 20:1592-1599, 1995.

16. Landreneau RJ, Hazelrigg SR, Mack MJ, et al. Postoperative pain-related morbidity: video-assisted thoracic surgery versus thoracotomy. Ann Thorac Surg 56:1285-1289, 1993.

17. Landreneau RJ, Wiechmann RJ, Hazelrigg SR, et al. Effect of minimally invasive thoracic surgical approaches on acute and chronic postoperative pain. Chest Surg Clin N Am 8:891-906, 1998.

18. McKinley W, Meade MA, Kirshblum S, et al. Outcomes of early surgical management versus late or no surgical intervention after acute spinal cord injury. Arch Phys Med Rehabil 85:1818-1825, 2004.

19. Rahimi-Movaghar V. Efficacy of surgical decompression in the setting of complete thoracic spinal cord injury. J Spinal Cord Med 28:415-420, 2005.

20. Rahimi-Movaghar V, Vaccaro AR, Mohammadi M. Efficacy of surgical decompression in regard to motor recovery in the setting of conus medullaris injury. J Spinal Cord Med 29:32-38, 2006.

21. Furrer M, Rechsteiner R, Eigenmann V, et al. Thoracotomy and thoracoscopy: postoperative pulmonary function, pain and chest wall complaints. Eur J Cardiothorac Surg 12:82-87, 1997.

22. Mathews HH, Evans MT, Molligan HJ, et al. Laparoscopic discectomy with anterior lumbar interbody fusion. A preliminary review. Spine 20:1797-1802, 1995.

23. Mayer HM. A new microsurgical technique for minimally invasive anterior lumbar interbody fusion. Spine 22:691-699; discussion 700, 1997.

24. McAfee PC, Regan JR, Fedder IL, et al. Anterior thoracic corpectomy for spinal cord decompression performed endoscopically. Surg Laparosc Endosc 5:339-348, 1995.

25. Mühlbauer M, Ferguson J, Losert U, et al. Experimental laparoscopic and thoracoscopic discectomy and instrumented spinal fusion. A feasibility study using a porcine model. Minim Invasive Neurosurg 41:1-4, 1998.

26. Olsen D, McCord D, Law M. Laparoscopic discectomy with anterior interbody fusion of L5-S1. Surg Endosc 10:1158-1163, 1996.

27. Regan JJ, Guyer RD. Endoscopic techniques in spinal surgery. Clin Orthop Relat Res 335:122-139, 1997.

28. Visocchi M, Masferrer R, Sonntag VK, et al. Thoracoscopic approaches to the thoracic spine. Acta Neurochir (Wien) 140:737-743; discussion 43-44, 1998

29. Beisse R. Endoscopic surgery on the thoracolumbar junction of the spine. Eur Spine J 15:687-704, 2006.

30. Kim DH, Jahng TA, Balabhadra RS, et al. Thoracoscopic transdiaphragmatic approach to thoracolumbar junction fractures. Spine J 4:317-328, 2004.

31. McAfee PC, Regan JR, Zdeblick T, et al. The incidence of complications in endoscopic anterior thoracolumbar spinal reconstructive surgery. A prospective multicenter study comprising the first 100 consecutive cases. Spine 20:1624-1632, 1995.

32. Dewald CJ, Millikan KW, Hammerberg KW, et al. An open, minimally invasive approach to the lumbar spine. Am Surg 65:61-68, 1999.

22

Total Disc Replacement Through the XLIF® Approach

Luiz Pimenta ▪ Thomas D. Schaffa ▪ Juliano T. Lhamby
Ihab Gharzeddine ▪ Etevaldo Coutinho

Total disc replacement (TDR) surgery is a revolutionary alternative to traditional fusion procedures for treating the pain and instability associated with degenerative disc disease. This procedure restores intervertebral disc height and neuroforaminal height while preserving spinal motion. TDR relies on the basic principle that by stabilizing the motion segment without eliminating motion, biomechanical changes at adjacent levels will be minimized and the occurrence of adjacent level degeneration will be reduced. To date, lumbar TDR surgery has been performed only through an anterior approach. This approach has a high learning curve and is fraught with possible complications such as the potential for vascular and visceral injuries as well as significant collateral damage to surrounding tissues. A complication rate of 38.3% has been reported in anterior fusion surgeries, including sympathetic dysfunction, vascular injury, somatic neural injury, sexual dysfunction, prolonged ileus, wound incompetence, deep vein thrombosis, acute pancreatitis, and bowel injury.[1] Studies of anterior TDR surgeries have reported similar approach-related complications.[2] By approaching the spine laterally, many of these potential risks can be reduced or avoided.

For a number of years the extreme lateral interbody fusion (XLIF, NuVasive®, Inc., San Diego, CA) approach has been advocated for fusion of the anterior column. Studies on the XLIF approach report few approach-related complications with no visceral or vascular injuries and minimal morbidity with rapid recovery. However, a low incidence of transient postoperative hip flexor weakness and anterolateral thigh numbness has been reported.[3-6]

In this chapter we discuss the advantages of the XLIF approach over the traditional anterior approach for TDR surgery (Box 22-1). The surgical considerations are outlined and early clinical results reviewed.

BOX 22-1   Benefits of a Lateral Approach to Lumbar TDR

■ Minimizes the risk of vascular and visceral injury

■ Avoids mobilizing the great vessels

■ Preserves the ALL and PLL, resulting in less stress on the facets

■ Permits a more forgiving device placement, because the midline is easy to identify on intraoperative fluoroscopy

■ Leaves safer surgical approach options if removal and revision become necessary

■ Allows hybrid constructs of TDR at L4-5 and fusion at L5-S1 for two-level L4-S1 pathology

■ Facilitates more rapid patient recovery because of less invasive surgical access

SURGICAL CONSIDERATIONS

INDICATIONS

The indications for lumbar TDR do not differ with approach and include degenerative disc disease without significant facet joint compromise. Because of obstruction by the iliac crest at L5-S1, placement of a TDR device laterally is limited to levels above L5-S1. We have treated multilevel pathologic conditions that include L5-S1 with a hybrid construct of lateral TDR at upper levels and ALIF fusion at L5-S1 (Fig. 22-1).

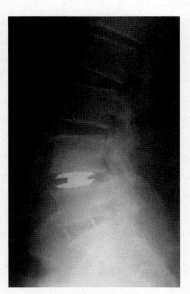

FIG. 22-1   Lateral radiograph showing a hybrid construct of lateral TDR at L4-5 and ALIF at L5-S1.

PATIENT POSITIONING AND RETROPERITONEAL ACCESS

The approach technique does not differ significantly from the standard XLIF approach for fusion procedures (see Chapter 8). The patient is placed on a radiolucent bending table in a true lateral decubitus position. The greater trochanter should be positioned over the table break and the table flexed to allow the space between the crest and the twelfth rib to open (Fig. 22-2, *A* through *C*). Lateral fluoroscopy is used to target the disc of concern, and the skin is marked over the direct lateral center of the disc space. Next, an incision is made just posterolateral to this direct lateral marking. The surgeon inserts a finger through this incision to dissect the retroperitoneal space and guide Dilators through the lateral incision site to the surface of the psoas muscle. NeuroVision® (NuVasive, Inc.) nerve avoidance is used with the blunt Dilators to gently split the psoas muscle fibers while avoiding injury to the nerves (Fig. 22-3, *A*). The exposure required for TDR device placement needs to extend more posteriorly than the exposure for a primary XLIF procedure, making NeuroVision an especially important part of this procedure.

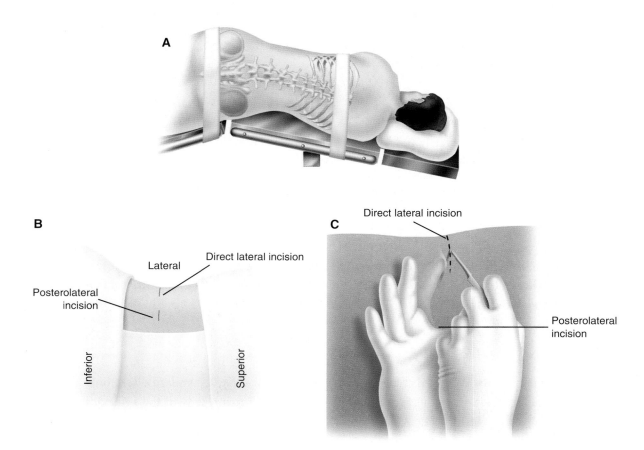

FIG. 22-2   **A,** Patient in lateral decubitus position on a bending operating table. **B** and **C,** Initial skin incisions.

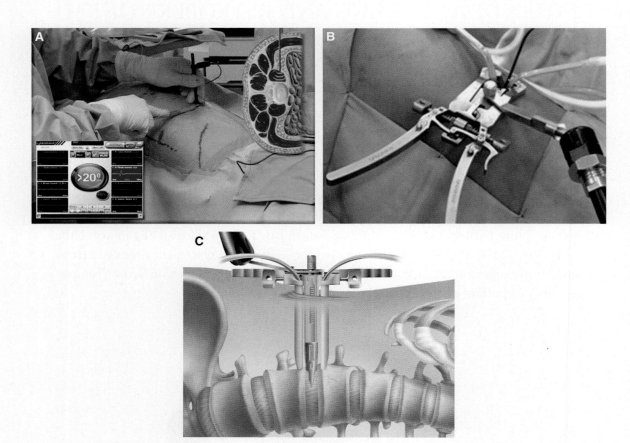

FIG. 22-3   **A,** To safely traverse the psoas muscle and avoid the nerves of the lumbar plexus, NeuroVision guidance uses discrete dynamic evoked electromyography. **B,** The MaXcess® Retractor (NuVasive, Inc.) is advanced over the disc space and spread to expose from superior to inferior endplates. **C,** MaXcess Retractor in place.

Dynamically stimulated electromyography (EMG) is recommended in all cases. Next, the MaXcess Retractor is advanced over the Dilators, rigidly locked to the surgical table, and expanded over the disc space (Fig. 22-3, *B* and *C*).

ANULOTOMY

An anulotomy is created at the lateral aspect of the disc. Next, standard discectomy and endplate preparation are performed, while maintaining the integrity of the anterior longitudinal ligament (ALL). The ALL not only provides an anterior restraint to extension, but also

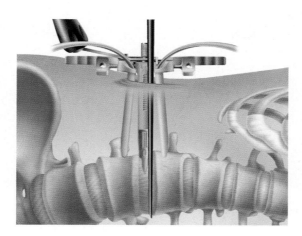

FIG. 22-4 To allow bilateral disc distraction and insertion of the TDR device across the ring apophysis, the contralateral anulus must be released.

to axial rotation. It has been shown that resection of the ALL leads to hypermobility of the segment and potential facet arthrosis at the same and adjacent levels.[7] It has been reported that removing both the ALL and posterior longitudinal ligament (PLL) increases horizontal translation by 33%, creating instability and increasing facet stress.[8] A finite element analysis of anterior TDR placement found that modeling the resuturing of the ALL had a strong effect on loading, and the authors concluded that reconstruction of the ALL would help to restore the biomechanics to normal.[9] Another study reported that preserving the ALL and placing the implant's axis of rotation posteriorly within the disc space may restore spinal stiffness in the sagittal plane and reduce facet loads to those of the intact condition.[10] The XLIF approach to TDR placement preserves the ALL and anterior annulus, unlike the anterior approach which requires resection of these structures. The resulting construct constrains the device from anterior expulsion, provides better ligamentotaxis and sagittal balance, and prevents excessive loading of the facet joints.

DISCECTOMY AND DEVICE PLACEMENT

A complete and thorough discectomy must be performed to the contralateral margin, and the contralateral anulus is released with a long Cobb Elevator (Fig. 22-4). This step ensures parallel distraction and proper coronal alignment and permits the placement of the device on both sides of the ring apophysis in its ideal position. Next, device Trials are used to perform sequential sizing of the device. The lateral TDR device is inserted as one assembly.

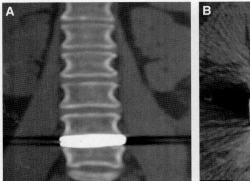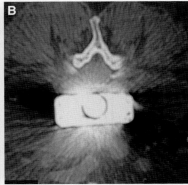

FIG. 22-5   A, Coronal and **B,** axial MR images showing the laterally placed TDR device with good endplate coverage.

The device, which provides surface area coverage of more than 50% of the endplate area, should span the ring apophysis on both sides for strong endplate support (Fig. 22-5). Studies of endplate strength have shown that the posterior endplate is stronger than anterior, and that the lateral margins are the strongest, whereas the center of the endplate, where most implants are currently placed, is the weakest area.[11] Laterally placed TDR and fusion devices can take advantage of the strongest regions of the vertebral endplates for initial and long-term stability.

Exact placement of the device in the midline for coronal stability and in a posterior location for range of motion is essential when performing anterior TDR surgery. However, accurate placement of devices from the anterior approach can prove to be difficult. The results of the Charité U.S. IDE trial showed less-than-ideal placement of the devices in 17% of patients and that ideal placement correlated with both improved ROM and clinical outcomes.[12] Lemaire et al[10] reported the results of a 10-year follow-up of a clinical series of patients who received Charité artificial discs. Twenty-five percent of the devices in this series were not centered in the frontal plane, and 40% were not in an ideal posterior location.[13]

In contrast, lateral device placement is less demanding. When a device is placed laterally the frontal midline is easily identified on intraoperative cross-table anteroposterior fluoroscopy, and central placement of the device is facilitated by aligning the midline device markings with the spinous processes. Furthermore, coronal balance is ensured because the device length spans the entire disc space, with easily identifiable landmarks of the lateral borders of the vertebrae (Fig. 22-6, *A*). The midline markers should align with the lateral center of the vertebral bodies in a lateral fluoroscopic view (Fig. 22-6, *B*). Lateral insertion of the device in the midline provides ideal placement and rotation, because the kinematic center of rotation is located posteriorly within the device.

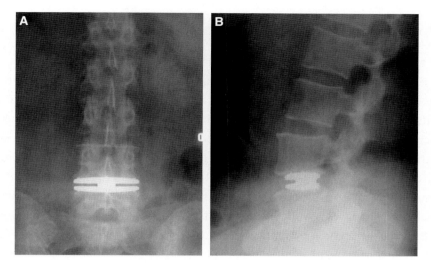

FIG. 22-6 A, An anteroposterior radiograph showing placement of a lateral TDR device in a 35-year-old woman with lower back pain that was unresponsive to treatment for 15 months. The device is placed in alignment with the midline and lateral margin. **B,** The lateral radiograph shows the device positioned centrally with the rotational center located more posteriorly.

POSTOPERATIVE MANAGEMENT

Because the XLIF approach requires less tissue disruption to access the spine, patients are typically walking within hours of surgery and discharged home after a single night's hospital stay, with minimal surgical pain and on minimal medications.

LATERAL APPROACH FOR REVISION SURGERY

As discussed in Chapter 17, the lateral approach is also used for revising primary anteriorly placed TDR devices. Anterior retrieval of a TDR device and revision to an ALIF is difficult, especially after the first 2 weeks postoperatively, because of scar formation and elevated risk of vascular injury, particularly at the level of the vascular bifurcation at L4-5.[14-16] The Charité U.S. IDE data showed that while the primary TDR procedure resulted in a rate of vascular complication of 3.4%, vascular injury occurred in 16.7% of the revision cases.[8] Although experience to date is limited, case reports describing the successful use of the lateral approach (which does not require anterior mobilization of the major vessels) to revise anteriorly placed TDR devices have been encouraging.[17]

Should removal and revision become necessary after primary placement of a lumbar TDR device from a lateral approach, several safer surgical approach options are available. The contralateral retroperitoneal approach can easily be performed, or an anterior (transperitoneal or retroperitoneal) approach can be more safely performed, because the primary procedure does not produce scars in or around the anterior vasculature.

CLINICAL EXPERIENCE

We have used the XLIF approach to implant lateral TDR devices in 36 patients who had discography-confirmed one- or two-level degenerative disc disease as part of a prospective nonrandomized clinical evaluation.[18] Patients averaged 42.6 years of age (range 22 to 60 years). Fifteen one-level, three two-level, and 18 hybrid TDR/ALIF cases were performed. The surgeries lasted about 1 hour on average and were performed through a 4 cm lateral incision. Patients had a blood loss of approximately 50 ml per level. No intraoperative or postoperative complications were encountered in this series. In all cases, postoperative radiographs show good device placement, with restoration of disc height, foraminal volume, and sagittal balance. All patients were walking within 12 hours of surgery, and most were discharged the next day. Three patients had a postoperative weakness of the psoas muscle (weakness to flexing at the hip); these instances resolved by the 6-week follow-up visit. One patient demonstrated a weakness of the leg ipsilateral to the approach side that lasted through the 3-month visit but resolved by the 6-month follow-up visit. One patient was found to have hypertrophy of the left quadriceps at the 12-month visit. Four patients (11%) had postoperative facet joint pain, all in hybrid cases. Patient pain and function improved dramatically short-term and improvements were maintained at 1- and 2-year follow-ups.

CONCLUSION

To date, experience with TDR through an XLIF approach is limited; however, midterm clinical results promise a safer and less invasive exposure and demonstrate good patient outcomes with maintenance of pain relief and functional improvement. This approach offers benefits that suggest an exciting new direction for TDR procedures (see Box 22-1).

REFERENCES

1. Rajaraman V, Vingan R, Roth P, et al. Visceral and vascular complications resulting from anterior lumbar interbody fusion. J Neurosurg 91(1 Suppl):60-64, 1999.
2. Blumenthal S, McAfee P, Guyer R, et al. A prospective, randomized, multicenter Food and Drug Administration Investigational Device Exemptions study of lumbar total disc replacement with the CHARITÉ artificial disc versus lumbar fusion. Part I: evaluation of clinical outcomes. Spine 30:1565-1575, 2005.
3. Diaz R, Phillips F, Pimenta L. Minimally invasive XLIF fusion in the treatment of symptomatic degenerative lumbar scoliosis. Proceedings of the NASS Twentieth Annual Meeting. Spine J 5(4 Suppl):131S-132S, 2005.
4. Ozgur B, Aryan H, Pimenta L, et al. Extreme lateral interbody fusion (XLIF): a novel surgical technique for anterior lumbar interbody fusion. Spine J 6:435-443, 2006.

5. Pimenta L, Schaffa T, da Silva Martins M, et al. eXtreme lateral interbody fusion. In Perez-Cruet M, Khoo L, Fessler R, eds. An Anatomical Approach to Minimally Invasive Spine Surgery. St Louis, Quality Medical Publishing, 2006, pp 641-652.

6. Wright N. Instrumented extreme lateral interbody fusion (XLIF) through a single approach. Proceedings of the NASS Twentieth Annual Meeting. Spine J 5(4 Suppl):S177-S178, 2005.

7. Denoziere G, Ku D. Biomechanical comparison between fusion of two vertebrae and implantation of an artificial intervertebral disc. J Biomech 39:766-775, 2006.

8. White A, Panjabi M. Clinical Biomechanics of the Spine, 2nd ed. Philadelphia: JB Lippincott, 2001.

9. Rohlmann A, Zander T, Bergmann G. Effect of total disc replacement with ProDisc on intersegmental rotation of the lumbar spine. Spine 30:738-743, 2005.

10. Dooris A, Goel V, Grosland N, et al. Load-sharing between anterior and posterior elements in a lumbar motion segment implanted with an artificial disc. Spine 26:E122-E129, 2001.

11. Grant JP, Oxland TR, Dvorak MF. Mapping the structural properties of the lumbosacral vertebral endplates. Spine 26:889-896, 2001.

12. McAfee P, Cunningham B, Holsapple G, et al. A prospective, randomized, multicenter Food and Drug Administration Investigational Device Exemptions study of lumbar total disc replacement with the CHARITÉ artificial disc versus lumbar fusion. Part II: evaluation of radiographic outcomes and correlation of surgical technique accuracy with clinical outcomes. Spine 30:1576-1583, 2005.

13. Lemaire JP, Carrier H, Sariali el-H, et al. Clinical and radiological outcomes with the Charite artificial disc: a 10 year minimum follow-up. J Spinal Disord Tech 18:353-359, 2005.

14. Bertagnoli R, Zigler J, Karg A, et al. Complications and strategies for revision surgery in total disc replacement. Orthop Clin North Am 36:389-395, 2005.

15. McAfee P, Geisler F, Saiedy S, et al. Revisability of the CHARITÉ Artificial Disc replacement: analysis of 688 patients enrolled in the U.S. IDE study of the CHARITÉ artificial disc. Spine 31:1217-1226, 2006.

16. Scott-Young M. Strategy for revision disc replacement surgery. Roundtbl Spine Surg 1: 1:23-72, 2005.

17. Pimenta L, Diaz R, Guerrero L. Charité lumbar artificial disc retrieval: use of a lateral minimally invasive technique. J Neurosurg Spine 5:556-561, 2006.

18. Pimenta L. Lateral TDR: evolution, development and early results. Presented at the Controversies in Motion Preservation Pre-Course, Spine Arthroplasty Society (SAS7), Berlin, May 2007.

Index

Depression, back pain and, 55, 128
Dermatomal pattern, radiculopathy with
    pain in, 58
Direct decompression, conditions that may
    require, 63, 64
Disc
    black, 131
    collapsed; *see* Degenerated/collapsed disc
    degenerated; *see* Degenerated/collapsed
        disc
    intervertebral, lumbar degenerative
        disease and, 42
    vacuum, 43, 48
Disc bulges, lumbar degenerative disease
    and, 43-44
Disc Cutters, XLIF thoracic spine surgery
    and, 234
Disc degeneration
    lumbar degenerative disease and, 51
    radiology of lumbar degenerative disease
        and, 43-46
Disc extrusions, lumbar degenerative
    disease and, 44
Disc herniation, 9-10
    recurrent, 160
    thoracic; *see* Thoracic disc herniation
Disc replacement, total; *see* Total disc
    replacement
Disc space narrowing, junctional disease of
    lumbar spine and, 144
Discectomy
    automated percutaneous, 8
    microendoscopic, 4, 7
    total disc replacement through the XLIF
        approach and, 279-280, 282
Discectomy/fusion, XLIF thoracic spine
    surgery and, 236-237
Discogenic/collapsed lumbar disease, XLIF
    for, 134-136
Discography
    degenerated/collapsed disc and, 132
    lumbar degenerative disease and, 41, 46
DRX, degenerated/collapsed disc and, 133
DSEPs, XLIF and, 107
Dynamic Stimulation Clip, XLIF and, 110

E

EBL; *see* Estimated blood loss
EHL; *see* Extensor hallucis longus
Electromyography (EMG)
    degenerative scoliosis and, 181
    lateral approach to thoracic disc hernia-
        tion and, 248
    in prevention of lumbosacral plexus
        injury, 121
    revision lumbar spine surgery using
        XLIF techniques and transpsoas
        technology and, 206, 207

spontaneous free-run, 106
    triggered, 106
    XLIF and, 94, 95, 101, 103, 106, 107, 109,
        112
Electrothermal therapy, intradiscal,
    degenerated/collapsed disc and, 133
EMG; *see* Electromyography
Endoscope, history of, 4
Endplate anatomy, XLIF and, 27
Endplate degenerative changes, lumbar
    degenerative disease and, 51
Epidural injections, degenerative spondy-
    lolisthesis and, 167
Equipment; *see* Instruments
Estimated blood loss (EBL), XLIF corpec-
    tomy and, 265
Extensor hallucis longus (EHL), degenera-
    tive spondylolisthesis and, 165
Extreme lateral interbody fusion (XLIF)
    advantages of, 28, 29
    after previous surgery; *see* Previous
        surgery, XLIF after
    applied anatomy of extreme lumbar
        interbody fusion and, 17-29
    basic concepts and, 17-29
    biomechanics of lateral arthrodesis and,
        31-40
    bone grafting options for lumbar spine
        fusions and, 75-83
    clinical application of
        after previous surgery, 153-161
        complex deformity and, 189-202
        degenerated/collapsed disc and,
            127-142
        degenerative scoliosis and, 177-188
        degenerative spondylolisthesis and,
            163-176
        junctional disease of lumbar spine
            and, 143-152
        revision lumbar spine surgery using
            XLIF techniques and transpsoas
            technology and, 203-216
    clinical evaluation of low back and leg
        pain and, 53-60
    complex deformity and, 189-202
    degenerated/collapsed disc and; *see*
        Degenerated/collapsed disc, XLIF
        and
    degenerative scoliosis and; *see* Degenera-
        tive scoliosis, XLIF and
    degenerative spondylolisthesis and; *see*
        Degenerative spondylolisthesis,
        XLIF and
    five key steps for performing, 87-103
    fundamentals of, 1-83
    historical background of minimally in-
        vasive spine surgery and, 3-15
    indirect decompression with, 61-73
        case example and, 67-71

clinical presentation and, 62-63
    conditions amenable to, 63
    mechanisms of treatment and, 63-66
    pathophysiology and, 61-62
junctional disease of lumbar spine and;
    see Junctional disease of lumbar
    spine, XLIF and
key steps for performing, 87-103
lateral arthrodesis and, 32, 38
lateral techniques and, 217-284
multilevel, for adult thoracolumbar de-
    formity, 194-197
outpatient, 217-220
    advantages of, 218-219
    open versus minimally invasive proce-
        dures and, 217-218
potential complications of, 117-126
    associated with ALIF and posterior
        methods of interbody fusion and,
        118-119
    avoidance of, 121-124
    neural anatomy and, 119-120
    observed complications of, 120-121
    patient selection and, 119
    related to approach, 119-120
    vascular anatomy and, 120
    visceral anatomy and, 120
principles of indirect decompression
    with, 61-73
radiology of lumbar degenerative disease
    and, 41-52
safety of, afforded by automated neuro-
    physiologic monitoring with
    NeuroVision and, 105-115
    anatomy and, 108
    anesthesia requirements and, 112
    experience with NeuroVision and,
        113-114
    neuroanatomy and, 106-107
    psoas traversal using NeuroVision
        and, 111
    types of intraoperative neuromonitor-
        ing and, 106-107
surgical technique and, 85-103
    anatomic landmark identification
        and, 90, 91
    closure and, 102
    disc space preparation and, 100
    implant placement and, 100-101
    implant sizing and, 100-101
    initial incisions and, 90, 91
    lateral plating and, 101-102
    operating room setup and, 88-90
    patient positioning and, 88-90
    posterolateral incision and, 92, 93
    postoperative management and, 103
    retroperitoneal access and, 91-92
    surgical considerations and, 88